David Ip
Orthopedic Principles –

David Ip

Orthopedic Principles
– A Resident's Guide

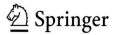 Springer

David Ip
MBBS (HKU), FRCS (Ed) Orth, FHKCOS,
FHKAM (Orthopaedic Surgery), LFIBA (UK)
Director of Division of Rehabilitation, Department of Orthopaedics
and Traumatology, Pamela Youde Nethersole Eastern Hospital,
Hong Kong
Deputy Governor, American Biographical Institute Research Association,
Deputy Director General, International Biographical Centre, Cambridge

ISBN 3-540-23259-1 Springer Berlin Heidelberg New York

Library of Congress Control Number: 2004113413

Springer is a part of Springer Science+Business Media

springeronline.com

© Springer Berlin · Heidelberg 2005
Printed in Germany

Editor: Gabriele M. Schröder, Heidelberg, Germany
Desk Editor: Irmela Bohn, Heidelberg, Germany
Production: Pro Edit GmbH, Heidelberg, Germany
Cover: Frido Steinen-Broo, eStudio Calamar, Spain
Typesetting: K + V Fotosatz GmbH, Beerfelden, Germany

SPIN 11013594   24/3130 Di   5 4 3 2 1 0 – Printed on acid-free paper

Dedication

This book is dedicated to:

- *My loving wife Esther* without whose support this book would not have been a reality

- *All my mentors,* including Professor John Leong, Professor Luk, and Drs F.K. Ip and S.H. Yeung

- *All my teachers* in different fields of orthopaedics, including Professors Jesse Jupiter, Charles Court-Brown, John Wedge, Rorabeck and William Harris

About the Author

Dr. Ip is a graduate of Hong Kong University Medical School. Since his graduation (1985), he developed an interest in the field of orthopaedics and traumatology. He is the fellow of multiple professional organisations, including the Royal College of Surgeons of Edinburgh and the Hong Kong College of Orthopaedic Surgeons. He has published multiple journal articles in peer-reviewed journals in the fields of total joint surgery, paediatric orthopaedics and traumatology. He is the winner of the International Health Professional of the Year 2004 Award and received the Universal Award of Accomplishment for Year 2004. He was also awarded the International Peace Prize by United Cultural Conventions of USA, among other awards that include the Man of the Year Award 2004, the Key Award (leader in science), Lifetime Achievement Award and 21st Century Award for Achievement, etc.

His biography has been included in famous biographical works, such as Marquis Who's Who in Science and Engineering, Marquis Who's Who in the World, Great Minds of the 21st Century, Leading Intellectuals of the 21st Century, 2000 Outstanding Scientists of the 21st Century and the Cambridge Blue Book.

His main interests include total joint replacement, osteoporosis and fragility fractures of the hip in elderly.

Foreword

The scope of orthopaedic knowledge has expanded to such a degree that it has become increasingly difficult to maintain a fundamental grasp of the required knowledge base. Add to this the time constraints of adult learning, with the student or practitioner facing ever-increasing demands on their time.

Dr. David Ip has laboured intensively to produce a much-needed resource of orthopaedic knowledge that will prove useful not only to those in training but also in the ever-increasing demand of certification and re-certification examinations.

Organized into eight chapters extending from basic science to every speciality of orthopaedic surgery – including hand, foot and ankle, sports medicine and spine, just to name a few with information provided in outline form – the reader will find it quite easy to locate information on a specific subject for direct patient care, conferences or rounds, or examination review. Alternatively, the organisation of each chapter facilitates on overall review of the subject matter. The chapters are well illustrated with 120 figures throughout the text.

By virtue of its succinct style of presentation of information, I am confident that this text will prove to be most useful to students and practitioners throughout the world.

Jesse B. Jupiter, M.D.
Director, Orthopaedic Hand Service
Massachusetts General Hospital
Hansjörg Wyss/AO Professor
Harvard Medical School

Preface

The aim of writing this book on orthopaedic principles was manifold. This book helps to arouse interest in the field of orthopaedics and highlight important points or concepts the reader might have overlooked during his reading of the subject matter in other large, thick standard textbooks. It is not meant to be a shortcut. The author feels that it is most useful to read this book after studying the standard texts and also useful to review the subject before professional examinations, grand rounds and vivas, even the long case of clinical examinations, since most examiners nowadays stress on asking clinical principles rather than digging into details of how to perform a difficult operation. The second major aim of this book was that it aims at a wide readership, including surgeons-in-training, practitioners, surgeons requiring re-certification and, in particular, surgeons in developing and under-developed countries where division into speciality or sub-speciality subjects is the exception rather than the rule. It may also prove useful for the orthopaedic surgeon who had specialised in a field for many years, but wishes to know the latest concepts of orthopaedic management in other fields of orthopaedics.

Lastly, the author wishes to express his gratitude to the world-renowned Professor Jupiter of Harvard University for writing a Foreword to this book. Happy reading!

Hong Kong, November 2004
David Ip

How to Use this Book

This section highlights the pearls to make reading of this book more fruitful for the reader. Please be reminded that the author expects the reader to know the classifications used for most of the common orthopaedic conditions mentioned in this book, the detailed description of which is outside the scope of this book.

Chapter 1 deals with orthopaedic basic science, with clinical examples taken from many of the common sports injuries. Other common sports injuries not mentioned, such as shoulder dislocation, etc., will be covered in a forthcoming textbook written by the same author on the field of Traumatology. Discussion of biomaterial science can be found in Chapter 6.

Chapter 2 deals with paediatric orthopaedics. The author recommends the reader to read textbooks written by Mercer Rang from the famous Hospital for Sick Children in Toronto before beginning clinical rotation to a paediatric orthopaedic service for training. Also, since this field of orthopaedics is sometimes more difficult to understand, this chapter has many illustrations.

Chapter 3 deals with hand surgery. The author strongly recommends the reader to read the books and articles published by Lister and Jupiter as a general reference. Quite lengthy description on management of the rheumatoid hand was given together with more illustrations, since this topic is more difficult to understand.

Chapter 4 deals with foot and ankle surgery. The author notices that many trainee surgeons consider gait analysis to be very difficult. This is not the view of the author. Gait analysis is an interesting yet important walk of orthopaedics, and a thorough understanding of pathological gait in different orthopaedic conditions is important. The books listed in the reference section for Chap. 4 provide a good basis for understanding this topic. Many an examiner expects the candidate to diagnose the patient just by looking at their gait.

Chapter 5 deals with spine surgery. There are many good articles on the degenerate spine, especially in the Japanese literature on the topic of cervical myelopathy, which the reader should know. There are also many good articles on scoliosis published by eminent professors such as Professor John Leong and Professor Luk and Cheung of Hong Kong University. Also the famous works of McMaster, Robert Winter and the Scoliosis Research Society should be noted.

Chapter 6 deals with total joint surgery. Owing to the size constraints of the book, it is impossible for the author to include a lengthy discussion on revision of total knee and total hip surgeries. I strongly advise the reader to read the works of Professor Rorabeck when it comes to revision of total knee surgery and the works of Rosenberg, Harris, Callaghan and Jasty – as well as Paprosky – when it comes to revision of total hip surgery.

Chapter 7 deals with orthopaedic infections. Infections in the presence of an orthopaedic implant is a common clinical problem as well as examination question. I strongly advise the reader to read the articles written by Gristina, Parry, Oga and also refer to the important animal studies coming from great works done in Case Western University.

Chapter 8 deals with tumour surgery. I advise the reader to read the books and articles published by Enneking. Limb salvage is quite a hot topic nowadays, but detailed discussions are outside the scope of this book. Many articles published in Clinical Orthopaedics and Related Research are worth reading, as are the great advances made in this field thanks to the marvellous works from the Mayo Clinic.

Contents

List of Abbreviations

AAI	atlanoaxial impaction
ABC	aneurysmal bone cyst
ABI	ankle brachial index
ACL	anterior cruciate ligament
AD	autosomal dominant
ADI	Atlas-Dens Interval
ADL	activities of daily living
AFO	ankle foot orthosis
AKA	above knee amputation
ALL	anterior longitudinal ligament
ALP	alkaline phosphatase
AMA	Austin Moore hemiarthroplasty
AP	anteroposterior
APL	abductor pollicis longus
AS	ankylosing spondylitis
ASD	atrial septal defect
ASF	anterior spinal fusion
ASIS	anterior superior iliac spine
ATR	angle of trunk rotation
AV	atrioventricular
AVM	arteriovenous malformation
AVN	avascular necrosis
BCC	body-centred cubic
BG	bone graft
BKA	below knee amputation
BP	blood pressure
BR	brachioradialis
Bx	biopsy

C.G	centre of gravity
C/F	clinical features
C/I	contraindication
CA	carcinoma
CCJ	calcaneo-cuboid joint
CE	centre-edge
CES	cauda equina syndrome
CIA	carpal instability adaptive
CIC	carpal instability complex
CID	carpal instability dissociative
CIND	carpal instability non-dissociative
CMC	carpal-metacarpal
CMCJ	carpal-metacarpal joint
CN	calcaneal-navicular
COM	centre of motion
CP	cerebral palsy
CPM	continuous passive motion
CR	close reduction
CRF	chronic renal failure
CRP	C-reactive protein
CSM	cervical spondylotic myelopathy
CVS	cardiovascular system
Cx	complication
D/P	distal phalanx
DDH	developmental dysplasia of the hip
DDx	differential diagnoses
DF	dorsiflexion
DIPJ	distal interphalangeal joint
DISH	diffuse idiopathic skeletal hyperostosis
DISI	dorsal intercalated segment instability
DJD	degenerative joint disease
DM	diabetes mellitus
DRUJ	distal radioulna joint
DVT	deep vein thrombosis
ECRL	extensor carpi radialis longus
ECU	extensor carpi ulnaris

EDC	extensor digitorum communis
EDL	extensor digitorum longus
EF	external fixation
EHL	extensor hallucis longus
EMG	electromyography
EOT	emergency operation
EPB	extensor pollicis brevis
EPL	extensor pollicis longus
ER	external rotation
ESR	erythrocyte sedimentation rate
F/E	flexion and extension
FB	foreign body
FCC	face-centred cubic
FCR	flexor carpi radialis
FCU	flexor pollicis ulnaris
FDL	flexor digitorum longus
FDP	flexor digitorum profundus
FDS	flexor digitorum superficialis
FF	forward flexion
FFC	fixed flexion contracture
FHL	flexor hallucis longus
FPB	flexor pollicis brevis
FPL	flexor pollicis longus
FTSG	full-thickness skin graft
Fu	follow-up
G/C	general condition
GCT	giant cell tumour
GCTTS	giant cell tumour of tendon sheath
GI	gastrointestinal
GN	gram negative
GT	greater trochanter
GU	genitourinary
HA	hydroxyapatite
HCP	hexagonal close packed
HK operation	Hong Kong Operation

HKAFO	hip-knee-ankle-foot orthosis
HO	heterotopic ossification
HTO	high tibial osteotomy
HV	hallux valgus
Hx	history
I/F	index finger
IB	Insall-Burstein
IFSSH	International Federation of Societies for Surgery of the Hand
IM	intramedullary
IPJ	inter-phalangeal joint
IR	internal rotation
IT	iliotibial
IVU	intravenous urogram
Ix	investigation
JOA	Japanese Orthopaedic Association
JRA	juvenile rheumatoid arthritis
L/F	little finger
LA	local anaesthesia
LBP	low back pain
LCL	lateral collateral ligament
LCS	low contact stress
LFT	liver function test
LL	lower limb
LLD	leg length discrepancy
LMN	lower motor neurone
LN	lymph node
LSJ	lumbosacral junction
LT	lesser trochanter
M/F	middle finger
M/L	medial and lateral
M/P	middle phalanx
MBKA	mobile-bearing knee arthroplasty
MC	metacarpal

MCL	medial collateral ligament
MCPJ	metacarpal-phalangeal joint
MEP	motor evoked potentials
MFH	malignant fibrous histiocytoma
MIC	minimum inhibitory concentration
MMA	methyl methacrylate
MPNST	malignant peripheral nerve sheath tumour
MPS	medical protection society
MRC	medical research council
MTPJ	metatarsal-phalangeal joint
MUA	manipulation under anaesthesia
MW	molecular weight
NCT	nerve conduction testing
NCV	nerve conduction velocity
NF	neurofibromatosis
NM	neuromuscular
NSAIDs	non-steroidal anti-inflammatory drugs
NV	neurovascular
NWB	non-weight bearing
OI	osteogenesis imperfecta
ON	osteonecrosis
OPD	outpatient
OPLL	ossification of posterior longitudinal ligament
OR	open reduction
ORIF	open reduction and internal fixation
OT	operation
P/E	physical examination
P/P	proximal phalanx
PA	posteroanterior
PADI	posterior atlantodens interval
PCA	porous coated anatomic
PCL	posterior cruciate ligament
PCR	polymerase chain reaction
PF	patello-femoral
PF	plantarflexion

PFJ	patello-femoral joint
PFMR	proximal femoral modular reconstruction
PID	prolapsed inter-vertebral disc
PIPJ	proximal interphalangeal joint
PL	palmaris longus
PLC	posterolateral complex
PLIF	posterior lumbar inter-vertebral fusion
PMMA	polymethyl methacrylate
PMN	polymorphonucleocyte
PMN	polymorphonuclear neutrophils
POP	plaster casting
PS	posterior stabilised
PSA	phosphate-specific antigen
PSF	posterior spinal fusion
PSIS	posterior superior iliac spine
PT	pronator teres
PTFE	tetrafluoroethylene polymer
PTT	tibialis posterior tendon
PVNS	pigmented villonodular synovitis
PWB	partial weight bearing
R/F	ring finger
RD	radial deviation
Rn	treatment
ROM	range of motion
RPS	regional pain syndrome
RSL	radioscapholunate ligament
RT	radiotherapy
S/E	side effect
SAC	'space available for the cord'
SCFE	slipped capital femoral epiphysis
SCJ	stenoclavicular joint
SED	spondylo-epiphyseal dysplasia
SIJ	sacroiliac joint
SL	scapholunate
SLJ	scapholunate joint or articulation
SNAC	scaphoid non-union with advanced carpal collapse

SNAP	sensory nerve action potential
SOL	space-occupying lesion
SPECT	single photon emission computed tomography
SSEP	somatosensory evoked potentials
SSG	split thickness skin graft
TA	tendo-achilles
TAL	tendo-achilles lengthening
TB	tuberculosis
TC	talocalcaneal
TF	tibio-fibular
TFC	triangular fibrocartilage
TFCC	triangular fibrocartilage complex
TFL	tensor fascia lata
THR	total hip replacement
TKR	total knee replacement
TL	thoracolumbar
TNJ	talo-navicular joint
TP	tibialis posterior
UD	ulnar deviation
UHMWPE	ultra high molecular weight polyethylene
UL	upper limb
UMN	upper motor neurone
USS	ultrasound
VBG	vascularised bone graft
VDRO	varus derotational osteotomy
VISI	volar intercalated segment instability
VSD	ventricular septal defect
WBCs	white blood cells

1 Orthopaedic Basic Science and Commmon Sports Injuries

Contents

1.1   Bone Structure and Function

1.1.1   Normal Function of Bone
- Protection
- Muscle attachment
- Leverage for motion
- Form and shape of body
- Mineral reserve: 98% of total body calcium
- Haemopoiesis role

1.1.2   Normal Structure
- Cells: osteoblast, osteocyte, osteoclast and osteoprogenitor cells
- Organic: collagenous and non-collagenous
- Inorganic: calcium hydroxyapatite
- Proteoglycans
- Water: 20%

1.1.2.1   Microscopic Types
- Trabecular: orientation determined by load according to Wolff's law; only 20% of skeletal mass is in trabecular bone, but it constitutes 80% of the surface area. High cellular activity at surface
- Harvesian system: at compact bone area, consists of central Haversian canal and circumferential collagen lamellae. Surface area greatly increased by canaliculi, lacunae and vascular channels
- Periosteal: deposited by cells at inner cambium layer of periosteum; collagen lamellae parallel to surface
- Subcortical: area of quite high bioactivity and active remodelling

1.1.2.2   Nomenclature
- Lamella versus woven bone: normal compact bone and trabecular bone are composed of lamellar bone (Fig. 1.1). Woven bone in a disorganised array is present in embryonic bone, in some stage of bone fracture healing and in some disease states like fibrous dysplasia
- Macroscopic type: compact bone versus trabecular bone

1.1.2.3   Bone Cells
- Osteoblasts
- Osteocytes

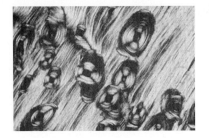

Fig. 1.1. Cross-section of lamellar bone

▨ Osteoclasts
▨ Marrow with pluripotential cells

1.1.2.3.1 Osteoblasts
▨ Functions
  – Synthesise matrix (collagen and non-collagenous proteins)
  – Work in unison with osteoclasts in bone modelling and remodelling
  – Mineralise bone (matrix vesicles production)
  – Control electrolyte flux between extracellular fluid (ECF) and the bone fluid
  [act via the receptor activator of NFκB (RANK)/RANK-L system to exert its action on the osteoclasts]
▨ Origin likely from undifferentiated mesenchymal cells in connective tissue and cambium layer of periosteum
▨ Locations in the bone
  e.g. endosteum, under periosteum, at ends of long bones with growth plate and on surface of newly formed trabecular bone
▨ Contain alkaline phosphatase that may be used as an indicator of bone formation
▨ Transient cells only

1.1.2.3.2 Osteocytes
▨ Functions
  – Possibly act as mechanoreceptor, via its multiple long processes
  – Cyclic loading releases chemical mediators, such as insulin growth factors (IGFs), causing osteoblast formation
  – Coordinate formation and resorption of bone

   – Help in minute-to-minute control of bone mineral homeostasis via exchange between cell and bone fluid compartment
- Origin
  - Incarcerated in bone matrix/lacunae during osteoid formation
  - Linkage with one another by fine cellular processes, hence increased surface area of bone matrix. Osteocytes are surrounded by ECF

1.1.2.3.3 Osteoclasts

- Functions
  - Bone remodelling and modelling (remodelling involves sequential action of osteoclasts and osteoblasts at same site. Modelling involves simultaneous action of osteoclasts and osteoblasts at adjacent locations)
  - Releasing calcium and digesting collagen
- Origin: From fusion of monocytes of macrophagic lineage in haemopoietic marrow
- Transient and very short lived

Mechanism of Action of Osteoclasts

First decalcify, then digest collagen via:
- First, adhere to bone surface to seal off a space
- Ruffled border formation with nearby clear zone with no organelle immediately adjacent to the ruffled border
- Endosomes move to ruffled border, transport protons into the dead space; decalcify bone by making pH 4
- Then, organic matrix degraded by acidic protease and pro-collagenase
- Note: osteoclasts have calcitonin receptors which will shrink the cell and not be able to form ruffled border

Regulation of Osteoclast Activity

General factors: parathyroid hormone (PTH), 1,25-dihydroxy vitamin D_3, calcitonin and others [oestrogen, androgen, growth hormone (GH)]
Local chemical factors: cytokines and growth factors
Local mechanical stimuli
(Note: PTH and vitamin D are unable to stimulate osteoclastic bone resorption in vitro in the absence of osteoblastic cells – there is no vi-

tamin D receptor on osteoclasts and doubtful for PTH. Calcitonin acts directly on osteoclasts since its receptor is present)

1.1.2.4 Collagen
- From 90% to 95% organic components
- Mostly type 1
- Fibrils in each lamella are in the same direction
- Adjacent lamellae are at 90° to each other, hence affording strength

1.1.2.5 CaPO$_4$ Hydroxyapatite
- Inorganic component constitutes 60–70% of the dry weight
- Calcium and phosphate as hydroxyapatite crystals
- Crystals contain labile carbonate and acid phosphate groups needed in interaction with surrounding ECF and organic matrix

1.1.2.5.1 Process of Mineralisation
- Site of mineralisation at the 'pores' on the collagen triple helix. Commence at the mineralisation front (at interface of osteoid and mineralised substance)
- Osteoblasts eject intracellular membrane bound vesicles (rich in sodium and sulphate) in rapid exchange with calcium and phosphate. Extracellular matrix vesicles act as foci of mineralisation
- Occur in the presence of PTH and activated D3

1.1.2.5.2 On Mineralisation
- If you want to take away calcium, you need also to take PO$_4$ with you from the bone
- If you want deposit calcium, you also need to give adequate PO$_4$ to the bone
- It follows, therefore, that if PO$_4$ is very low, it is very difficult to deposit enough calcium to have good bones

1.1.2.6 Other Substances in the Bone
- Water – 10%; importance of water content
- Other substances

1.1.2.7   Other Non-Collagenous Proteins
- Integrin – helps binding of osteoclasts
- Osteocalcin – modulates bone formation and absorption
- Osteonectin – modulates mineralisation process
- Osteopontin
- Bone sialoprotein
- Cytokines
- Growth factors, e.g. transforming growth factor-β (TGF-β)

1.1.2.8   Non-proteins
- Complex saccharides
- Lipids

1.1.2.9   Growth Factors
- Bone morphogenetic protein (BMP)
- Transforming growth factors
- Fibroblast based
- Platelet-derived growth factors

1.1.2.10   Bone Circulation
- Sources:
    - Nutrient arterial system
    - Periosteal system
    - Metaphyseal
    - Epiphyseal system (child)
- Arterial supply of the cortex is centrifugal. Direction is reversed in a displaced fracture that disrupts the endosteal nutrient arterial system
- Venous flow is centripetal. The cortical capillaries drain from sinusoids to emissary venous system

1.1.2.10.1   Nutrient System
- Supplies inner two-thirds of cortex
- Nutrient artery enters the medullary cavity, sending arterioles proximally and distally
- High pressure, hence centrifugal flow

1.1.2.10.2   Periosteal System
- Extensive network covering the entire shaft
- Supplies outer one-third of cortex
- Low pressure system
- Important in children and required for growth in width

1.1.2.10.3   Metaphyseal System
- Anastomoses with the nutrient artery system
- In child, supplies zone of provisional calcification of the growth plate

1.1.2.10.4   Epiphyseal System
- Present in children
- Supplies the resting, germinal, proliferating and upper hypertrophic zones of the physis

1.1.3   Biomechanics of Bone
- Bone can be thought of as a biphasic composite material, one phase being the mineral, the other phase being the collagen and ground substance
- The combination is stronger for their weight than either substance alone
- Normal bone: resistance to compression is greater than tensile, which is greater than shear

1.1.3.1   Viscoelasticity
- Bone is also viscoelastic, like other connective tissues such as cartilage, tendons, etc. The viscoelasticity of a tissue is a time-dependent property where the deformation of material is related to rate of loading
- Bone loaded at a higher rate is stiffer and more brittle and may sustain higher load to failure. It also stores more energy before failure with a higher rate of loading

1.1.3.2   Concept of Bone as a Two-Phase Material
- Explains some adaptations such as increase in strength especially at high strain rates like running, or even higher strain rates like impact
- Marrow (and fat) flows under pressure at a high strain rate along the maze of trabeculae

1.1.3.3 Anisotropism

- Bone is anisotropic, thus having different mechanical properties when loaded along different axes
- Caused by different bony structure along its longitudinal and transverse axes
- Human long bones are stronger in compression than tension, but weakest in shear

1.1.3.4 Coupling of Bone Formation and Destruction

- Coupling process: under normal circumstances, if more bone forms, more bone will be destroyed; if more bone is destroyed, more bone will form, etc.
- Uncoupling occurs in osteoporosis and some other pathological conditions that affect bone (e.g. osteopetrosis, etc.)

1.1.3.4.1 Bone Remodelling and Wolff's Law

Wolff's Law:

- Bone has the ability to adapt by changing its size, shape and structure in response to the mechanical demands placed on the bone. (Form follows function)
- Bone is being laid down where needed and resorbed where not needed
- Remodelling can be external (changed external shape of the bone) or internal structure (mineral content and density)

1.1.3.4.2 Possible Mechanism Explaining Wolff's Law

- Compression side of a long bone is piezoelectric negative, which stimulates osteoblasts; tension side is piezoelectric positive, which stimulates osteoclasts

1.1.3.4.3 Application of Wolff's Law

- Disuse leads to periosteal and sub-periosteal bone resorption
- In the presence of an implant, stress shielding/protection of bone occurs, thus there is less bone density in the stress shielded area, since the implant shared the imposed load upon the bone leading to resorption of the surrounding bone
- Prolonged weightlessness in space can cause bony resorption as well

1.1.4   Normal Protective Mechanisms Against Trauma

- Importance of muscle contractions to counteract the load application to bone and offer a protective effect (fatigue fracture has more tendency to occur with muscle fatigue upon prolonged strenuous exercise)
- Ability of normal bone to remodel and repair its defects help prevent fatigue fracture
- With ageing, bones increase their area moment of inertia by distributing even more bone tissue in the periphery away from the central axis by increasing the diameter of the medullary cavity

1.1.5   Fatigue Fractures

- Caused by cyclic applications of a load below the ultimate strength of the bone
- Only occur when the rate of remodelling is outpaced by the loading process
- Likelihood of fatigue fracture depends on the amount of load, frequency of loading and number of repetitions

1.1.6   Bone Healing

1.1.6.1 Stages of Bone Healing

- Fracture haematoma formation
- Soft callus formation
- Hard callus formation
- Remodelling

1.1.6.2 Initial Stages

- After the initial haematoma formation and acute inflammation dominated by neutrophils that secrete cytokines (brings in multipotent cells, angiogenesis and phagocytes)

1.1.6.3 Effect of Hypoxia After Fracture

- Hypoxia after fracture is due to interruption of vascular supply
- It is thought that hypoxia, resultant acidity and changes in pH cause the neutrophils to release the cytokines – one effect of which is to bring in more angiogenesis

1.1.6.4   Soft Callus
▨ Forms from an initial cartilage model
  – Various growth factors stimulate chondroblasts that secrete matrix
  – Mineralisation later occurs in the presence of phosphates and pro-teases
  – Later replaced in favour of bone formation

1.1.6.5   Hard Callus
▨ By osteoprogenitors at cambrium layer a short distance from the fracture but not at the fracture site itself – forms by intra-membranous ossification

1.1.6.6   Remodelling Phase
▨ After the repair phase, can remodel for up to two years
▨ Slow change of woven to lamellar bone
▨ Cutting cones (Fig. 1.2) only occur in secondary bone healing, usually only at the stage of remodelling

1.1.6.7   Healing in Special Situation
▨ Rigid fixation: AO principle of interfragmentary compression and absolute rigidity. Primary bone healing results, involving direct osteonal remodelling
▨ Gap: depends on the gap size. Whether bone or other connective tissue, like cartilage/fibrous, form depends on the strain theory put forward by Parren. Bone cannot form if the strain is too high
▨ Intramedullary (IM) nail: healing by mainly external callus formation
▨ Distraction osteogenesis is a special case: bone formation by intra-membranous ossification if given adequate rigidity

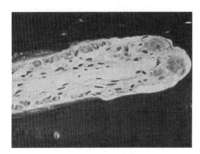

Fig. 1.2. Cutting cone

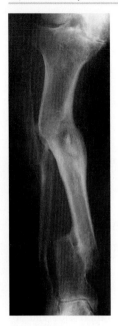

Fig. 1.3. Natural healing by external calluses

[By contrast, natural healing by callus can be strong, although often malaligned. (Fig. 1.3)]

1.1.6.8 'Primary Bone Healing'
▦ Primary bone healing – direct osteonal remodelling – cutting cones at cortical bone and vascularity and osteoblasts at its trailing end to re-create the Harversian model

1.1.7   Metabolic Bone Disease

1.1.7.1 Introduction
▦ To really understand the role of bone in calcium and phosphorus metabolism and in metabolic bone disease, one must note that bone is really an extension of the extracellular space
▦ The surface area of exchange is much increased by the hydroxyapatite crystals – dimension 200×100 angstroms

1.1.7.2 Basic Rules of Calcium Metabolism

- Bone formation and destruction is coupled
- Unlike PO_4, calcium difficult to get across cells and need transport system – affected by PTH that creates 'holes' in cells and 1,25-dihydroxy vitamin D to provide calcium-binding proteins inside cells

1.1.7.3 Normal and Abnormal Calcium and Phosphate Metabolism

1.1.7.3.1 Calcium

- Function: neuromuscular conduction/activation, coagulation cascade, enzyme co-factor and formation of the rigid mineral content of bone
- Daily requirement: total body calcium 1100 g, 98% of which is in bone and teeth. Requirement of adult 1000 mg, adolescent 1300 mg
- Absorption from gastrointestinal (GI) tract include: active transport in duodenum and facilitated diffusion in jejunum. Active transport requires both vitamin D and PTH. PTH is needed for transport across the cellular membrane and to stimulate production of 1,25-dihydroxy vitamin D_3, while vitamin D helps form proteins to bind calcium inside cells
- Of dietary calcium, 35% is absorbed. Excretory routes include both the GI tract and kidneys. In the kidney, two-thirds is reabsorbed in the proximal tubule, one-third adjustable absorption in the distal tubule

1.1.7.3.2 Calcium Regulation (Homeostasis)

- Minute-to-minute control (rapid process)
  - Involves transfer of calcium from bone surface to ECF in response to PTH. Involves osteocytes and osteoblasts, especially the former
- Draining from bone reserve (slow process)
  - Really a balance between osteoblastic bone formation and osteoclastic resorption
- Hormonal control

1.1.7.3.3 Details of Hormonal Control

- PTH: stimulated by low [Ca]. Acts by decreasing renal excretion and stimulating 1,25-dihydroxy vitamin D, hence increasing GI absorption of calcium. Acts on osteoclasts to release calcium from bone mainly indirectly via osteoblast cells

- Calcitonin: stimulated by high [Ca]. Acts by decreasing the number and activity of osteoclasts. Osteoclasts have calcitonin receptors and calcitonin will shrink the osteoclast in in vitro experiments
- The role of vitamin D was mentioned. Other hormones include GH, cortisol etc., but are not the main players

1.1.7.3.4 Effect of Phosphates and Magnesium on Calcium Metabolism

- Phosphates: stimulate PTH production, bind to calcium rendering it inert. Insoluble calcium phosphate crystals deposit to bone and are removed in stool
- Magnesium: if [Mg] low, suppresses PTH secretion even if [Ca] is low
- Drugs: substances like thiazide diuretics can increase calcium excretion

1.1.7.3.5 Other Issues Concerning Calcium

- Concentration of ionised calcium in blood depends on:
  - pH: e.g. acidosis decreases protein binding and causes increased ionised calcium, etc.
  - Albumin concentration: decrease of [albumin] by 1 g/dl changes protein-bound calcium by 0.8 mg/dl. Thus, hypercalcaemia may be missed in cases of hypoalbuminaemia
- The reader is referred to physiology texts as regards causes and management of hypercalcaemia and hypocalcaemia

1.1.7.3.6 Phosphorus

- Functions: component of cell membrane, messenger for hormone adenosine monophosphate (AMP), energy transfer (adenosine triphosphate/adenosine diphosphate), components of fats and proteins
- Daily requirement: 800 mg
- Distribution: total body contains 600 g; 90% in bone and teeth as reservoir, 10% intracellular
- Absorption: in duodenum and small bowel as inorganic phosphate, depends on amount taken

1.1.7.3.7 Homeostasis

- PTH stimulated by high [P]: acts by increasing urinary excretion and decreasing absorption. Also increases mobilisation from bone and stimulates increased 1,25-dihydroxy vitamin D

▓ Increased 1,25-dihydroxy vitamin D in turn increases phosphate absorption in the gut

▓ Other regulators: e.g. GH increases renal absorption, calcitonin decreases its excretion in urine

1.1.7.3.8 Appendix 1

Role of Vitamin D in Calcium and Phosphate Metabolism

  UV light converts dietary pro-vitamin D_2 and D_3 to cholecalciferol

  Then undergoes 25- and 1-hydroxylation at the liver and kidney respectively (in cases with high calcium, mainly 24,25-dihydroxy vitamin D will be made in the kidney)

  Acts on targets by diffusion through cytoplasmic membrane; bound to cellular protein and transported to the nucleus

  In bone, stimulates both osteoblasts and osteoclasts, increases mineralisation and resorption and increases collagen production

  Kidney: like PTH, vitamin D increases calcium absorption. However, unlike PTH, increases phosphate absorption

  GI tract: synthesis of calcium-binding proteins helps calcium absorption and increases phosphate absorption

Role of PTH in Calcium and Phosphate Metabolism

  Produced in parathyroid gland, prepro-PTH made from mRNA, changed to pre-PTH in rough endoplasmic reticulum, then PTH in Golgi apparatus and packed for secretion

  Acts as a sensitive control of [Ca]

  Mechanism: most actions via membrane receptor attachment, in turn activating cAMP and protein kinase and increasing intracellular calcium

  Bone: (short-term) induces increased permeability of osteocyte cell membrane to calcium, promotes exchange between calcium and ECF. (Longer term) induces osteoclasts (via osteoblasts) to mobilise calcium from bone

  Kidney: increased calcium but decreased phosphate absorption, increased 1,25-dihydroxy vitamin D

  GI tract: increased calcium and phosphate absorption via increased vitamin D

Role of Calcitonin in Calcium and Phosphate Metabolism

Produced from the C cells of thyroid as a large precursor, then cleaved into 32 amino acids

Stimulated by increased [Ca]

Mechanism: binds to cell membrane receptor and activates adenyl cyclase

Bone: shrinks osteoclasts, prevents ruffled border formation and inhibits formation of osteoclasts

Kidney: decreases absorption of calcium and phosphate

GI tract: uncertain, storage of calcium in peri-lacunar space after meal

1.1.7.3.9 Appendix 2

Types of Rickets

Common types include:

- Nutritional: supplements needed
- Vitamin D-resistant rickets: PO_4 lost in urine – PO_4 and vitamin D needed in treatment (Rn)
- RTA: Needs alkaline in Rn
- End organ non-response: needs activated 1,25-dihydroxy vitamin D_3
- Renal rickets: loss of the normal natural adjustments of calcium absorption and PO_4 excretion – Rn not easy, consult renal physician

Adult Osteomalacia

Massachusetts General Hospital study: 27% of patients coming in for hip fracture with osteomalacia

Sometimes co-exists with osteoporosis

Looser's zones and milkman's lines at the concave side of the long bone if present are characteristic

1.2 Cartilage Structure and Function

1.2.1 General Important Features

- Ability to withstand great compressive forces despite being very thin – only a few millimetres
- Ability to withstand sudden high loading, e.g. at stance phase of gait, even distribution of stress, hence diminished damage to subchondral bone
- Very low friction due in part to fluid mechanics
- Partial thickness (PT) defects usually do not heal
- Full thickness (FT) defects do not heal if subchondral bone not penetrated and heal with fibrocartilage if subchondral bone penetrated
- Fibrocartilage, though it has good tensile strength, cannot withstand high compressive stresses

1.2.2 Why Is Cartilage Near to a Perfect Machine?

- Very low coefficient of friction
- Joint is self-renewing, self-lubricating and even works better under load
- This is mainly because of a form of lubrication in which water present in cartilage as a gel is extruded with pressure on the joint and lies within a fine filamentous fibrous layer (lamina splendens) on the cartilage surface. The situation is like water rubs on water, thus an almost frictionless system

1.2.3 Biomechanics

- Collagen component of cartilage resists shear and tensile stresses
- Proteoglycans with high negative charge entrap water and resist the very high compressive loads despite cartilage being a very thin structure
- Proteoglycans determine the 'permeability' of the matrix

1.2.4 Other Features

- No nerves, blood vessels or lymphatics
- Paucity of cells – adapt to anaerobic metabolism (functions at 8% O_2)
- Overall 'low' metabolic rate because of paucity of cells, but individual cells can be quite active
- Biomechanical properties depends on MATRIX.

(Cartilage contains an anti-angiogenic factor that inhibits vascular invasion and is an inhibitor to many chondrolytic proteineases)
- (Growth factors normally present, such as TGF/IGF, help keep proteases in check)

1.2.5   Structural Anatomy in Layers
- Superficial (lamina splendens): high collagen, low proteoglycans, cells parallel to surface
- Transitional (middle zone): more glycans and larger collagens, sheroidal cells
- Deep layer: largest collagen fibrils, complex network of proteoglycans and hyaluronic acid, cells radially aligned
- Calcified cartilage: mineralised matrix, cells small. Between zones 3 and 4 is the 'tide mark'
  (Mankin thinks that just below the lamina splendens is a 'fibrous layer' likened to the skin of cartilage – helps prevent ingress of particles that are too large or have wrong charge or chemical configuration and prevents egress of wanted materials)
  (Bulkwater divides the matrix into three regions: pericellular, territorial and inter-territorial)

1.2.5.1 On a Microscopic Scale
- Haematoxylin and eosin stain looks like homogeneous matrix
- Cells sparse and lonely – division apparently ceases after growth in length ceases – but since cellularity remains quite constant, experts like Mankin think that these chondrocytes might be quite 'immortal'

1.2.5.2 Structure of Cartilage
- H_2O: 80%
- Cells (probably no direct cell-cell contact)
- Collagen-type 2 (6, 9, 10, 11)
- Non-collagen proteins: glyco-proteins
- Proteoglycans (hyaluronic acid/protein core, connected are one or more glycosaminoglycans chains): some liken its action as a spring, others say most important to lock water in place.
  (In cartilage, two major classes of proteoglycans: large aggregating proteoglycan monomer (or aggrecans) and small proteoglycans, including decorin, biglycan, etc.)

- (Collagen fibres of cartilage not anchored into bone; but the cartilage tissue is 'keyed' into the irregular surface of bone like a jigsaw puzzle)

1.2.6   Nutrition: Two Barriers to Diffusion
- Synovial linings
- Different layers of cartilage

1.2.7   On the Potential for 'Healing'
- Unlike adult cartilage, foetal cartilage can heal spontaneously (seen in foetal lamb animal studies)
- PT defects – transient cell reaction in the edge of lesion, usually does *not* heal (except in the rare case when mesenchymal cells can be induced to migrate from the synovial membrane across the articular surface into the defect)
- Osteochondral lesions heal with fibrocartilage: combined type 2 and 1 collagen, not tough enough to withstand high compression stresses
- Salter had shown a positive effect of continuous passive motion (CPM) on cartilage healing (e.g. in studies with periosteal grafts) – immobilization is detrimental to cartilage repair and development

1.2.8   General Management of Chondral Defects
1.2.8.1 Natural History of Chondral Defects
- (Arthroscopy 1997) – In over 30,000 knee arthroscopies for knee injuries, a chondral lesion was found in 60%
- Other studies report 23% when associated with anterior cruciate ligament (ACL) injuries, increasing to 54% with chronic ACL injuries
- But, exact natural history of isolated lesions *not known for certainty*

1.2.8.2 Diagnosis of Chondral Defects
- With an arthroscope
- Magnetic resonance imaging (MRI)
- Others [physical examination (P/E) not too reliable]
- New method: Finland originated the use of articular cartilage stiffness tester/probe (trade name ArtScan) – potentially useful since cartilage softening is one of the first signs of the degenerative process – seems

proportional to the degree of superficial loss/re-distribution of collagen/proteoglycans.

Artscan may be more objective than a simple probe

1.2.8.3 Essential Steps in Managing Chondral Defects

- Find aetiology
- Adequate description of the lesion: location, depth, size (Frank Noyes classification)
- Degree of containment and any kissing lesions
- Assess ligament integrity
- Any limb malalignment: if not corrected, will ruin any repair of cartilage defects
- Status of meniscus
- Cruciates integrity: (e.g. ACL-deficient knees subjected to multiplanar shear forces)

Also ensure proper rehabilitation protocol – most cases need CPM and period of protected weight bearing

1.2.8.4 Details of Assessment Methods of Chondral Damage/Defects

- Noyes four-point scale (to this, may add checking for any kissing lesion): location, depth, description and diameter
- Outerbridge: four types (only depth of involvement stressed here, originally Outerbridge meant to assess chondromalacia, *not* chondral defects)
- Bauer and Jackson: descriptive, e.g. linear crack/stellate/flap/crater/fibrillation/degrading
- ICRS (International Cartilage Repair Society): with detailed forms to be filled in

1.2.8.5 Role of MRI

- MRI not too useful for diagnosis, especially poor in diagnosis of PT defects
- Most used sequence being 'fat suppressed three-dimensional T1-weighted gradient echo technique'
- Bone bruise now believed by some experts as indicator of possible significant cartilage injury

▨ New advances: spectroscopic imaging with view-angle tilting; spec-tral-spatial 3-D magnetisation transfer; high-resolution short echo time spectroscopic imaging, etc.

1.2.8.6 General Options for Managing Chondral Defects

▨ Supervised neglect
▨ 'Chondro-protection'/debridement and curettage [mainly for relief of say, knee osteoarthritis (OA) symptoms]
▨ Fixation of chondral fragments (especially if osteochondral)
▨ Stimulation of healing – drilling, abrasion, micro-fracture techniques
▨ Autologous osteochondral transfer
▨ Autologous chondrocyte culture/reimplantation (ACI)
▨ Periosteal and perichondrial transplantation
▨ Use of allografts and growth factors
▨ Future – regeneration and gene therapy

1.2.8.6.1 Supervised Neglect

▨ Increasing evidence that especially FT defects may lead to OA
▨ Although some defects remain asymptomatic for considerable period and true incidence not known for sure

1.2.8.6.2 'Chondro-Protection'

▨ Hyaluronic acid: animal studies claim protective effect; mechanics – unknown. Probably provides lubrication
▨ Glucosamine and chondroitin sulphate: since OA results when carti-lage breakdown exceeds synthesis of chondrocytes, providing exoge-nous glucosamine increases matrix production and alters natural course. While chondroitin sulphate is the most abundant glucosami-noglycans in articular cartilage, may inhibit many degradative en-zymes in synovial fluid in OA

1.2.8.6.3 Lavage and Debridement

▨ Pain relief in OA cases from removal of loose intra-articular debris, inflammation, mediators, enzymes. Changing the ionic environment of the synovial fluid
▨ Paper by Robert Jackson in the States: relief in 50% at 3.5 years – seems better if mechanical debridement added
▨ Drawback: cannot treat the chondral defect

1.2.8.6.4 Subchondral Drilling

▦ Advocated by Pridie 1959

▦ Aim at repair by formation of fibro-cartilage and/or a little hyaline cartilage (animal studies noted that hyaline nature lost at 8 months)

▦ Drilled in pin-point fashion, results in fibrin clot formation

1.2.8.6.5 Microfracture Technique

▦ Advocated by Richard Steadman of Colorado

▦ Procedure: Steadman believes that removal of the calcified layer is very important and damage to the subchondral bone should be avoided

▦ Arthroscopic awl used to make many holes (microfractures) in the exposed subchondral bone; 3–4 mm apart; depth of about 4 mm

▦ Goal: a blood clot rich in pluripotential marrow elements to form and stabilise while it covers the lesion. The technique provides a rough surface that clot can adhere to – less thermal necrosis

▦ Tissue produced: hybrid of hyaline and fibro-cartilage, with viable chondrocytes in lacuna – but, the good results deteriorate over time, because of poor wear character of the repair tissue. (Proper post-op rehabilitation and ± joint unloading procedures are important)

1.2.8.6.6 Abrasion Arthroplasty

▦ Advocated by Johnson 1981

▦ Extension of the drilling procedure, except that a superficial layer of subchondral bone 1–3 mm thick is removed to expose intra-osseous vessels with added debridement of the cartilaginous defect to an edge containing normal looking tissue

▦ (There have been some arguments about the depth of drilling and also as to whether the debridement of the sclerotic lesion should be intra-cortical or cancellous.)

▦ Tissue formed is mainly fibro-cartilage

1.2.8.6.7 Perichondral Transplant

▦ Theory: previous animal experiment – neochondrogenesis possible with autologous perichondrial grafts sutured or glued with cambium layer facing the joint

- It was demonstrated that perichondrium taken from the cartilaginous covering of the rib could be placed in a joint where it will develop into hyaline cartilage
- Drawback: 60% graft failure at a mean of 6 years with symptom recurrence

1.2.8.6.8   Periosteal Transplantation

- This technique (tried by O'Driscoll) may not yet be ready for very wide general use
- Involves harvest of periosteal graft from proximal tibia and suture into the defect with cambrium layer facing up; recipient area must debride down to subchondral bone
- O'Driscoll results fair, occasional failures

1.2.8.6.9   Autologous Chondrocyte Implantation

- Idea: cultured chondrocytes placed into defects and a periosteal flap used to retain the gel
- Swedish experience – 14 of 16 patients with femoral condyle transplant had good results at 2 years. Claims near normal hyaline cartilage regenerated (N Engl J Med 1994/ Brittberg). Resulted in hyaline-like cartilage
- (Cultured chondrocytes harvested from patients replanted in 3–4 weeks time; important that the cambium layer of the periosteum is facing the joint, as it may serve as a source of growth factors or cells in the new matrix.)

Further Comments on ACI

- Unanswered questions – long-term efficacy not known, initial success in rabbits not reproduced in canine model; what are the biomechanical properties of this surface, any reproduction of the tide mark?
- So far, no evidence to suggest clinical outcome better than repair-stimulating techniques. It is expensive. It is possible that the clinical application may be ahead of time

1.2.8.6.10   Osteochondral Autograft Transplantation

- Only for osteochondral defects (forms hyaline cartilage)
- Contraindication: deep and large subchondral defects, since limited availability and difficult to restore contour of large defects

▨ Best used in: FT 10–20 mm, i.e. smaller lesions
▨ Main reason for long-term survival of the hyaline cartilage is preservation of the tide mark and as bone carrier
▨ The bone base acts as an anchor – enables secure fixation and integration with nearby bone – likely that nutritional pattern not affected

Details of Osteochondral Autograft Transplantation

Donor: along the outer edge of the lateral femoral condyle, above the sulcus terminalis (exposed to less contact pressure because this area has a convex articular surface similar to the central weight-bearing area of the femoral condyles and is seldom worn out, even in OA)

Alternative donor: just adjacent to the superolateral margin of the intercondylar notch – in the notchplasty and roof area of ACL reconstruction

Sized by sizers, harvesting perpendicular to the surface, driven to 15 mm depth – if not, will not be flush and graft will not be circular. Before extracting, rotate clockwise and anti-clockwise and fracture base of cancellous bone. Never use power; thus preserve cells. Recipient tube driven into subchondral bone to depth of 13 mm. Ensure perpendicular and flush with surface. (P.S. Cartilage between grafts are fibro-cartilage, donor in second look usually covered by fibrous tissue/fibrocartilage)

Complication: haemarthrosis, pain, graft fracture, condyle fracture, loose bodies, avascular necrosis (AVN) if too many harvested from one area

Osteochondral Autograft Transplantation: 10-Year Result

One recent study: 3% donor morbidity – includes deep infections and claims that serial scope shows 90% congruent gliding surfaces

1.2.8.6.11   Other Potential Methods

Transforming Growth Factors

Recent experiment of the use of timed release of TGF-β in PT defects reported that the cells migrated into the defect from synovial tissue and formed a fibrous matrix. (Trans Orthop Res Soc 1994)

For FT defects, potential to use in future since it has the potential to stimulate the restoration of an articular surface superior to that formed by current repair-stimulating techniques

Artificial Matrices

- In animal experiments, fibrous polyglycolic acid, collagen gels and fibrin have proved effective matrices for the implantation of cells and fibrin has been used for timed release of growth factors
- Brittberg/Muckle (JBJS-Br 1990) reported use of woven carbon fibre pads – 77% good results in 3 years

Allografts

- Current rationale for fresh osteochondral allografts – clinical and experimental evidence of maintenance of viability and function of chondrocytes – 95% at 5 years, 77% at 10 years, 66% at 20 years; histological evidence that the bony part of these grafts can be replaced by host bone in a uniform fashion in 2–3 years
- Successful reports by Allan, Gross and Garrett in the setting of traumatic defects and osteochondritis dessicans (OCD)

1.2.8.6.12   Appendix

Regulation of Synthesis and Degradation of Cartilage

- Since there are no nerves or blood vessels, it looks logical that protein synthesis may be regulated by mechanical forces and there is ample evidence to suggest that the key player in altering synthetic activity is 'intermittent hydrostatic pressure'. (Other agents, e.g. drugs and change in cation distribution may also be at work)

Effects of Cartilage Loading

- Normal cartilage is subjected to: (1) static and (2) dynamic peak stresses
- Physical stimuli, e.g. deformation of cells and matrix, fluid flow, hydrostatic pressure, electrical streaming potentials, altered intracellular pH and ion composite
- Static compression may inhibit collagen aggrecan and small proteoglycan synthesis
- Dynamic compression may *stimulate* synthesis of macromolecules and dynamic shear stimulates collagen synthesis

1.2.8.6.13   Progression to OA

- No data on natural history for isolated chondral defects
- It seems that FT cartilage defects continue to progress and deteriorate, though at a slow rate (recent serial MRI follow-up studies)
- Common occurrence in traumatic knee haemarthrosis in one series (Shelbourne)
- Severe defects: most believe will progress to OA
- Even milder cases can sometimes occur, e.g. experimental evidence that disruption of the superficial zone can contribute to OA from altered biomechanical behaviour of tissues
- Bone bruise in MRI, e.g. common in ACL injuries, is believed by many to represent cartilage/subchondral bone damage – might progress to OA

1.3   Comparison of Ageing versus OA: Features of the Osteoarthritic Process

- Stage 1: (from high impact loading, etc.) disrupted matrix macromolecular structure – results in more water, less proteoglycan aggregates
- Stage 2: chondrocytes detect the tissue damage and release mediators that stimulate a cellular response – both anabolic/catabolic activities increased, and more cells (explains why in some cases the process may improve/abort/revert). Histology: 'clones of proliferating cells surrounded by newly synthesised matrix molecules is a hallmark'
- Stage 3: progression of cartilage loss and abated anabolic response
- Subchondral area: increased density, cyst forms, cyst cavities with myxoid/fibrous/cartilage tissues, appearance of regenerating cartilage within and on subchondral bone surface. End stage, thick dense bone on bone articulation
- Osteophytes: around the periphery of joints – marginal at the 'cartilage-bone interface' and along the insertions of the joint capsule (capsular osteophytes). Most marginal osteophytes with cartilaginous surface that resemble normal articular cartilage look like extension of the joint surface
- Why osteophytes form: probably a response to the degeneration of the articular cartilage and the remodelling of subchondral bone; including

the release of anabolic cytokines that stimulate cell proliferation and formation of osseous and cartilage matrices

1.3.1   Definition of Primary Osteoarthritis

- The process involves progressive loss of articular cartilage accompanied by attempted repair of the cartilage; remodelling and sclerosis of subchondral bone, with or without forming subchondral cysts and marginal osteophytes
- More in weight-bearing joints and hand joints; theoretically any synovial joints

  (Possible role of chondrocyte senescence was also suggested by recent papers)

1.3.2   Other Features

- Inflammation *not* a major component
- More primary OA with ageing
- Normal life-long joint use differs from cartilage of people with OA
- Rate of OA progression varies – can be very slow or very fast; a few improve spontaneously!
- Involves all the tissues that form the synovial joint – cartilage, subchondral/metaphyseal bone, synovium, ligament, capsule, muscles

1.3.3   Differential diagnosis Causes of Secondary OA

- Trauma (e.g. intra-articular fracture)
- Instability (e.g. cruciate insufficiency)
- Cartilage abnormal (med, acromegaly)/sometimes abnormal bone remodeling (e.g. Pagets)
- Osteonecrosis (with collapse)
- High-impact loading
- Neuropathic (decreased proprioception, unstable, intra-articular fracture, increased joint loading)
- Infection-related cartilage destruction
- Metabolic crystals deposits: haemochromatosis (mechanics unknown), haemophilia, ochronosis, calcium pyrophosphate
- Rare syndromes (Gaucher, Stickler)

1.3.4   Normal and Excessive Joint Use versus Degeneration

▦ Moderate activity may not accelerate OA in normal joints

▦ Regular activity needed to maintain joint – cyclic loading of cartilage stimulates matrix synthesis, but prolonged static loading or no loading motion degrades the matrix and later degeneration sets in

▦ Special occupations have more risk of OA, e.g. heavy weight lifting, labourers, farmers, miners, users of pneumatic drills

▦ Normal ageing with superficial fibrillation – does not appear to cause symptoms or to affect the function of the joint

▦ Isolated cartilage defects can cause pain, effusion and mechanical dysfunction. Untreated can fail to heal and may progress to joint degeneration

▦ Many procedures for osteochondral/chondral defects can be rendered *not* useful if in the setting of already global OA changes

1.4   Osteochondritis Dessicans

1.4.1   Differential Diagnosis
from Traumatic Osteochondral Fracture

▦ OCD

▦ Traumatic osteochondral fracture

▦ Others: osteonecrosis, osteochondroses and hereditary epiphyseal abnormalities

1.4.2   Nature of OCD

▦ A focal bone cartilage lesion featured by separation of an osteochondral fragment from the articular surface – by definition, involves *both* bone and cartilage elements

▦ Typical sequence: from an initially intact lesion, to a partially loose fragment, to a detached lesion

▦ Main difference from osteonecrosis: separates from a normal vascular bone bed, as opposed to osteonecrosis with an avascular bone bed

1.4.3   Other Features

▦ Common in adolescent and young adult, rare less than 10 years old or greater than 50 years old

- Prognosis: depends on age and other factors (better if small lesion, in classic position, stable on arthroscopic exam or MRI)
- Most common affected joints: knee, elbow, ankle
- For the knee, most common classical area – lateral part of the medial femoral condyle

1.4.4   Possible Aetiology of OCD
- Trauma
- Repeated microtrauma from impingement of the tibial spine
- Stress fracture with no injury
- Vascular (ischaemic event)
- Defects of ossification

1.4.5   Classification
- Juvenile form
- Adult form
  [differential diagnosis (DDx) is before and after closure of epiphysis]

1.4.6   Main Rn Options
In general: non-operative for intact lesions and operative in unstable lesions
- Excision (weight-bearing joints treated with removal of sizeable OCD fragments that are detached tend to do poorly)
- Some are amenable to fixation
- If cannot fix: consider cartilage repair techniques, e.g. subchondral drilling; allograft, osteochondral autograft transplantation (OATS), ACI, perichondral (open) and periosteal (open) resurfacing

1.4.7   Clinical Significance of OCD
- If defect in weight-bearing part of knee joint, degeneration of affected compartment later possible
- Loose bodies, if present, can cause locking
- For OCD, important to realise that age has important influence on prognosis

1.4.8   Types and Prognosis

▪ Juvenile: open physis – better prognosis, more likely healing (one study however say it is not always benign, 50% incidence of X-ray signs of arthrosis at average 30 years follow-up)

▪ Adult: closed physis – worse prognosis, less healing potential (adult form can be difficult to diagnose from traumatic osteochondral fracture, but the latter can be an isolated lesion or with ligament/meniscus injuries)

(Pure chondral lesions occur more often in older adults, whereas osteochondral fractures and OCD more in children and younger adults)

1.4.9   Why Occur at the Classic Location?

▪ Classic location – lateral aspect of the medial femoral condyle and possible role of trauma/impingement

▪ Why this site? – Smillie (and Fairbank) think could be the result of repeated impingement of the tibial spine on the medial femoral condyle during tibial internal rotation

1.4.10   Clinical Features

▪ History: trauma history in 50% cases, OCD in child usually athletically active child; symptoms vague – e.g. pain, crepitus, stiff, recurrent knee effusions, and/or mechanical symptoms

▪ P/E: Wilson test – pain on progressive extension of the knee from 90° to 30° knee flexion with the tibia in internal rotation and relieved by external rotation

1.4.11   Diagnosis and Investigation

▪ Most seen initially on X-ray (including a tunnel view is helpful)

▪ Bone scan – sensitive in diagnosis and follow-up of OCD lesion in children since indicates blood flow (and hence potential of healing). Less useful in adult form of OCD

▪ MRI: helps diagnosis of associated meniscal and ligamentous injuries and helps to determine the size and degree of displacement of chondral lesions and the integrity of overlying cartilage

1.4.12   Factors Affecting Decision Making

▪ Amount of subchondral bone attached to the cartilage – important indicator of healing potential

- Age: affects also the healing potential
- Others: size of lesion, location (especially weight-bearing)
- Diagnosis: e.g. OCD versus trauma versus hereditary epiphyseal anomalies

1.4.13 Management Schemes
- Group 1/Juvenile: trial of conservative Rn appropriate for skeletal immature cases, success rates from 50% to 90% reported
- Group 2/Adolescent: assessment of remaining growth potential is most important
- Group 3/Adult: management can be quite similar to adult osteochondral fracture

1.4.14 Management
- Pure chondral small lesion/small osteochondral defects can initially be treated in the immature conservatively
- Success of conservative Rn may depend on adequate subchondral bone attachment (theoretically, if no subchondral bone attached to the fragment, there is little chance for the articular lesion to heal)

1.4.15 Operative Rn
- Arthroscopic drilling and fixation
  - Based on the theory that the lesion is regarded as a fracture nonunion, works by penetration of the subchondral bone to initiate inflammatory cascade
  - Types: antegrade versus retrograde drilling, an undesirable consequence of antegrade drilling, is the creation of permanent drill holes in the articular surface that fill with fibrocartilage [retrograde drilling with bone graft (BG) sometimes advocated for in situ lesions with intact overlying articular cartilage]
  - Fixation of osteochondral lesions increase the likelihood of maintaining joint congruity during healing and potential to allow early range of motion (ROM; by means of K-wires, Herbert, Acutrak) – important to bury screw head
- Abrasion chondroplasty and microfracture
  - Again, stimulation of cartilage regeneration by penetration of the subchondral bone to release pluripotential stem cells

- Subchondral drilling – fibrin clot formation – stem cell migration – chondrocyte differentiation – repair the defect
- Histology: fibrous or mixed fibro- and hyaline cartilage. (Many experts think this tissue does not last more than 1 year, i.e. long-term effect of the inferior repair tissue uncertain)
- Microfracture avoids heat necrosis, awl to create multiple micro-fractures 3–4 mm apart, (rougher surface for attachment of the fibrin clot). Histology: mixed fibro- and hyaline cartilage, as above

▪ Autograft: mosaic-plasty and ACI
- Mosaic – transport cylindrical osteochondral plugs from new woven bone (NWB) areas to the osteochondral defect – first performed in Hungary for lesions in knee and talus
  Donor from supracondylar ridge of the femur or intercondylar notch, plugs up to 8.5 mm in diameter
  Use press-fit method
  Histology: hyaline cartilage with fibrocartilage in between
  Indication – osteochondral defects less than 45 years old, open method for large lesions, arthroscopic for smaller defects
  Post-op: NWB from 6 weeks to 8 weeks allows bone union and prevents graft subsidence
- ACI
  Harvest, culture, periosteal flap, then inject cells as mentioned
  Disadvantage – cost, tenuous fixation of periosteum to the chondral surface
  Indication – some say may be good for pure chondral injuries and not if significant bone loss

▪ Allograft
- Best use in traumatic injuries; not good for OCD
- Histology: Allograft replaced by host bone in 2–3 years by creeping substitution, but percentage of viable chondrocytes varies. Decreased a lot after cryotherapy, but fresh grafts – 99% at 1 year and 38% at 6 years
- Allan Gross group claims 85% success rate with fresh grafts and sometimes combined with realignment osteotomy. Rn of bipolar defects was less successful, however
- Side effects: immune reaction, size matching, availability, disease transmission

– On the issue of immunity – although articular chondrocytes are immunogenic, humeral antibodies *cannot penetrate* intact articular cartilage matrix; hence, rejection is usually insignificant (tissue typing and immune suppression not usually deemed necessary)

1.4.16   Other Methods
▩ Realignment osteotomy – since malalignment can cause excess stress on the injured joint surface and prevent healing of chondral defects
▩ Arthroplasty (uni/total) – not for the initial Rn of the adolescent and young adult

1.5   Tendon Basic Science

1.5.1   Tendon Structure
▩ Cells: 20%
▩ Water: 70%
▩ Collagen type 1
▩ Small amount of proteoglycan/glycoprotein as 'cement' function and small amount of elastin
▩ Collagen arrangement absolutely parallel – can withstand high tensile stress
▩ Weak area is musculotendinous junction
▩ Rupture risk depends on muscle force generation, cross-section ratio between muscle and tendon, eccentric muscle force and any weakness in the tendon proper

1.5.2   General Features
▩ Low blood supply
▩ Low metabolic rate and demand (tendon is predominantly an extra-cellular tissue)
▩ Therefore, can stand high tensile loads, since low metabolic demands
▩ The drawback is that healing is slow

1.5.3   Function
▩ Anchors muscle to bone
▩ Withstands large tensile stresses
(Adaptations can occur with age, exercise and disuse)

1.5.4   Anatomy

▦ Follows the blue-print of connective tissue: 'mesenchymal cell in a supporting matrix', with cells making the matrix
   - Tenocytes (longitudinally aligned)
   - Matrix contain proteins – collagen type 1 and elastin; ground substance – water and glycoproteins

1.5.5   Structural Hierarchy

Collagen secreted as trophocollagen → microfibrils (after cross-linked), molecules overlap as quarter-stagger/striations → fibril → fascicle (with crimp structure) → tendon (covered with paratenon)

1.5.5.1   Junctional Zones

▦ MTJ (musculotendinous junction): how the tension generation by muscle fibres transmits from intracellular contractile proteins to extracellular cartilage: 'The collagen fibrils insert into recesses formed between the finger-like processes of the muscle cells' – this folding increases the contact area, thus less force/area
   - But still the weakest link is in the muscle-tendon-bone unit (e.g. after eccentric loads in young sportsman)
▦ Osteotendinous junction (OTJ): with four zones, viz:
   - Tendon
   - Fibrocartilage
   - Mineralised fibrocartilage
   - Bone
   (Border distinct between fibrocartilage and mineralised fibrocartilage called 'cement line' or tide-mark – place where avulsion fracture occurs)

1.5.6   Structure versus Function Correlation

▦ Elastin contributes to tendon flexibility
▦ Ground substance gives structural support and diffusion of nutrients and gases – the proteoglycans regulate matrix hydration and contain glycosaminoglycans
▦ Collagen aligned in the direction of stress, orderly and parallel. But at rest, fibres are wavy with crimped appearance
▦ Low metabolic rate withstands high tensile stresses
▦ Tenocytes squeezed in between collagen

(The low metabolic rate enables it to remain under tension for long periods without risk of ischaemia and necrosis)

1.5.7   Blood Supply
- Perimysial at MTJ
- Periosteal at OTJ
- Paratenon – major supply
  Paratenon vessels enter the tendon substance and passing longitudinally within the endotenon sheath form a capillary loop network
- Tendons enclosed in synovial sheaths are supplied by vinculae
- Vascularity compromised at junctional zones and areas of friction/torsion/compression – no capillary anastomosis: [e.g. (1) supraspinatus near its insertion, (2) Tendo-achilles (TA) – where the combined tendon of Gastrosoleus undergoes a twist that raises stresses across this site]

1.5.8   Nerve Supply
- Innervation mainly afferent
- Nerve endings mostly at MTJ
- Four types of nerve endings:
  - Free – pain reception
  - Golgi – mechano-reception
  - Paccinian – pressure sensors
  - Ruffini

1.5.9   Biomechanics
- Tendon is the strongest component in the muscle-tendon-bone unit
- Tensile strength is one-half that of stainless steel (e.g. 1 cm^2 cross-section can bear weight of 500–1000 kg)

1.5.10   Force–Elongation Curve
- *Less useful* than the stress–strain curve because, unlike the stress–strain curve, not only depends on the mechanical behaviour of the tissue; shape of curve also depends on the length and cross-sectional area (more cross-sectional area, larger loads can be applied; longer the tissue fibres, greater the elongation before failure)

1.5.11 Stress–Strain Curve

▪ Four regions: (1) toe region, (2) linear region, (3) microfailure and (4) macrofailure occurs

- Toe: disappears at 2% strain as the crimpled fibres straighten. Non-linear in shape
- Linear portion: tendon deforms in linear fashion due to the intermolecular sliding of collagen triple helices. This portion is elastic/reversible and the tendon will return to original length when unloaded, if strain is less than 4%. Slope is elastic modulus
- Micro-failure: collagen fibres slide past one another, intermolecular cross-links fail and tendon undergoes irreversible plastic deformation
- Macroscopic failure: occurs when tendon stretched greater than 10% of its original length. Complete failure follows rapidly once the load-supporting ability of the tendon is lost and the fibres recoil into a tangled, ruptured end

1.5.11.1 Viscoelasticity

▪ The stress–strain behaviour of tendon is *time-rate dependent*

▪ The sensitivity to different strain rates means that tendon is viscoelastic

▪ Hence, exhibits associated properties of 'stress–relaxation' (decreased stress with time under constant deformation) and creep (increased deformation with time under constant load)

▪ At higher rates of loading, tendon becomes more brittle – exhibits a much more linear stress–strain relationship prior to failure (under these circumstances, the ultimate strength is greater, energy absorbed (toughness) lesser and more effective in moving heavy loads. At slow loading rates, tendon is more ductile, undergoing plastic deformation and absorbing more energy before failure)

1.5.11.2 Storage of Energy

▪ During movement, part of the kinetic energy created by muscle is transiently stored as 'strain energy' within the tendon. This gives the tendon the capability to passively transfer the muscle force to bone, as well as control the delivery of the force. A stronger, stiffer tendon exhibits a higher energy-storing capacity – but if pre-stretched, its energy absorbing capacity is reduced and risk of rupture is higher should added loading occur

1.5.12   Tendon Failure

1.5.12.1 Terminology: Concentric, Isometric, Eccentric Contractions

- Under a given load, the tension generated across the tendon depends on the type of muscle contraction
  - Concentric: the MTU (musculotendinous unit) shortens in length, resulting in positive work
  - Isometric: the MTU length remains constant while resisting force and no work is generated
  - Eccentric: the MTU lengthens in response to load resulting in negative work

1.5.12.2 Sites of Tendon Injury

- MTJ – the weakest link; especially during eccentric contractions, since maximum tension is created in such contractions (greater than isometric/concentric types by threefold) and especially if speedy – hence, increasing the speed of eccentric contraction will increase the force developed
- If the loading rate is slow, bone breaks and avulsion fracture likely occurs. If loading is fast, more likely to cause tendon failure (especially if degenerated to start with)

1.5.12.3 Other Terms Concerning Injury Mechanics

- Direct: penetrating, blunt, (thermal-chemical)
- Indirect: acute tensile overload (macro-traumatic partial/complete tear), chronic repeated insult (micro-traumatic subthreshold damage – cause can be exogenous, e.g. acromial spurs, or endogenous)
  - Acute tensile failure when strain beyond 10%
  - But lesser strain can cause the same if pre-existing degeneration (Chronic repeated overload occurs when fails to adapt to repeated exposure to low magnitude forces less than 4–8% strain)

1.5.12.4 Four Types of Micro-Traumatic Tendon Injury

- 'Tendinitis': tendon strain or tear
- 'Tendinosis': intra-tendinous degeneration

- 'Paratenonitis': inflamed paratenon only
- 'Paratenonitis with tendinosis'

1.5.12.5 Three Phases of Tendon Healing
- Inflammation: fibrin links collagen, chemotactic to acute inflammatory cells – leukocytes, monocytes and macrophages; clear damaged tissue
- Repair: macrophage as coordinator of migration and proliferation of fibroblasts, tenocytes ± endothelium. These cells secrete matrix and form new capillaries, replace clot with granulation tissue. Type 3 collagen produced, type 1 later around second week
- Remodeling: started at third week, scar maturing, collagen more densely packed and oriented. The scar never has same properties – final tensile strength 30% less; biochemical and mechanical deficiencies will persist

1.5.12.6 Rehabilitation
- Knowledge of the *phased* healing response allows the proper time frame whereby to introduce our rehabilitation programme
- From first few days to end of week 2 – inflammatory response, significant decrease in tendon tensile strength, type-3 collagen deposition – our programme here should avoid excess motion, as excess stress in this time *disrupts* the healing instead of promoting it
- From the second to third week, this is the repair phase. Gradual introduction of motion, and prevention of excess muscle and joint atrophy
- In the rehabilitation phase there is remodelling and progressive stress can be applied; but note that tendons can require 10–12 months to reach the normal strength levels

1.5.12.7 The Scar
- Much collagen 3 persists in the scar with thinner, weaker fibrils and fewer cross-links
- Collagen – deficient in content, quality and orientation

1.5.12.8 Effects of Use, Disuse and Immobilisation
- Use: will slowly hypertrophy – more action of tenoblast, accelerated collagen synthesis, more collagen thickness and cross-links, improved stress orientation of fibres, larger diameter and total weight

▪ Disuse: opposite changes
▪ Immobilisation: tendon atrophies, seen only after a few weeks. These adaptations are more rapid than changes after exercise

1.5.12.9 Clinical Example: Ruptured Tendo-Achilles. (Described in the Section on Foot and Ankle Surgery)

1.6   Ligament Basic Science

1.6.1   General Functions
▪ Neurosensory role
▪ Stabilising joints
(Mechanical behaviour is like other viscoelastic soft tissues, but with adaptations that allow joints to be flexible, yet stable)

1.6.2   Important Features
▪ Different ligaments heal differently
▪ ACL, in particular, often fails to show any healing response
▪ Medial collateral ligament (MCL) seems to have much better healing potential, perhaps because of its environment, nutrition sources and other intrinsic advantages

1.6.3   Anatomy
▪ Types 1±3 collagen
▪ Non-linear portion represents unwinding of the collagen
▪ Two main types of ligament–bone attachments
  – Like femoral attachment of MCL – attaches via fibrocartilage, then bone
  – Like MCL tibial attachment (indirect variety) – attaches to periosteum/bone through Sharpley's fibres
▪ Water is from 60% to 70% of total weight
▪ Collagen is 80% of dry weight (90% type 1, others mainly type 3)
▪ Proteoglycans are 1%, but their hydrophilic nature plays an integral part in viscoelasticity
▪ Elastin resists tension by reverting from globular to coiled form under stress
(other content: minor amount of actin and fibronectin)

1.6.4   Gross and Microscopic Structure

- Gross; white, shiny band-like
- Hypocellular, a few fibroblastic cells interspersed within the tissue matrix
- Under polarised light, the fibrils have a sinusoidal wave pattern or crimp which is thought to have significance in the non-linear functional properties

1.6.5   Biomechanics

- Viscoelastic behaviour
- Stress–strain behaviour is time–rate dependent
- During the cycle of loading and unloading between two limits of elongation, the loading and unloading curves of a ligament follow *different paths* – the area enclosed by the two curves is called area of hysteresis, which represents the energy loss
- Other viscoelastic behaviour
  - Stress–relaxation – decrease in stress when subjected to constant elongation
  - Creep – a time-dependent elongation when subjected to a constant load

1.6.5.1 Viscoelasticity (Using ACL Reconstruction as Illustration)

- The phenomenon of stress–relaxation predicts that the initial tension applied to the graft in ACL reconstruction can decrease from 30% to 60% over the course of surgery; however, it has been shown that cyclic stretching of patella tendon grafts prior to graft tensioning reduced the amount of stress–relaxation. Hence, preconditioning a graft will lessen the loss of tension after its fixation
- Although stress–relaxation is reduced via pre-conditioning, the replacement graft continues to demonstrate cyclic stress–relaxation, e.g. a large number of cyclic loads like running reduces stress in the graft with each elongation cycle; fortunately, this behaviour is recoverable
- Also, cyclic stress–relaxation contributes to prevention of graft failure, the viscoelastic behaviour also illustrates the importance of warm-up exercise before physical testing to decrease maximum stresses in the ligament

1.6.5.2 Shape of the Stress–Strain Curve
- Non-linear toe area
- Linear area
- Ultimate tensile strength
- Area under curve is energy absorbed

1.6.5.3 Effect of Strain Rate
- Savio Woo's group seem to think that strain rate plays a relatively minor role with respect to mechanical properties
- Other workers, however, believe that strain-rate sensitivity is important, the ligaments becoming slightly stronger and stiffer at higher loading rates

1.6.5.4 Site of Ligament Rupture and Age
- Young age: ligament-bone junction (e.g. rabbit MCL model, all tears before skeletal maturity at tibial insertion area)
- After growth ceased and physis closed: the ligament-bone junction is no longer the weakest link
- Older age: mid-substance tear more common; there is also overall decrease in tensile strength of the ligament

1.6.5.5 Healing of the Injured Ligament
- Inflammation
- Matrix and cell proliferation
- Remodelling
- Maturation

1.6.5.6 Factors Affecting Healing
- Systemic factors
- Local factors – especially immobilisation versus early motion
- Prolonged immobilisation can cause joint stiffness and damage healthy ligament by synovial adhesions
  (Cooper 1971 JBJS: immobilisation of a joint can lead to sharp decline in ligament-bone junction strength, especially in the collateral ligament that inserts via the periosteum)

1.6.5.7 Effect of Immobilisation and Exercise

▓ Rabbit model, structural properties of MCL decrease dramatically at 9-week immobilisation, the elastic modulus and ultimate tensile strength of MCL is also reduced; histological evaluation shows marked disruption of the deeper fibres that attach the MCL on the tibia by osteoclastic absorption in the subperiosteum. Resorption was prominent especially in the femoral and tibial insertions – the structural properties are slow to recover

▓ Ligament substance recovers more quickly from immobilisation than the insertion areas. Takes months of rehabilitation for full recovery

1.6.5.8 Example 1: Isolated MCL Injury

▓ Operative versus conservative results comparable, but both are inferior to the natural ligament (although adequate for most knee functions)

▓ MCL was shown to heal spontaneously and yielded good knee function – though tensile strength reached only 60% at 1 year

▓ No major difference between the operative and the conservative groups at 6 weeks. The healed MCL is adequate for knee function due to the larger cross-section area of the healed ligament

▓ Gap versus in-contact healing in laboratory experiments: in-contact healing yielded slightly better results

1.6.5.9 Example 2: MCL and ACL Injury

▓ Still debated whether need to repair grade 3 MCL tear in subjects needing ACL reconstruction

▓ Currently, there are some laboratory experiments in support of comparable results with conservative versus operative Rn

▓ Checking the overall limb alignment for any other associated ligamentous injury is very important

▓ In cases of ACL tear with Grade 3 MCL injury, it may be wise to treat the MCL conservatively for a period (most heal with conservative Rn) before proceeding to ACL definitive reconstruction

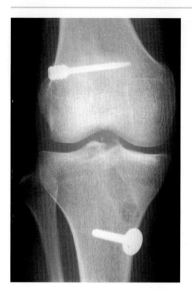

Fig. 1.4. Post-operative X-ray after right ACL reconstruction

1.6.5.10 Example 3: ACL Reconstruction (Fig. 1.4)

- Pre-conditioning is advisable for the graft
- At 6 weeks laboratory experiment in Savio Woo's lab bone-patella-tendon-bone (BPTB) incorporation good, slower incorporation for soft tissue graft
- Recommend going slower if soft tissue (hamstring) graft was used since it incorporates slower, also future use of growth factors possible to speed healing
- Recent robotic experiment in laboratory – strain maximum post-op in knee extension; hence, some suggest avoid full knee extension in post-op rehabilitation after ACL reconstruction

1.6.5.11 Appendix: Growth of Ligaments

- Interstitial growth – pericellular addition of collagen and other matrix
- In some ligaments, active vascular outer layer of 'periligament' identified in the rabbit in laboratories
- Ligament growth also affected by nearness to growth plates and degree of ligament strain

1.6.5.12   Related Topic: Important Aspects of ACL Reconstruction

1.6.5.12.1   Normal ACL Function
- Resists anterior tibial translation
- Resists rotatory motion
- Helps resist varus/valgus stresses

1.6.5.12.2   The Two ACL Bundles
- Anteromedial (AM) bundle
- Posterolateral (PL) bundle

1.6.5.12.3   Natural History of ACL Tear
- Not totally sure, but can predispose to OA, especially if associated with meniscus injury hence, close monitoring if treated conservatively
- 'Rule of thirds'
  One-third of patients – adequate compensation
  One-third – Inadequate compensation – give up sporty activities
  One-third need operation (OT) for frank instability

1.6.5.12.4   Partial ACL Tear: Diagnosis and Natural History
- Diagnosis – clinical not always accurate, arthroscopic probing is said to be best in assessment
- Natural history of partial ACL tear:
  If 25% torn, unlikely to progress
  If 50% torn, 50% progressed
  If 75% torn or more; 86% progressed

1.6.5.12.5   Concept of Laxity versus Instability
- All depends on symptomatology. absent in pure laxity and if symptoms present (i.e. with a feeling of joint about to dislocate or very unstable) then there is instability
- Hence, not every case with laxity will have instability symptoms

1.6.5.12.6   Physical Assessment
- Lachman test most sensitive
- Anterior drawer test
- Pivot shift test

Check also for concomitant injuries, including the secondary stabilisers, e.g. anteromedial restraints, PL restraints, etc.

1.6.5.12.7 Common Case Scenarios that Require Operative Intervention

Acute/chronic ACL with repairable meniscus

Acute less than 3 months with no meniscus injury – these cases tend to operate if age less than 20 years, sporty, greater than 5 mm side-to-side difference

(Chronic) ACL greater than three months – followed rehabilitation protocol, but started to give way

Used to cope with ACL non-operative programme but new injury with non-reparable meniscus tear – consider reconstruction and ± partial meniscectomy

(Some tests said to help predict whether one can cope with ACL injury, e.g. the cross over hop test)

1.6.5.12.8 In Non-Operative ACL Cases; Why Sometimes Still Need to Operate

ACL stump impingement → persistent effusion, loss of end extension, pain with hyper-extension at inferior pole of patella → arthroscope: looks like cyclops, Rn by removal of the cyclops

May predispose to meniscus tear – if repairable tear, consider repair and ACL reconstruction. If not reparable, partial meniscectomy

Predisposes to OA, but differential diagnosis from instability needed

1.6.5.12.9 Summary of Usual Factors to Consider Before Proceeding with OT

Degree of athletic level (e.g. number of sporting hours)

Whether secondary stabilisers can compensate

± Objective translation with respect to opposite knee

Compliance with rehabilitation and reasonable expectations

1.6.5.12.10 Contraindications to Reconstruction

Sepsis (absolute)

Degenerative joint disease (DJD)

Poor compliance

1.6.5.12.11 Operative Timing

- Avoid acute reconstruction (danger of arthrofibrosis when tissues inflamed)
- Wait until:
  - Restored ROM
  - Swelling subsided and haemarthrosis (that can limit rehabilitation progress and cause recurrent effusion and quadriceps inhibition) subsided
  - Full extension achieved
  - Good active leg control (if not, difficult to regain full flexion and to maintain patella mobility)

1.6.5.12.12 Pearls to Success

- Patient selection + OT timing + indications (especially never to forget about secondary stabilisers like PL and anteromedial areas clinical assessment)
- Graft selection (autograft/allograft/synthetic)
- Intraoperative technical side → tunnel placement (most common error especially femoral side), graft fixation, tensioning – how much and at what knee flexion angle, etc.
- Post-op rehabilitation, dangers of over-aggressive
- In less than a 6-week to 9-week period, will see success of graft incorporation or not (so called ligamentisation)
- DDx of failure of reconstruction, e.g
  - Instability – attention not paid to factors mentioned above or to new trauma (even after incorporation)
  - Others – arthrofibrosis

1.6.5.12.13 Stages of Healing of ACL Autografts

- Vascular necrosis
- Revascularisation
- In-growing cells, macrophages
- Replacement of graft collagen
- Fibre alignment and cross-linking
- New collagen fibres, fibroblasts
  (P.S. Allografts commonly show delayed cell re-population, incomplete graft replacement by scar tissue and lesser mechanical properties)

1.6.5.12.14 Graft Types – Autograft
- BPTB
- Double-looped hamstrings
- Others
    - Iliotibial (IT) band – in extra-articular cases
    - Quadriceps tendon (tried by experts like Fulkerson, etc.)

1.6.5.12.15 Graft Selection
- More BPTB in high-demand labourers that do not need to kneel and do not have patello-femoral joint (PFJ) symptoms
- More hamstring reconstruction in lower demand cosmesis-conscious female patients and/or those with PFJ problems or pain or work/religion requires kneeling

1.6.5.12.16 Hamstrings Autografts
- Pearls to success
    - During the first 6 weeks, tendon fixation devices must provide more fixation than patellar tendon bearing (PTB) devices because the formation of the tendon-tunnel interface is slower
    - Perfect tunnels – no roof impingement or posterior cruciate ligament (PCL) impingement
    - Equal tension four strands (maximise stiffness) – align each strand in parallel, avoid braiding
    - Proper rehabilitation
- Roof impingement causes loss of extension and increased anterior laxity. Rn: roof/wall plasty (tibial tunnel posterior and parallel to roof with knee in full extension)
- If there is PCL impingement, will increase anterior laxity and loss of flexion (put tibial tunnel at 65° in coronal plane between medial and lateral spines)

1.6.5.12.17 Pros and Cons of Hamstring Grafts
- Pros: of adequate stiffness if double-looped/quadripuled types; some studies report cosmetic and donor site may regenerate (viability not greatly dependent on revascularisation, but more on synovial diffusion)
- Cons: tendon healing slower than bone at 3 weeks (picks up at 6 weeks); more difficult revision, usually with enlarged tunnels (may

need grafting and reconstruction a few months later after the BG is incorporated)

1.6.5.12.18 BPTB Grafting
- Pros: strong, available, bone healing good, good track record
- Cons: patello-femoral symptom, patella fracture
  (P.S. Some experts like Shelbourne have also tried the use of contralateral BPTB grafting)

1.6.5.12.19 Allograft
- Advantages: no donor site problem; some studies claim reasonable result, although many experts reserve allograft for use more in revisions and reconstructions after multiple knee ligament injuries and in elective reconstruction after knee dislocation
- Disadvantages: delayed maturation; disease transmission (need 2.5 Mrads); sometimes with lesser mechanical properties (especially after irradiation)

1.6.5.12.20 Synthetic Graft
- Poor track record
- Not for routine use

1.6.5.12.21 Causes of ACL Reconstruction Failure
- General contraindication: sepsis
- Failure of DDx
  - Technical: nonanatomic tunnel, inadequate notchplasty, inappropriate tension, graft fixation failure, inadequate graft material
  - Biological: failed ligamentisation, infection, arthrofibrosis, infrapatella contraction
  - New trauma
  - Secondary stabiliser injuries not tackled: rotatory instability; malalignment, varus or valgus instability

1.6.5.12.22 Importance of Proper Tunnel Placement
- Dictates isometry of graft over a ROM
- ACL graft can tolerate only a small amount of strain before deforming

1.6.5.12.23 Femoral Tunnel: Possible Faults

▪ Anterior placement – (1) tensioned in extension → tight on flex; (2) tensioned in flexion → too lax
▪ Too posterior placement – (1) tensioned in extension → lax in flexion; (2) if tension in flexion → loss of extension
▪ Vertical 12 o'clock placement – rotation part of the instability remains with persistent pivot shift

1.6.5.12.24 Tibial Tunnel Possible Faults

▪ Too anterior: impinges graft on knee extension (sometimes more tension if flexed)
▪ Too posterior: too lax on flexion
▪ Medial/lateral: impingement (wall), synovitis, laxity

1.6.5.12.25 Tibial Tunnel Positioning

▪ Some authors (JBJS 1993) proposed tibial tunnel should be inclined posterior to Blumensaat's line – a line that joins the roof of the notch in a lateral full extension X-ray of the knee

1.6.5.12.26 Tunnel Size Changes with Time

▪ Especially hamstring autografts due to micromotion – may need bone grafting if subsequent revision ACL reconstruction is needed

1.6.5.12.27 Injury to Secondary Stabilisers Not Addressed

▪ PL stabilisers
▪ Anteromedial stabilisers

1.6.5.12.28 Inadequate Notchplasty

▪ Large enough to avoid impingement and allows full ROM
▪ Notice that graft often larger than native ACL
▪ Impingement can cause cyclops lesion and loss of extension (Impingement, in general, causes blood flow and cellular ingrowth) – good graft with low signal on MRI, impinged one with area of high signal on MRI

1.6.5.12.29 Graft Fixation Pearls

▪ Important, since takes more than 6–12 weeks before graft incorporates

- BPTB failure can result from bone block advancement or sometimes lost fixation if tibial interference screws are used
- Hamstring graft failure can occur with improper positioning of endoscopic fastener or poor soft tissue interference fixation

1.6.5.12.30 Suggested Graft Tension in BPTB and Hamstring Autografts
- PTB: from 5 pounds to10 pounds, 10–15° knee flexion
- Hamstring: from 10 to15 pounds, 20–30° knee flexion
  - Why graft needs to be cycled – to preload it before fixing (75% of viscoelasticity returns to graft if tension drops for even 1 min)

1.6.5.12.31 Drawbacks of Too Much and Too Little Tension
- Too much: decreased vascularity, delayed incorporation, later degeneration (Am J Sport Med)
- Too little: laxity

1.6.5.12.32 Post-op Rehabilitation Phase
- Graft is weakest in early rehabilitation period
- The design of the post-op rehabilitation protocol depends on our understanding of the time frame of the different stages of graft incorporation

1.6.5.12.33 Does 'Ligamentisation' Really Mean New Durable Ligament?
- Our collagen substitute placed into the knee must undergo remodelling to become incorporated as 'organised scar tissue' that functions as a check to instability
- This ligamentisation is a misnomer, as real new ligament is *not* created
- Difference: native ligament is able to provide stability with different loads over a ROM with large and small fibres diameter of different lengths
- The collagen in the graft are uniform in length and parallel in orientation, unlike those of the native ligament

1.6.5.12.34 Failure of ACL Reconstruction
- 8% of primary ACL reconstruction fails
- Revision surgery is 80% effective
- Common problems

- Dilated tunnels
- Stretched out
- Failed fixation
- New ruptures
- Missed 2° secondary stabilisers failure, e.g. posterolateral complex (PLC)
- Concomitant injury, e.g. Meniscus
- Limb malalignment

1.6.5.12.35 Future of ACL Reconstruction

- Less morbidity of soft tissue grafts but greater tunnel motion may dictate a slower rehabilitation protocol
- Gene therapy is a powerful tool to enhance the process of graft incorporation
- In future, a more anatomic ACL, e.g. double bundle (AM and PL) reconstruction
- Hopefully, with above advances, the current 5–25% failure of ACL reconstruction will be a thing of the past (and the higher incidence of OA in the ACL-reconstructed knees)
- Also, more physiological loading in our rehabilitation protocols – performed at higher flexion angles of the knee to reduce the in situ forces in the ACL graft

1.6.5.12.36 Features of ACL Injury in Females

Introduction

- From two to five times more common than in males
- Prevention is better: by means of organised sports at a younger age (e.g. hip/knee muscle strength, neuromuscular (NM) training, landing strategies, agility/reaction skills, training proprioceptive reflex at a younger age)
- PTB results comparable, mild increased laxity (include KT testing) after hamstring grafts (less return to pre-injury level)

Problems and Their Solutions

- Wider pelvis and more genu valgum: control valgus moment at knee (other anatomic considerations: more laxity, less thigh muscle, narrower femoral notch, increased tibial torsion)

- Mainly recruit quadriceps to stabilise knee: retrain the NM pattern for them to use more hamstrings
- Low hamstring/quads ratio: as above; train better co-contraction of the two muscle groups
- Slower to regenerate muscle force: faster speed and reaction time training is needed
- Less developed thigh muscles: consider training hip muscles to assist stabilisation
- Greater knee flexion when jumping, landing and cutting
- Poorer dynamic stabilisation pattern: enhance NM control
- Less muscle endurance: training to enhance the endurance

1.6.5.12.37 ACL Reconstruction in the Skeletally Immature
- Consider reconstruction if the child is unable to avoid re-injury
- Delay until growth is near complete if possible (females 14 years old, males 15 years old and less than 1.5 mm of growth left)
- Patients under 12–14 years, avoid drilling across the epiphyseal plate (Note: extra-articular type of reconstruction may not be adequate enough for active youths)

1.6.5.13   PCL Injury

1.6.5.13.1   Anatomy
- Anterolateral (AL) part is main bundle
- Posteromedial (PM) bundle
- Two variable meniscofemoral ligaments (Humphrey and Wrisberg) originate from the posterior horn of the lateral meniscus and contribute fibres to the PCL

1.6.5.13.2   Biomechanics Considerations
- AL bundle stronger
- If PCL only sectioned: posterior translation 11 mm
- If PLC only sectioned: posterior translate 3 mm only
- PLC and PCL sectioned: posterior translate 30 mm; thus, the two are synergistic
  PCL in situ forces are increased by hamstrings, decreased by quadriceps and popliteus action

1.6.5.13.3   Mechanism of Injury

- Posterior blow to proximal tibia with foot plantar flexed – the foot position is important only because it changes the force vector (if the foot is dorsiflexed, the ground force will contact the patella and distal femur, but with the foot plantar flexed, the ground force intersects with the proximal tibia)
- Hyperflexion knee injury
- Combination of forces

1.6.5.13.4   PCL Isometry Issues

- PCL is not an isometric ligament
- Anterolateral single bundle reconstruction alone may still produce laxity in terminal extension (graft tensioned in 70–90° flexion in single bundle reconstruction)

1.6.5.13.5   Physical Assessment

- Most sensitive and specific test: **posterior drawer test** → supine flex the knee 70–90° and first assess the tibial starting point. The tibia normally has an anterior step-off of 10 mm. If the tibia is posteriorly subluxed (as in PCL injury), then the starting point may be even with, or even posterior to, the medial femoral condyle. Displacement beyond this suggests complete PCL injury or combined injury
- Quadriceps active test: for suspected combined ACL/PCL cases
- Tests for PLC: (1) Dial test (prone, knees together) external rotation (ER) more than 15° than the other leg suggestive, i.e. record thigh-foot angles. (2) ER recurvatum test. (3) PL drawer test not only at 90°, but also at 30°
- Importance of gait assessment: check for gait anomalies like varus thrust (with lateral compartment opening up) in chronic PCL/PLC injuries. If these gait anomalies are associated with underlying varus alignment of the knee, then a bony procedure, e.g. high tibial osteotomy (HTO), should precede any consideration for soft tissue reconstruction

1.6.5.13.6   Imaging

- Acute cases – look for: fibula avulsion fracture (arcuate), medial Segond fracture, posterior sagging, lateral joint space widening and PCL avulsion fracture

- Others: lateral X-ray with a posterior directed force
- MRI: in particular, can assess PLC but not always easy
- Chronic cases: scanogram, weight-bearing lateral and look for degeneration of the PFJ and medial compartment

1.6.5.13.7   Arthroscopic Findings

- Direct signs of PCL tear: torn fibres, laxity (not as dramatic as ACL since mostly hidden)
- Indirect sign: floppy ACL (since tibia translated)
- PLC signs: suggested by lateral joint opening ('drive through' sign); check popliteus tendon integrity at same time

1.6.5.13.8   Management

- Grade 2 (less than 10 mm): conservative, de-emphasise hamstring during rehabilitation
- Operation considered for
  - Higher-grade PCL tears
  - Combined PCL and PLC injuries
  - Bony avulsed PCL fracture: direct post approach
  - Associated meniscal and chondral injuries
  - Combined ACL/PCL or above, i.e. functional knee dislocation

1.6.5.13.9   General Rn Principles

- Identify and treat all pathology
- Protect neurovascular bundles
- Accurate tunnels
- Anatomic graft insertion sites
- Strong graft
- Minimise graft bending
- Tension appropriate
- Use secure primary and, if necessary, back up graft fixation
- Structured post-op programme (initially put in extension brace, less strain on graft; protected prone ROM exercise, quadriceps rehabilitation and de-emphasise hamstring, etc.)

  Overall goal is to reproduce the normal anterior tibial step-off, restore the restraint to posterior displacement and repair any PLC tear

1.6.5.13.10 PLC Injuries

Feature
- Isolated PLC injury rare
- Many are associated with PCL injury, especially in high energy trauma cases – not uncommon to diagnose PCL injury but miss concomitant PLC injury

Anatomy
- Superficial layer: IT band, biceps femoris
- Deep layer: lateral collateral ligament (LCL), fabellofibular ligament, arcuate ligament, popliteus muscle complex (including the popliteofibular ligament)

Posterolateral Complex
- Most important components of this PLC are:
  - Popliteus tendon
  - Popliteofibular ligament (that portion of the popliteus tendon attached to the fibula head instead of the muscle belly). This ligament is important to resist PL rotation and varus rotations
  - LCL

More on Isometry Issues with Special Reference
to PLC Reconstruction Issues
- The fibula head is isometric to the lateral femoral epicondyle through a functional ROM
- Implication: a graft taken from any position of the fibula head to the lateral femoral epicondyle will remain supportive through a functional ROM (so does the natural popliteofibular ligament)
- Grafts, however, that attach to PLC of the tibia instead of the fibula head are not isometric and are less strong in resisting ER stresses because of the difference of the lever arms (with the lever arm to the posterior fibula head 50% greater)

Options and Illustrations of PLC Reconstruction
- Option 1/advance/recess the lateral epicondyle – only works if the soft tissues are stretched only
- Option 2/biceps tenodesis, a popliteus bypass, a free graft reconstruction to fibula head, or combined

- Option 3/chronic ones sometimes need to attach not only at posterior fibula head, but to the PL tibia as well (here a graft with bone block is secured to the epicondyle and tissues are attached to both the fibula head and PL tibia)
- Option 4/HTO – it is essential to restore a proper mechanical axis at the knee for chronic reconstruction to work

1.7   Meniscus

1.7.1   Epidemiology
- USA annual 60 per 100,000 cases
- Males more, two- to threefold
- Peak age 20–30 years
- Greater than fourth decade, most are degenerative tears

1.7.2   Anatomy
- Collagen: from 60% to 70% dry weight, major collagen is type 1; others: types 2, 3, 5 and 6
- Elastin and non-collagenous proteins
- Cells: called fibrochondrocytes, because of appearance
- Fibro-cartilaginous like matrix

1.7.3   Fibre Orientation in the Meniscus
- Compressive loads get dispersed by the circumferential fibres, while the radial fibres act as fibres to resist longitudinal tearing
- Random network of fibres on the surface to help distribution of the shear stresses

1.7.4   Overall Function
- Absorption shock
- Transmission of force
- Decreasing of contact stress
- Help in joint stability – e.g. medial meniscus, if injured further, increases anteroposterior laxity in ACL deficient knee
- Proprioception
- Possibly limiting of extremes of flexion/extension

▦ (Note: medial menisectomy in ACL deficient knee results in an increase in anterior tibial translation of 60%, especially at 90° knee flexion)

1.7.5   General Features
▦ Medial meniscus more fixed than lateral with extensive meniscocapsular attachment (a thickening of which is MCL) – overall, tears are more common to occur on the medial side
▦ Lateral more circular – near a perfect semicircle – and more mobile
▦ Posterior horn ± mid-portion more prone to tear
▦ Lateral side common in acute tears, but medial more common in chronic tears
▦ Tear is common in association with ACL injury and tibial plateau fracture

1.7.6   Post–Total Menisectomy: Fairbank's Changes
▦ Joint space narrows, osteophyte formation, squaring of the femoral condyles – underlines the importance of joint protection by preservation of the meniscus

1.7.7   Meniscus Vascular Supply
▦ Birth: wholly vascular; 9 months: only outer two-thirds vascular
▦ Greater than age 10 years/adult: only 3–4 mm from peripheral attachment (or in other words, the peripheral 10% to 30% portion)
▦ Methods of trephination/abrasion to increase vascularity sometimes used
▦ The synovial fringe near the rim confers no added vascularity
▦ Source of blood supply: superior and inferior branches of the medial and lateral geniculate arteries – forms a perimeniscal capillary plexus
▦ Meniscus also avascular near the popliteal hiatus

1.7.8   Nutrition and Neural Innervation
▦ Though inner two-thirds of adult meniscus not vascular, nutrition by diffusion and mechanical pumping
▦ Neural endings (myelinated and non-myelinated) mostly at the outer portion, i.e. peripheral part painful

1.7.9   Anatomic Variants, Especially for the Lateral Meniscus

- Some very mobile lateral menisci are only attached to the femur at its posterior aspect by: ligament of Wrisberg and, to a lesser extent, ligament of Humphrey – less stability
- A handful of cases with rather loose anterior horns attachment (from 5% to 15%)

1.7.9.1   Classification of Meniscus Tear (by Aetiology)

- Traumatic
- Degenerative

1.7.9.2   Classification of Meniscus Tear (by Pattern)

- Vertical longitudinal: association with bucket handle most common variety – 80% according to Metcalf
- Horizontal tear: association with meniscal cysts (also known as cleavage tears)
- Radial tear
- Oblique: e.g. parrot beak
- Complex: multiplanar, degeneration type under this heading

1.7.9.3   Appendix to the Different Types of Tears

- Vertical longitudinal tear: complete (bucket handle) or incomplete and mostly in young. Mostly associated with ACL tear
  - (Bucket handle tear usually begins in posterior horn; can vary in length from less than 1 cm to greater than two-thirds of the meniscus. Often unstable and common cause of locking.) The *medial meniscus* is usually affected because of its more secure attachments to the tibial plateau and is susceptible to shear injury. Incomplete tears also affect posterior horn and can be found on both the superior and inferior surfaces of the meniscus
- Oblique: often called flap or parrot beak tears, can occur in any location but most at post/mid-portion – propagation can occur if the free torn edge of the flap catches in the joint
- Complex: older age greater than 40 years; often check for associated degeneration not only of meniscus, but for chondrosis
- Radial tear: (or called transverse tear), most are in posterior or middle one-third, medial or lateral meniscus. May propagate across the entire meniscus if the edges catch within the joint. Complete radial

tears disrupt the circumferential fibres of the meniscus resulting in a loss of load-bearing function
- Horizontal: believed to begin in inner margin of the meniscus and extend towards the capsule. Mechanism likely from shear forces generated by axial compression. More in the elderly

1.7.10 Diagnosis
- Combination of history, P/E and X-ray should have accuracy approaching that of MRI
- Although individual test taken, alone not too accurate (not even with McMurray since low sensitivity, if considered alone, according to Shelbourne)
(Block to extension is commonly the result of a displaced bucket handle meniscal tear and usually requires acute surgical Rn)

1.7.10.1 Pros and Cons of MRI
- Overall accuracy nowadays: 95%
  - Advantages:
    non-invasive, no radiation, high accuracy in good hands, can see some concomitant joint pathologies, can assess the knee in multiple planes
  - Disadvantages:
    cost, false positive, e.g. grades 1 and 2 change sometimes interpreted as a real tear, sometimes confusion in Ddx from intermeniscal ligament and fat pad

1.7.10.2 MRI Grading of Meniscal Tear
- Only grade 3, if present, reliably predicts a real tear
- Grades 1 and 2 have an intra-meniscal signal that does not abut on the free edge

1.7.10.3 Diagnosis by Arthroscopy: Gold Standard
- Gold standard to confirm diagnosis:
  - Better able to see posteromedial and PL compartment
  - At the popliteal hiatus, direct probing will help access hypermobility which can occur after popliteomeniscal fasciculi disruption

1.7.10.4 Indication for Arthroscopy

- Symptoms affect daily activity
- Positive physical findings
- Failure to respond to non-surgical Rn
- No other causes of knee pain identified on X-ray or other imaging studies

  (In the setting of ACL, meniscal tears need to be tackled in the same go. Surgical timing is most often dictated by issues related to ACL, e.g. ROM, quadriceps function and associated ligamentous injuries, but loss of motion may sometimes necessitate urgent/early OT)

1.7.11   Meniscal Repair

1.7.11.1 Indication for Meniscal Repair

- Complete vertical longitudinal tear – especially greater than 1 cm long
- Tear within peripheral 10–30% of the meniscus or within 3–4 mm of the meniscocapsular junction
- Tear unstable, displaced by probing
- Tear with no secondary degeneration or deformity
- Active patient
- Tear associated with concomitant ligamentous instability or unstable knee

1.7.11.2 Groups that Do Not Need Intervention

- Short, stable, less than 1 mm vertical longitudinal tear
- Stable, partial, less than 50% thickness tear at superior or inferior surface
- Small less than 3 mm radial tear
  - (In a stable knee, tears may heal spontaneously or remain asymptomatic – the technique of simple rasping and trephination may enhance the healing potential of these tears and should be considered. About 10% with stable tears need added Rn over a 2- to 10-year period in one study)

1.7.11.3 Groups that Need Partial Menisectomy

- Remove unstable fragments
- Eliminate locking or catching and decrease the pain
- Always strive to preserve as much viable tissue as possible to minimise the effect on joint mechanics

1.7.11.4 Important Factors Affecting Repair Ability

- Vascularity
- Tear pattern
- Quality of meniscal tissue
- Concomitant ligament injuries and lower limb alignment are important

1.7.12 Meniscal Cysts

- From 1% to 10% of meniscal pathology
- High correlation with meniscal tear, especially horizontal ones and lateral meniscus
- Contains gel-like material like synovial fluid
- P/E: cyst at, and sometimes below, the joint line; more prominent at 30–40 degree knee flexion

1.7.13 Discoid Meniscus

1.7.13.1 Features

- Usually lateral side
- Complete/incomplete/Wrisberg types
- Wrisberg subtype due to deficient posterior tibial attachment, can look like normal meniscus

1.7.13.2 Physical Assessment

- Snapping/popping: classic (most are the hypermobile Wrisberg type); snapping occurs upon extension
- Click, effusion, McMurray
- Incidental finding: most common, most belong to complete/incomplete types – picked up by MRI

1.7.13.3 Mechanism of Clunk in Discoids

- Occurs on knee extension
- Because on extension, the lateral joint space is more and the displaced (usually Wrisberg) meniscus pops back into the space

1.7.13.4 Investigation

- X-ray: enlarged lateral joint space (mostly in complete/incomplete types), flattened lateral femoral condyle, (flattened) tibial spine

- Role of MRI in diagnosis: most books quote 'easy' diagnosis by seeing full space on all sections, but Wrisberg type more normal looking, can be more tricky to diagnose
- Role of arthroscopy: especially good to diagnose Wrisberg and other types, can assess any tears, can probe for stability, can repair, can resect with remaining 4–6 mm peripheral rim, sometimes central saucerisation

1.7.13.5   Theories of Aetiology
- Smillie: part of meniscus fails to involute, not easy to explain mostly normal looking Wrisberg type. Recently doubted by Ogden from knee dissections at various foetal stages
- Kaplan: 'developmental', claiming the unstable types caused by repeated microtrauma during development
- More favoured nowadays: 'congenital'; evidence from the twin studies and in Wrisberg type, born with deficiency of posterior tibial attachment

1.7.13.6   Traditional Classification (Wantabe)
- Complete
- Incomplete
- Wrisberg

1.7.13.7   New Classification (Jordan)
- Stable or unstable
- Symptomatic versus asymptomatic
- Whether there is tear or not

1.7.13.8   Overall Management Guideline

1.7.13.8.1   Rn Group 1: Stable and Asymptomatic (No Tears)
- Left alone
- Many such cases are never discovered in the whole lifetime

1.7.13.8.2   Rn Group 2: Stable Symptomatic with Tear
- Trim to preserve peripheral rim 4–6 mm at least, central saucerisation
- If very peripheral tear, repair if possible

1.7.13.8.3   Rn Group 3: Unstable Asymptomatic (No Tear)
- Prophylactic removal can predispose to OA, especially if young
- Best option, possible elective reconstruction, but rather controversial

1.7.13.8.4   Rn Group 4: Unstable Symptomatic No Tear
- If Wrisberg, in the past, some suggested total meniscectomy
- Now tend to reattach and reconstruct

1.7.13.8.5   Rn Group 5: Unstable Symptomatic with Tear
- Trim to a peripheral rim of 4–6 mm
- ± Reconstructive measures to stabilise the meniscus

1.7.13.9   Overall Aim of Rn
- Avoid total meniscectomy
- Repair peripheral longitudinal tears
- Trimming down to peripheral 4–6 mm rim sometimes needed
- Sometimes done together with central saucerisation
- Attempts to stabilise Wrisberg type evolving
  (P.S. No long-term studies, many experts say not sure of exact incidence since many are asymptomatic)

1.8   Muscles

1.8.1   General Comments

1.8.1.1   Muscles

1.8.1.1.1   Pathway of Contraction
- Central nervous system (CNS) control
- Spinal cord (SC) and nerve roots
- Peripheral nerve/plexus
- Motor unit
- Neuromuscular junction (NMJ)
- Muscle structure versus function
- Note on MTJ
- Contraction coupling

Motor Unit: Number of Muscle Cells Innervated by a Single Motor Neuron, from 10–2000

- All or none
- In big, two-jointed muscles: ratio high
- Fine co-ordination, e.g. eye muscles: ratio is small

Motor End Plate

- Wasted away after too long denervation (2 years)

NMJ: Release of Acetylcholine (ACh) Across Synapse on Arrival of Impulse

- Negative inhibition either competitive, e.g. curare that binds ACh receptors, or non-competitive, e.g. depolarising agent such as suxamethonium
- Reversal agents include, for example, neostigmine which prevents ACh breakdown and reverses non-depolarising agents

Muscle Structure Hierarchy

- Start with sacromere (between two Z lines)
- → Myofibril → muscle fibre → fasicle → muscle
- A/'Skeleton' of each muscle fibre is endomysium – the sacroplasmic reticulum, rather like endoplasmic reticulum, is calcium rich
- T-tubes penetrate, help spread action potential
- B/Exo-'skeleton'; with perimysium around each fascicle and epimysium around each bundle of muscle

MTJ

- Weak link between muscle and tendon
- Especially injured in eccentric exercises
- Although sometimes it is either the muscle proper which is partial or complete tear, or sometimes tendon itself (tendon has stronger tensile strength than muscle)
  [P.S. Tendon more likely injured with greater muscle force (eccentric); also depends on any weakness of the tendon and ratio of cross-section of muscle versus tendon]

Contraction Coupling
- Z-lines are locations of actin
- 'Zone of Actin': I band
- 'Zone of Myosin': A band
- Normal resting state: portion of myosin prevented from binding to actin by troponin–tropomyosin; release of calcium causes uncovered strategic sites and binding occurs. Then, calcium is pumped back into the sarcoplasmic reticulum

1.8.2   Clinical and Rehabilitation Issues

1.8.2.1   Types of Muscle Fibre and Effect of Training
- Type 1 – slow acting, red in colour since aerobic with much mitochondria – involved in endurance activities
- Type 2 into A and B
- These are explosive, fast-acting, anaerobic metabolism; white in colour since less myoglobin – involved in resistance training like weightlifting

1.8.2.2   Terminology
- Isotonic: same force (use machine)
- Isometric: no change in muscle length, simulate many daily activities like leg presses and good training in the early rehabilitation phase after ACL and PCL reconstruction
- Isokinetic/fixed velocity: usually by machine, since fixed velocity needed
- Concentric contraction: muscle shortens and force is produced proportional to the load applied
- Eccentric contraction: muscle lengthens and force generation is less than the external force

1.8.2.3   Response to Injuries
- Notice little regenerate potential except in newborn
- Delayed muscle soreness: after unaccustomed exercise (especially eccentric)
- Partial muscle rupture: especially two-jointed muscles, especially MTJ – wait until heals before returning to sport. Prevent further injuries by warm-up exercises and stretching

- After healing, contraction only 60% as forceful, but has full ability to shorten
- Complete muscle rupture: heals by scar, is only 50% as forceful and has 80% ability to shorten
- 'De-training'
  - Even strong athletes cannot maintain muscle mass after 2 weeks of no training

1.8.2.4 Proprioception
- Muscle spindles: sensory structures within muscles that help regulate tension and act as proprioceptive organ
- Primary afferent annulospiral ending – response to stretch
- Secondary afferent flower spray – response to tension

1.9   Neural Injury

1.9.1   Nerve Anatomy
- Discussion of the details of nerve anatomy is beyond the scope of this book; the reader is referred to standard neuroanatomy texts

1.9.2   What Happens After Nerve Injury
- Retraction
- Inflammation and factors are secreted to attempt to stimulate neurites
- Degeneration

1.9.3   What Happens After Nerve Injury: Microscopic
- Distal part of severed nerve: Wallerian degeneration (after Waller who first described the phenomenon), survival of nerve fibres occurs only if still remain connected to nerve cell body – starts on day 3
- Proximal part of severed nerve: cell body becomes basophilic (chromatolysis), nucleus moves to periphery, swollen (changes in proximal segment only as far as the next node of Ranvier)
- Activation of Schwann cells close to injured site: takes few weeks to clear debris, axonal sprouts start as early as day 1 (nerve growth factors help this process if the perineurium is disrupted)
- Self-repair does not occur with gaps of more than 2 mm

1.9.4   Outcome
- Sprouts make distal connection then nerve fibre matures (increased axon and myelin thickness)
- Neurites that fail to make distal connection die back and are lost; if the perineurium is not disrupted, then the axons will be guided along the original path at 1 mm/day

1.9.5   Seddon Classes of Nerve Injury
- Neuropraxia: most are compressive in aetiology → local conduction block/demyelination – heal by repair of demyelination, especially of the thick myelin nerves
- Axonotmesis: mostly traction ± severe compression cases → Wallerian degeneration, prognosis not bad since will regenerate and not mis-wire (sensory recovers better since sensory receptors live longer, especially in more proximal injuries)
- Neurotmesis – complete cut, no recovery unless repaired – yet can mis-wire, hence reduced mass of innervation

1.9.6   Sunderland Classification (Six Types)
- Neuropraxia: no Tinel sign
- Axon: both epi- and perineurium intact, Tinel +, progresses distally
- Axon: only epineurium injured, Tinel +, progresses distally
- Axon: perineurium injured, Tinel + but Tinel not progressing distally
- Neurotemesis
- Neuroma in continuity (i.e. partly cut nerve, the remainder can be first/second/third/fourth degree of injury)

1.9.7   Feature of the Sunderland Classification
- Accounts for injuries between axonotmesis and neurotemesis – based on involvement of perineurium

1.9.8   Assessing after a nerve injury
- Motor: assess power and diagnose level of injury
- Sensory: mapping and pattern recognition
- Autonomic: e.g. wrinkle test
    - [Reflex sympathetic dystrophy (RSD) in 3%, featured by swelling, porosis, sweating, pain, etc.]
    - Tinel sign may be present

- Reflexes are not a good guide to injury severity; of course, lost if afferent or efferent limb affected, but sometimes absent in partial injuries as well

1.9.9   Autonomic Changes After Nerve Injury

■ Three major losses – vasomotor, sweat, 'pilomotor'
  - Test pilomotor – loss of wrinkle of denervated skin when immersed in water
  - Test sweating – rub smooth pen against side of finger/ninhydrin test – due to diminished sweating
  - Vasomotor – observation: initial 2 weeks pink, then pale and mottled skin

1.9.10   Checking for, and the Importance of, the Tinel Sign

■ Start distal and proceed to proximal percussion when you test for Tinel sign
  - + Tinel: regenerating axonal sprouts that have not completed myelinisation
  - Distally advancing Tinel: seen in Sunderland types 2 and 3; good sign but does *not* alone indicate complete recovery
    (Note: type 1 Sunderland with no Tinel sign, types 4 and 5 Sunderland no Tinel unless repaired)

1.9.11   Motor and Sensory Charting

■ Motor
  - Grade 0 – nil
  - Grade 1 – flicker
  - Grade 2 – not against gravity, can contract
  - Grade 3 – against gravity
  - Grade 4 – some resistance
  - Grade 5 – normal
    (Motor end plate lasts only 12 months after denervation)
■ Sensory
  - S0 – nil
  - S1 – pain recovers
  - S2 – pain and touch returning
  - S3 – pain and touch throughout autonomy zone
  - S4 – as S3 and S2 – point discrimination returning
  - S5 – normal

1.9.12 Investigations

▦ Role of nerve conduction testing (NCT)/electromyography (EMG) in diagnosis of neurapraxia and axonotmesis
▦ Presence or absence of a progressing Tinel sign

1.9.13 NCT

▦ Aim
  – Check motor/sensory responses of peripheral nerves
  – Check conduction velocity
  – Locate site(s) of compression or injury
  – Together with EMG, may diagnose denervation from myopathy
  – Other related studies, e.g. f-wave studies, etc.

1.9.13.1 Terminology

▦ Latency: time between stimulus onset and response, amplitude – size of response, velocity $V = d/t$
▦ Motor response: nerve over motor point, ground over an inactive muscle, stimulate where the nerve is superficial, turn on stimulator until compound muscle action potential (CMAP) obtained, later maximise potential
▦ Sensory response: CMAP has lower amplitude than motor, $V = d/t$
▦ Somatosensory-evoked potentials (SSEP): stimulate peripheral sensory nerves and measure on the scalp – for study of brachial plexus and spinal cord monitoring

1.9.13.2 Timing of NCT

▦ Ideal time after injury: 2 weeks
▦ Reason: needs from 7 days to 10 days to have absence of sensory conduction (and 3–7 days to get an absent distal motor potential); starting from 2 weeks after the injury, usually can detect denervation changes

1.9.13.3 EMG

▦ What changes do we expect after nerve cut?
▦ Answer: at first normal, then, positive sharp waves as from day 5 to day 14; later, at 2 weeks, spontaneous denervation fibrillation
▦ Implication: good sign if no denervation fibrillation at 2 weeks

▓ Another important use of EMG: diagnosis of neuropathic muscle atrophy from myopathy

1.9.14 Primary versus Delayed Repair of Nerves: Clinical Scenarios
▓ Open clean wound: primary repair
▓ Open wound but poor general condition: repair in 1 week, moist dressing first
▓ Gross contamination: debride, tag nerve ends, repair in less than 3–6 weeks
▓ Closed injury: many are observed since a lot of cases are incomplete, can follow-up with NCT
▓ Closed injury and fracture: only explore if fracture needs open reduction, otherwise follow-up clinically and with NCT
▓ Nerve injury after casting or manipulation: advice exploration

1.9.15 Repair Methods
▓ Epineurial
▓ Perineurial
▓ Combined (epi- and perineurial repair)
▓ In practice, fasicular repair not possible in all cases (each fascicular group is made up of fibres to a particular branch occupying a constant position at the nerve ends)

1.9.16 After Repair
▓ Somewhat controversial as to duration of immobilisation
▓ Upper limb: plaster for 4 weeks, then gradually extend over next few weeks
▓ Lower limb: 6 weeks is usual
  – But, rigid splinting may not be justified if prognosis of nerve function doubted (some advocate mobilisation of distal joints with passive exercises to maintain motion while nerve recovers)

1.9.17 Assessing Return of Neural Function
▓ Motor recovery from more proximally innervated muscles: e.g. test brachioradialis (BR)/extensor carpi radialis longus (ECRL) in early radial nerve recovery
▓ Distally progressing Tinel (especially type-2 and -3 injuries)

– [Note: motor end plates waste away in 1 year, muscle atrophied by 2–3 months, sensory function (erratic) can return in up to 2 years]

1.9.17.1 Assessing Return of Motor Power
- M0: nil
- M1: see contraction proximally
- M2: see contraction proximally and distally
- M3: muscle against resistance
- M4: some independent movements possible
- M5: normal

1.9.17.2 Assessing Return of Sensation (General Recovery Sequence: Pain > Touch > Vibration > Two-Point/Stereognosis)
- S0: nil in nerve autonomous area
- S1: deep pain in auto area
- S2: some pain and touch in autonomic area
- S3: pain and touch over whole autonomic area
- S4: two-point returns
- S5: normal

(Two point discrimination best correlation to final function)

1.10   Growth Factors in Orthopaedics

1.10.1   Clinical Relevance and Introduction
- Most experiments done in animals, interactions complex. Clinical trials mostly not yet quite available, with some exceptions
- Applications:
  - Medicine: e.g. GH defects
  - Orthopaedics:
    Enhancement in fracture healing and role in normal bony healing
    Enhancement of fusion OTs and Rn of bone defects
    Possible future use in osteoporosis
    Distraction osteogenesis
    BMP-related clinical diseases, possible future role of inhibition of heterotopic ossification (HO) by antagonists
    Future role in management of osteolysis around total joint implants

1.10.2   Clinical Studies of BMP

- Several reports of bone-derived BMP preparations available
  - In non-union and segmental defects, e.g. Corr 1998 with the use of human BMP; no controls
  - Periodontal defects
  - Established tibial non-unions (reported by Ortho Research Soc 1998) and human recombinant BMP (reported in J Ortho Trauma 2000 by Swiontowski)
  - Boden planning a pilot study with BMP and cages (to be published in Spine)
    (Note: existence of BMP first suggested by the work of Urist: bone formation in muscle pockets given demineralised bone matrix. Nowadays – different BMPs have been purified and now creating a recombinant library)

1.10.3   Clinical Case One: Fracture Healing

- No human studies, animal studies of fracture models
  - BMPs potent stimulators of bone formation in models of rat/rabbit/sheep/monkey/pigs, but they need a *carrier* to be effective in low doses. Also implicated in bone healing after radiotherapy (RT), cartilage repair
  - TGF-β and fibroblast growth factor (FGF) are mitogenic for bone cells
  - FGF also angiogenic
  - Role of IGF-I less certain, however, promising results reported by a few investigators

1.10.4   Clinical Case Two: Oestrogen-Related Osteoporosis

- Intermittently administered PTH said to have positive effect to increase bone mineral density (BMD)/bone formation and reduce fracture rates (J Clin Investigation)/Finklestein
- Some rat experiments, positive effect of IGF-I; needs more investigation

1.10.5   Clinical Case Three: Age-Related Osteoporosis

- Pending the result of long-term studies on IGF-I to increase bone formation

▧ Short-term administration of the above shows positive stimulant effect

(Note: there is decline in IGF-I with ageing)

1.10.6   Clinical Case Four: Idiopathic Osteoporosis
▧ Current data insufficient to define role of IGF-I

1.10.7   Clinical Case Five: Anorexia Nervosa
▧ Importance: anorexia nervosa may prevent these usually adolescent girls from achieving peak bone mass; causes profound and at times irreversible osteopaenia in adulthood. There is evidence of increased bone resorption in this condition

▧ Oestrogen alone in this group cannot prevent accelerated bone loss

▧ Nutrition factors may play a role and IGF-I is believed by investigators to be implicated. More data needed, but short-term administration of the IGF-I has been shown to increase bone formation in these girls

1.10.8   Clinical Case Six: Distraction Osteogenesis
▧ Role of vascular endothelial growth factor (VEGF) stressed in several studies

▧ BMP role – now believed to be important, exact details pending further investigation

(It is likely that mechanical factors influence BMP gene expression at sites of distraction osteogenesis through a yet to be understood process and that BMPs are components of the complex signals required during the repair paths)

1.10.9   Clinical Case Seven: BMP-Related Clinical Condition
▧ Fibrodysplasia ossificans progressiva – with heterotopic ossification as a series of lumps in muscles of the neck and back; later limitation of motion since heterotopic bone replaces skeletal muscle, tendon, ligament and fascia; most can still reach adult age, usually die of pneumonia, and bone forms from cartilage model. BMP-4 expression detected in cultured fibro-proliferative cells and tissue specimens. Most are from new mutations: ± autosomal dominant. Histology without immune-stain looks like juvenile fibromatosis. However, linkage analysis shows mutation at chromosome 4 and not at the BMP-4 gene: possible that signalling pathway is affected

- Future possible use of drugs that block the pathway of BMP-4 for Rn in HO cases
- Acremesomelic dysplasias – more in Brazil
- Hunter-Thompson chondrodysplasias

1.10.10   Clinical Case Eight:
To Enhance Bony Fusion and Use with BG

- Mostly animal studies; sparse clinical studies
- Most animal models use bone-defect greater than a critical size – reason: these will not heal short of surgical intervention
- Carriers: hydroxyapatite/calcium phosphate materials had success history. Other possible carriers – other constituents of normal bone matrix, e.g. demineralised bone matrix, purified collagen and newer synthetic polymers made from polylactic acid
- Example of a clinical study not of bone defect but in anterior spinal fusion in the presence of cages, e.g. J Spinal Disorders – but most people agree in fact that the spinal fusion models have so far been confined mostly to animal models

1.10.11   Clinical Case Nine:
Prevention of Osteolysis in Implanted Devices

- BMPs may be useful either at the time of device placement (accelerating/augmenting fixation) or during revision surgery

1.10.12   Clinical Case Ten: Osteopetrosis

- A few cytokines implicated in its aetiology. Example: in mice studies, interferon alpha 1b – macrophage colony stimulating factor (M-CSF), vitamin D binding protein-macrophage acting factor (DBP-MAF)
- A recent study suggests the above interferon plus calcitriol has been shown to increase survival

1.10.13   Special Details of Different Factors in Bone Healing

1.10.13.1   TGF-β

- The superfamily of TGF-β genes includes TGF-β, BMP, inhibin-activin subfamilies
- Initially produced from platelet in the haematoma, later by chondrocyte, osteoblast, etc.

- Role: help form granulation tissue, attract macrophages and stimulate chondrocytes and osteoblasts

1.10.13.2   Bone Morphogenic Protein
- Osteoinductive
- BMP-4 detected before cartilage/bone forms in the fracture haematoma
- During the intra-membranous bone forming process, BMP-2 and BMP-4 are expressed
- During endochondral process: BMP-2, BMP-4, BMP-7
- The interactions of different BMP complexes suggests a bone-healing cascade

1.10.13.3   Insulin Growth Factor
- Exact role to be determined

1.10.13.4   Fibroblast Growth Factor
- Angiogenic properties
- Mitogenic properties of chondrocytes

1.10.13.5   Platelet-derived growth factors
- In fracture haematoma
- Role: mitogenic for mesenchymes, modulates blood flow locally

1.11   Osteoporosis

1.11.1   Definition: WHO Criteria
- Normal: BMD less than or equal to 1 SD – young adult average
- Osteopaenia: BMD greater than 1, less than 2.5 SD
- Osteoporosis: BMD greater than or equal to 2.5 SD
- Severe osteoporosis: BMD greater than or equal to 2.5 SD and having fragility fracture

1.11.2   Pathogenesis
- Uncoupling of bone formation and resorption
- Decreased bone mass
- Deterioration of micro-architecture
- Fragility fracture risk increased (Fig. 1.5)

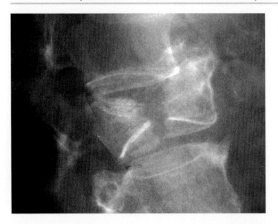

Fig. 1.5. Osteoporotic fracture of the lumbar spine

1.11.3 Caution in Interpretation of WHO Criteria

■ Original aim: focus on checking prevalence in populations, *not* diagnosis in individuals

■ Attempted to 'reconcile the prevalence of osteoporosis created by the chosen density with lifetime fracture risk'

■ Data based on dual- and single-photon absorptiometry and dual-energy X-ray absorptiometry (DEXA) of the posteroanterior (PA) lumbar spine, proximal femur and radius
(WHO also pointed out the importance to differentiate the diagnostic and prognostic use of BMD measures)

1.11.4 Pitfalls in Interpretation of T Score

■ There is a growing consensus that the WHO criteria are not uniformly applicable to all skeletal sites as measured by all techniques

■ The committee of Scientific Advisors of the International Osteoporosis Foundation suggested reserving the WHO criteria for measurements of the proximal femur
  - (Some authors have recently attempted to identify T score cut-off that results in acceptable sensitivity and specificity at other non-spine non-hip sites – not yet received very wide acceptance, however)
  - (Beware of marked differences noted as a percentage of women diagnosed as having osteoporosis by means of different DEXA devices; diagnostic disparity also exists even when using a single device to different regions)

1.11.5 Caution About Interpretation of T Scores from Peripheral Sites

▓ Thus, the derived fracture risk varies dramatically from device to device, and care should, in general, be exercised in interpretation of T scores, especially scores generated from the use of peripheral sites as opposed to hip and spine. Some have recommended that central DEXA, particularly at the hip, be used for diagnostic and Rn decisions and have cautioned against the use of T scores derived from peripheral devices for diagnosis

1.11.6 Cautions in Interpretation of Z Scores

▓ Caution an unusually low Z score: check secondary causes of osteoporosis, e.g. thyroid, renal, PTH excess, osteomalacia, tumour, blood disorders like myeloma
▓ A common treatable cause of osteoporosis is hyperthyroidism
▓ A common cause of non-response to alendronate is inadequate calcium and vitamin D intake as in occult osteomalacia

1.11.7 Suggested Method for Diagnosis and Assessment of Fracture Risk

▓ Women less than 65 years old
PA spine (L1–4 or 2–4)
Proximal femur
▓ Women older than 65 years
Proximal femur (since spine readings inaccurate from osteophytes and sometimes from compression fracture)
± Forearm/heel – can sometimes be used

1.11.8 Rn Guidelines: Word of Caution

▓ Guidelines for the Rn of osteoporosis *cannot be universal* because of cost-effective use of available medical resources, which vary dramatically from country to country. The decision is a societal one and is affected by health-care planning and the budgets of local government. As some experts pointed out in the past, 'Widespread BMD testing with long-term pharmacological therapy for osteoporosis prevention or Rn will only be feasible in the most wealthy of societies'

1.11.9 Monitoring of Rn

- Always either PA spine or proximal femur
- Never peripheral sites
- Same device and same site each time
- DEXA mostly used
- Use of bone markers still experimental
  Frequency: once per year (unless in patients with chronic steroid usage)

1.11.10 Pros and Cons of BMD as a Monitor
(or Use Alternative: the Bone Markers)

- The precision of BMD and the (somewhat controversial) relationship between magnitude of BMD changes and magnitude of fracture reductions were mentioned as arguments for monitoring with BMD. Arguments against monitoring include the finding that, among women taking alendronate, most who lost bone in the first year gained bone in the second. Furthermore, it should be pointed out that there are no studies showing that women randomised to therapy are more likely to adhere to therapy when BMD is monitored

1.11.11 Traditional Teachings of Two Main Types of Osteoporosis

- Postmenopausal
- Senile

1.11.12 Clinical Assessment

- Age is very important
- Height
- Weight: low body weight independent risk
- Maternal fracture history: important risk factor
- Drug history: especially steroids and dilantin, etc.
- Menstrual history
- Social history: smoking and drinking
- Diet and general nutrition
- Past health: especially history of gynaecological OTs and endocrine disease, previous osteoporotic fracture in patient, coronary heart disease (CHD)/breast disorders
- Previous and current osteoporotic Rn

1.11.13   Management of Osteoporosis

The reader should know that the strategies for prevention versus Rn are very different

1.11.13.1   Prevention versus Rn

- Whether for prevention or Rn of osteoporosis, most if not all agents available are anti-resorptive agents
- These agents work by decreased bone turnover and increased BMD, thus lesser fracture
- Even a 2–3% small increase in BMD may produce decreased spine and non-vertebral fracture risk

1.11.13.2   Categories of Agents with Examples

- Prevention only: oestrogens
- Rn only: calcitonin
- Prevention and Rn:
  - Bisphosphonates
  - Raloxifene

1.11.13.3   What Makes Bisphosphonates so Different?

- Alendronate (and risedronate) not only (1) prevent bone loss, but (2) the increase of bone mass and positive bone balance appears to continue (no clear plateau) even more than 1 year after stopping alendronate
- In contrast, oestrogens and calcitonin also increase bone density for 1–2 years and then plateau – but provide little protection after stopping

1.11.13.4   The Opposite of the Anti-resorptive Agents Are Formative Agents

- FDA has just approved the use of pulsatile PTH therapy, though not yet in wide general use
- Research agents: PTH peptides, fluoride, strontium, anabolic steroids, GH, insulin-like factors
- Pulsatile PTH Rn is the more promising among the different agents

1.11.13.5 Individual Agents

1.11.13.5.1 Calcium and Vitamin D
- All Rn regimes rendered futile if there is not adequate calcium
- Helps prevent bone loss, especially in elderly – especially in institutions
  - Most studies have not shown fracture reduction, but reduction or prevention of bone loss
  - Though one study says it does by Dawson-Hughes in NEJM

1.11.13.5.2 HRT as a Preventive Agent
- Two very important studies (on fracture risks)
  - HERS [oral oestrogen and progestin – no definite decrease in fracture (if not more fracture) – do not reduce myocardial infarction [MI]/cardiovacular system (CVS) morbidity]
  - WHI [women's health initiative]
    Important large RCT with more than 16,000 women shows a hip fracture risk after 5.2 years
    Trial stopped early due to an increase in cardiovascular events in the HRT group
- HRT increases in bone density are accepted
- New advice from some experts
  - Better taper off HRT, especially in cases of CHD and breast cancer
  - Oestrogen sometimes used to decrease menopausal symptom, but not in osteoporosis reduction

Latest Results of the WHI Study
- It took three decades to get this formal RCT done, which involved more than 16,000 patients and compared oestrogen/progestin with placebo
- The study ended prematurely in May 2001 because HRT caused a higher incidence of: heart disease (30%), breast cancer (26%), cerebrovascular accident (CVA) (40%) and pulmonary embolism (110%)
- Morbidity far greater than the benefits of less hip fracture (–34%) and colon cancer (–37%)

1.11.13.5.3 Calcitonin as a Therapeutic Agent

(Miacalcin nasal spray)

- Increases spine BMD (2%)
- Lowers spine fracture risk (30%)
- Proof study: dosage = 200 I.U. daily
  The 200 I.U. dose said to be optimal to reduce fracture risk
  No effect on hip and other non-spine fracture
  Another important use: pain control after acute vertebral fracture, acting via its central action

1.11.13.5.4 Raloxifene – as a Preventive and Therapeutic Agent

- Selective oestrogen receptor modulator (SERM)
- Both hip and spine: increased BMD (3%)
- Decreased spine fracture only (40%)

Studies Concerning the Use of SERM

- Raloxifene has been developed specifically to treat osteoporosis and the multiple outcomes of raloxifene evaluation (MORE) study was designed to specifically evaluate the efficacy of raloxifene in women
- A total of about 7700 women around the world were randomised to receive either 60 mg (marketed dose), 120 mg or placebo. The study showed a modest increase in BMD (about 2.5% at the spine) and a reduction of about 35% (with the 60-mg dose) in vertebral fractures throughout 3 years. However, there was no evidence of a reduction in non-vertebral or hip fractures in the 3 years of the trial or during a 1-year extension

1.11.13.5.5 Bisphosphonates: Result at 10 Years)

- Increased spine (8%), hip (4%) BMD
- Decreased fracture risk by 50% each of spine and hip (at 1 year)

Nature and Mechanics of Bisphosphonates

(Second Generation: Alendronate, Third Generation: Risedronate)

- Pyrophosphate analogues by nature bind to exposed bony mineral surfaces
- Ingestion by osteoclasts prevents ruffled border formation
- Other actions (at selected doses will not affect mineralisation; and/or less apoptosis of osteoblast/osteocytes)

Details of Bisphosphonates

Contraindications:

- Oesophageal problems (not with risedronate) sometimes less with re-challenge
- Patient cannot stand/sit-up for various reasons
- Drug sensitivity
- Low [Ca] with renal failure

Uses:

- Prevention and Rn of osteoporosis
- Possible role (animal model) in total joint osteolysis
- IV administration, e.g. pamidronate in malignant hypercalcaemia

Dose:

- As prevention: 5 mg q.d., or 35 mg per week
- As Rn: 10 mg q.d., or 70 mg per week

Administration: glass of water on empty stomach in morning before eating and drinking, remain upright for 0.5 h

Potential disadvantage: decreased micro-repair of bone, and bones may be more brittle with chronic use

1.11.13.5.6 Combination Therapy

- HRT and alendronate: with 20% additive effect
- Other combinations: minimal effect
- Experimental: intermittent PTH and bisphosphonates

1.11.13.5.7 Experimental Agents

PTH: Two Main Actions

- Helps calcium homeostasis: maintains serum calcium for proper cell function – across three areas: gut, bone and kidney
- Controls and modulates cells active in the remodelling cycle → increases the size, activity and working life of osteoblasts and strengthens the trabeculae – sometimes even bypassing local mechanostatic limits
  [Given continuously – bone is lost; given intermittently – works via TGF-β, decreasing apoptosis of osteoblasts]

  - Action stops on withdraw – but this might be blocked by alendronate; said to be good for steroid cases
  - Some initial reports of associations with osteosarcoma in animals, but now thought to be dose and species related; trials are resumed

Is the Use of PTH Promising?

■ It is currently uncertain as to how PTH will best be used clinically (e.g. by itself, in combination with anti-resorptive agents or followed by anti-resorptive therapy)

■ Lindsay and co-workers reported that during 18 months of observational follow-up there was a lower incidence of vertebral fractures among women who had originally been randomised to PTH. This study, together with that from Papaioannou and co-workers, challenges the popularly-held belief that any gains in BMD or strength from PTH will be lost soon after cessation of therapy

■ However, the inferences that can be drawn from these observational data are limited, because the patients were using a variety of therapies during the observational periods and these therapies were self-selected

1.11.14   Appendix

1.11.14.1   Key to Osteoporosis

■ Uncoupling between bone formation and destruction (H. Mankin)
■ Normal adult bone mass reached at around 20 years of age

1.11.14.2   Causes of Secondary Osteoporosis

■ Steroid (depress osteoblasts and stimulate osteoclasts) methotrexate (MTX; unknown mechanics)
■ Rheumatoid arthritis (RA; disuse, interleukin, drugs)
■ Hormonal causes
■ Disuse and post-trauma
■ Idiopathic transient
■ Others, e.g. RSD

1.11.14.3   Causes of Idiopathic Osteoporosis

■ Traditionally divided into two major groups:
  – Postmenopausal
  – Senile – men and women
    Newer concept – both types have one thing in common – decline in sex hormones, especially oestrogen – in both sexes in the latter type

1.11.14.4 Possible Pathomechanics of Idiopathic Group

- Uncoupling of bone-remodelling process, decreased bone formation no matter whether the overall turnover is normal/increased/decreased in a given osteoporotic individual
- Possible genetic factor (likely polygenic)
- Peak bone mass
- Role of sex hormones just mentioned

1.11.14.5 Role of Possible Genetic Basis

- Research from U.K. recently found that peak bone mass is probably not environmentally determined and is probably under genetic control. Studies of twins suggest that spine and hip peak bone mass is from 70% to 80% heritable
- There is, in addition, some suggestion that bone geometry and quality are highly heritable
- Although there are a number of interesting candidate genes related to osteoporosis, it seems likely that osteoporosis is a polygenic disease, and most of the genes related to osteoporosis remain to be discovered
- One example of a gene of current interest is the collagen 1A1 gene (*COL1A1*), which seems more strongly related to fracture risk than to BMD

1.11.14.6 Epidemiology in USA

- In the United States alone, approximately 10 million individuals (8 million women and 2 million men) have osteoporosis, and 18 million more have osteopaenia, placing them at increased risk for the most serious consequence of the condition – fracture. Dr. Einhorn had done many great works in reviewing the determinants of bone strength, which include bone mass, bone size, bone structure and bone microarchitecture. He noted that it is becoming increasingly clear that factors *other than* bone mass are important in determining bone strength and the changes that occur in bone strength as a result of osteoporosis Rn

1.11.14.7 Comparing Trends in US/Europe versus Asia

- Rates of both hip and vertebral fractures are similar in Europe and North America
- Although hip fracture rates are generally lower in Asia, vertebral fracture rates are similar to those in North America

- Recent data show that the incidence of hip fracture is rising significantly in both Hong Kong and Singapore, while that of some other Asian countries, such as Thailand, has a less obvious change, but the incidence might pick up later

1.11.14.8 Epidemiology from Asia

- Recent studies from the Chinese University of Hong Kong suggested that by the year 2050, of the 3.2 million hip fractures annually, more than 50% of them will occur in Asia. This shift is primarily attributed to the increase in the number of elderly people in Asia
- There are few data about vertebral fractures in Asia, but the data that do exist suggest that vertebral fracture prevalence is at least as high in Asia as in the United States or Europe
- Studies have consistently shown that BMD is lower in Asia, suggesting that population-specific T scores should be used

1.11.14.9 Trend in Hong Kong

- Hip fracture incidence is estimated to have increased 3.3% per year in Hong Kong between 1966 and 1989, compared with only about 1% per year in the United States, and there is every indication that it is still on the increase

General Bibliography

Bulkwalter J, Einhorn T, Simon S (eds) (2000) Orthopaedic basic science, 2nd edn. American Academy of Orthopaedic Surgeons

Favus MJ (1999) Primer on the metabolic bone diseases and disorders of mineral metabolism, 4th edn. Lippincott Williams & Wilkins, Philadelphia

Selected Bibliography of Journal Articles

1. Peterson L, Brittberg M et al. (2003) Articular cartilage engineering with autologous chondrocyte implantation. A review of recent developments. Foot Ankle Clinic 8:291–303
2. Brittberg M, Lindahl A et al. (1994) Treatment of deep articular defects in the knee with autologous chondrocyte implantation. New Engl J Med 331:889–895
3. Muckle DS, Minns RJ (1990) Biological response to woven carbon fibre pads in the knee. A clinical and experimental study. J Bone Joint Surg Br 72:60–62

4. Finkelstein JS, Klibanski A et al. (1998) Prevention of estrogen deficiency related bone loss with human parathyroid hormone: a randomized controlled trial. JAMA 280:1067–1073

5. Boyan BD, Schwartz LD, et al. (1992) Effects of bone morphogenic protein on the expression of glycosaminoglycans, collagen, and alkaline phosphatase in nonunion cell cultures. CORR 278:286–304

6. Salter RB, Simmonds DF et al. (1980) The protective effect of continuous passive motion on the healing of full thickness defects in articular cartilage. An experimental investigation in the rabbit. J Bone Joint Surg Am 62:1232–1251

7. Shelbourne KD, Jari S et al. (2003) Outcome of untreated traumatic articular defects of the knee. A natural history study. J Bone Joint Surg Am 85A[Suppl 2]:8–16

8. Laros GS, Cooper RR et al. (1971) Influence of physical activity on ligament insertions in the knees of dogs. J Bone Joint Surg Am 53:275–286

2 General Paediatric Orthopaedics

Contents

2.1   Generalised Disorders

2.1.1   Skeletal Dysplasia

2.1.1.1   Definition of Terms

- Dysplasia: The term implies a generalised abnormality in growth and development
- Dysostosis: Denotes maldevelopment of a single bone or body segment
- Dystrophy: Defined as a disorder, usually congenital, of the structure or function of an organ or tissue due to its "perverted nutrition". It includes agenesis, atrophy, hypertrophy, hyperplasia and metaplasia

2.1.1.2   Other Terminology

- Of limb shortening:
  - Rhizomelic, i.e. proximal short
  - Mesomelic, i.e. middle short
  - Acromelic, i.e. distal segment short
- Descriptive terms:
  - Diatrophic: Twisted
  - Campomelic: Bent limb
  - Metatrophic: Changing
  - Hyphomelic: Bend forward

2.1.1.3   Classification (Rubin)

- Epiphysis: hyperplasia (e.g. Trevor)
  - Hypoplasia [spondylo-epiphyseal dysplasia (SED), multiple epiphyseal dysplasia (MED), pseudo-achondroplasia]
- Physis: hyperplasia (e.g. endochondromatosis)
  - Hypoplasia (e.g. achondroplasia)
- Metaphysis: hyperplasia (e.g. multiple exostoses)
  - Hypoplasia (e.g. osteopetrosis)
- Diaphysis: hyperplasia (e.g. diaphyseal dysplasia)
- Hypoplasia [e.g. osteogenesis imperfecta (OI)]
  Others: e.g. osteopathia striata (Fig. 2.1)

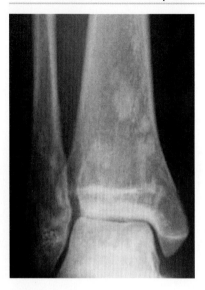

Fig. 2.1. Osteopathia striata

2.1.1.4 History
Do not forget also to ask about:
- Family history
- Birth history
- Pedigree

2.1.1.5 Physical Examination
- Adult height (exact) and percentile (adult height is an important diagnostic feature since adults affected by specific dysplasia show little variation in height: e.g. 3.5 ft diastrophic dwarf, 4 ft in achondroplasia; 4.5 ft in hypochondroplasia)
- Proportional/not proportional (e.g. of proportional ones: constitutional, endocrine, malnutrition, chromosomal disease, and prenatal dwarf)
- Ratio of arm span: height (i. short-limbed, e.g. achondroplasia; ii. short trunk e.g.. SED; iii. long trunk and limbs, e.g. Marfan syndrome)
- Ratio of upper and lower segments (lower segments between symphysis to foot; rest of height is upper segments) (Upper: lower segment normal ratio decreases from 1.6 in infant to near 1 in adults)

▨ Dysmorphic features
▨ Clinical deformity
  [distal upper limb (UL) to proximal 75% usually; distal lower limb
  (LL) to proximal 82%]

2.1.1.6 Investigation
▨ X-ray (XR): skull, pelvis, lumbar spine, hands/wrists, knees
▨ Laboratory work: e.g. endocrine tests, genetic tests
▨ Pathology/histological anomalies: e.g. some dysplasia have special mi-
  croscopic abnormalities – pseudoachondroplasia, diastrophic dwarf-
  ism, kniest

2.1.1.7 General Goals of Treatment
▨ Accurate diagnosis (Dx)
▨ Genetic counsel
▨ Psychological support
▨ Symptomatic treatment:
  – Orthopaedic: e.g. prevent deformity, stabilise lax joints, support
    brittle bones, correction of leg length discrepancy (LLD), joint re-
    construction
  – Others: dental, eye consult, etc.
▨ Hormonal
▨ ±Gene therapy

2.1.1.8 Specific Dysplasias

2.1.1.8.1 Osteogenesis Imperfecta (Fig. 2.2)
▨ A hereditary condition featured by tendency to have multiple fractures from mutation and changed structure of type-1 collagen. Associated with involvement of other body tissues, such as poor dentition,
  laxity of ligaments, eye (cornea thinned), etc.
▨ The fracture callus in OI – heals and appears early; is identical to the
  rest of the skeleton, i.e. easily deformed with weight-bearing and muscle actions

Silence Classes
  Type 1: mildest, autosomal dominant (AD), blue sclera, normal life
  expectancy

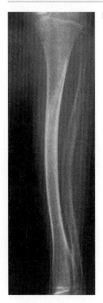

Fig. 2.2. Gracile bowed tibia in osteogenesis imperfecta

- Type 2: autosomal recessive (AR), lethal with death at very young age (stillborn or shortly after birth), mortality from pulmonary insufficiency and thoracic wall injury, blue sclera
- Type 3: severe AR, deformity usual, wheelchair bound, normal sclera, short stature, moulding of forehead creates a characteristic sunset appearance of faces due to apparent lowering of cornea and exposes sclera above
- Type 4: AD, severity intermediate between types 1 and 3, short stature, life expectancy usually decreased

Differential Diagnosis
- In newborn: heritable chondrodystrophies, congenital lethal hypophosphatasia
- In children: child abuse, idiopathic juvenile osteoporosis, childhood hypophosphatasia, endocrinopathy induced osteopaenia
- In adult: hypophosphataemic rickets, malabsorption, secondary causes of osteoporosis

Workup

- History:
  - Family and family tree
  - Perinatal
  - Past history of fractures and their treatment
  - Past history of dislocation(s) and their treatment
  - Other system: dentition, eye, hearing, cardiovascular system (sometimes valvular heart)
  - Activities of daily living (ADL)

Physical Assessment

- Head: "triangular" shape
- Eye
- Hearing aid
- Posture plus ligament laxity
- Deformity and old scars
- Dislocated joints
- Scoliosis and sagittal balance
- UL/LL neurology
- Cervical spine
- General exam

Radiological Assessment

- Skull – wormian Bone, look for platysbasia
- Scoliosis and/or kyphosis
- Vertebra plana/collapse
- Gracile bone, bent thin and very narrow medulla in severe cases; flared metaphyses (if present) caused by defective modelling
- Trefoil pelvis, protrusio is common; perhaps cause for fracture
- In severe cases, the epiphysis contains whorls of matrix (popcorn sign)
- Callus/intramedullary (IM) rod may be present (e.g. Bailey rod); refer to the Sofield operation

Special Test if Dx Not Sure

- Culture of skin fibroblasts in skin punch biopsy

Overall Treatment Goals
- Maximise function
- Minimise disability
- Less-dependent ADL
- Greatest possible mobility
- Overall health

Non-operative Treatment
- Mainstay of treatment
- Light-weight braces can be of help in external support to promote stance and locomotion
- Even vacuum pants and pneumatic trouser splint

Other Non-Operative Treatment
- Medical – physiotherapy: strengthen muscles, assess cardiopulmonary
  - Dental visit each 3–6 months
  - May need bracing for scoliosis
  - Ensure adequate calcium and vitamin D; there is some evidence the second generation bisphosphonates may reduce bone loss and possibly fractures

General Surgical Principles
- Avoid surgery in patients less than age 2 years of age
- Avoid plate and screws in favour of IM devices
- Gentle technique for muscle preservation and minimise bleeding
- Rehabilitation after operation important and in general. Therapy to restore joint motion and muscle strength is important following fracture, etc.
- Treatment of fracture in mild cases may resemble that of other children

Timing and Indication of Surgery
- Indication: recurrent fracture or deformity that impairs function, optimal age for surgical intervention controversial
- Mostly accepting deformity from closed treatment until age 5 years and then proceeding to corrective osteotomies

Techniques of Deformity Correction

- Closed osteoclasis with traction by pneumatic splints
- Close reduction (CR) and IM nailing
- Multiple corrective osteotomy with IM nailing (e.g. Sofield operation in the femur)
- Osteotomies with elongating rods (e.g. Bailey Dubow rods)

Spinal Deformity in OI

- Pathogenesis:
  - Soft and brittle bone
  - Compression vertebral collapse
  - Ligamentous laxity
  - Occurs in majority of severe cases,
  - If greater than 80 will contribute to pulmonary insufficiency
- Role of bracing:
  - Not effective since soft deformed rib cage and truncal shortening may worsen rib cage deformity and not effective in controlling curve progression
  - May consider if pure kyphosis

Management of Scoliosis in OI

- Any curves greater than $40°$ likely to progress
- Mostly use posterior approach, despite the soft bone the posterior arch usually still adequate for fixation
- Correction and stabilisation with rods anchored in every vertebra sometimes necessary

Future

- Gene therapy?
- To tackle the frequent glycine mutation of the type-1 collagen

2.1.1.8.2 Achondroplasia

- Featured by frontal bossing, mid-face hypoplasia, short limbs rhizomelic. Can present as spinal claudication in later life
- AD inheritance, but many are new mutations
- XR: flattening of anterosuperior aspect of the lumbar vertebra, progressive decrease in inter-pedicular distance on AP lumbar XR; extremities can show "ball and socket" epiphysis, flared metaphyses, besides short bones

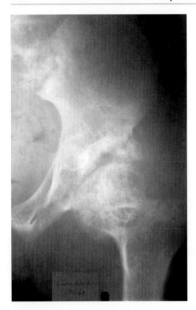

Fig. 2.3. Hip affection in multiple epiphyseal dysplasia

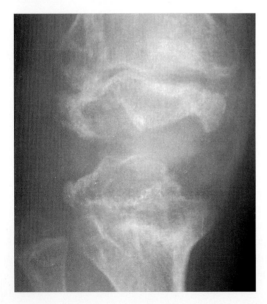

Fig. 2.4. Knee affection in multiple epiphyseal dysplasia

2.1.1.8.3 Spondylo-epiphyseal Dysplasia
- Rare, AD
- Mainly affects the trunk (axial skeleton) and large proximal joints (hip and shoulder). The former can cause scoliosis; the latter can produce premature OA

2.1.1.8.4 Multiple Epiphyseal Dysplasia (Figs. 2.3, 2.4)
- Variable Inheritance,
- Mainly affects the long bones epiphysis
- Skull and axial skeleton normal
- Frequently just short for the age of the child, not necessarily a dwarf

2.1.1.8.5 Dysplasia Epiphysialis Hemimelica (Trevor's Disease)
- Featured by osteocartilaginous exostoses coming from the medial or lateral half of the epiphysis of a single limb
- More in males, and LL more affected

2.1.1.8.6 Diaphyseal Aclasis (Multiple Exostoses) (Figs. 2.5–2.7)
- AD mostly
- Cartilage capped exostoses point away from the joint
- Not truly "diaphyseal" as the name implies, for the exostoses are next to epiphysis
- Malignant change can occur if lesions found in the flat bones of pelvis or the scapula

2.1.1.8.7 Ollier's Disease (Endochondromatosis) (Fig. 2.8)
- Featured by multiple endochondromata of bones
- Mostly unilateral or aymmetrical affection if bilateral bony involvement occurs, giving rise to limb deformity, LLD
- Affected limbs are short, and sarcomatous transformation can occur in middle to old age
- Association with multiple haemangiomata is called Maffuci's syndrome

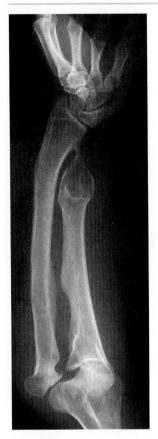

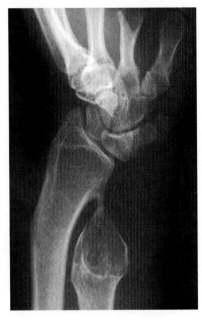

Fig. 2.6. Multiple exostoses affecting the forearm close up

Fig. 2.5. Multiple exostoses affecting the forearm

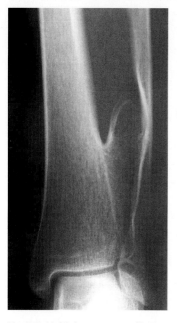

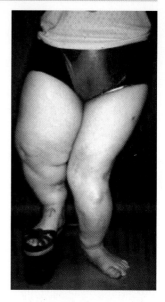

Fig. 2.8. Ollier's disease

Fig. 2.7. Multiple exostoses affecting the ankle

2.1.2   Cerebral Palsy

2.1.2.1   Definition

▓ Group of non-progressive, motor (mainly) impairment syndromes secondary to lesions or anomalies of the brain from foetal to around age 2 years
  – [But its manifestations can change over time with growth, development and maturation]
▓ Can have defects in sensation, cognition, seizure, gastrointestinal/genitourinary problems, etc.

2.1.2.2   Aetiology

▓ Intrinsic abnormal central nervous system (CNS) structure (e.g. chromosomal, metabolic disease)
▓ External insult (e.g. infection, ischaemia)

2.1.2.3 Classification

▓ Geographical Classification (Gage)
- Diplegic (1/3 cases)
- Hemiplegic (30%)
- Dyskinetic (15%)
  All three types may walk
- Quadriplegic (one-quarter of cases)
  Most will not walk

2.1.2.4 General Basic Concepts

▓ Bleck's criteria: Communication >ADL >mobility
(e.g. if completely no contact with the outside world, avoid operating if possible)
Pattern of spasticity rather different even in the same anatomic class (e.g. diplegic)

2.1.2.5 Art of Treatment of Cerebral Palsy

▓ More mature gait pattern of normal child reached at 4 years; main reason for not operating (unless forced to) at less than 5–7 years old is that we do not want to do anything irreversible

▓ One common reason of recurrence of deformity is: spastic muscle grows more slowly than bones

2.1.2.6 Determining the Goal of Operation is Important

▓ Mild diplegics – goal is ambulation; avoid tendo-Achilles lengthenings (TALs) – use gastrocnemius recessions, hamstring lengthening at times, iliopsoas recessions sometimes, varus derotation osteotomy for significant internal rotation (IR), and rectus femoris transfers (to the semitendinosis) if lack of knee flexion in swing phase of gait. Sometimes split tibialis anterior transfer for equinovarus on swing and split tibialis posterior (TP) transfer for equinovarus on stance. Many may require adductor tenotomy/release for the usually associated adductor tightness; avoid obturator neurectomy

2.1.2.7 Goal in the More Severe Diplegics

▓ Still keep them as functional as possible in their childhood – although they may end up in a wheelchair (or can get by with a walker or stander) in adulthood due the changes in the weight-strength ratio, i.e. as they become bigger, their engine is not enough to propel them

2.1.2.8   Timing of Operation

▦ In most cases operate (if operation needed) on those around age 7–8 years; (preferably not after 12 years of age, since operation works less well after that age)

▦ Prior to age 4–5 years and if deformity is dynamic, botox is sometimes useful – each injection can last for months, not for cases with generalised spasticity. Inject at various lengths of the muscle. Some units have started to use electromyography (EMG)/ultrasound (USS) to ensure the injection goes to the desired muscle group

2.1.2.9   Those in Most Severe End of Spectrum of Diplegics – Mimic Total Body

▦ Here, may be forced to do surgery early

▦ If deformities still dynamic and patient is young, may consider posterior selective rhizotomy for global spasticity

▦ Some can have windswept legs. See later discussion

▦ Needs more careful physical exam, rule out possible triplegia, etc.

2.1.2.10   Principles in Total Body

▦ First of all, avoid operation if no contact with outside world

▦ Three very common vexing problems:
   – Severe scoliosis with pelvic obliquity
   – Impending/completed hip dislocation
   – Windswept deformities

2.1.2.10.1   Problem 1: Scoliosis with Pelvic Obliquity

▦ General golden rule is:
   – If scoliosis and hip contracture → tackle hip first (exception: if the maximum curve is quite extra-pelvic, wherein surgery to the hip is difficult to assess correction intraoperatively)
   – If the pelvis is part of the curve → fuse to sacrum with stable construct such as the Galverston technique

2.1.2.10.2   Problem 2: Windswept Deformities

▦ EMG studies support that the pathogenesis usually involves three of the four muscle groups active (i.e. abductor and adductor on one side plus adductor of the other side – but the other side abductor not active)

- Implication
  - Prone to recurrence of deformity
  - Bony surgeries on both sides usually may be required
  - Adequate release of adductor on one side and very minimal only release of adductor on the side with active abductor tone – if not, one ends up with abduction deformity
  - If varus derotational osteotomy (VDRO) is planned – one side IR, the other side external rotation (ER)

2.1.2.10.3 Problem 3: Impending Hip Subluxation

- Frequently for these cases, there is a roughly 2-year window of opportunity to tackle the impending dislocation
- Parents must be told there is a 30–40% chance of being symptomatic with pain if left untreated
- Treatment mostly involves both femoral varus derotational osteotomy and pelvic surgery: most of these lack posterolateral coverage, so-called triplane posterolateral actabuloplasty may be needed. Subluxation cases usually no degeneration yet. But acetabulum sometimes does wear away quickly, especially posteriorly, and may need 3D computed tomography (CT) scan preoperatively for assessment
  [Note: Acetabulum widely believed to remodel up to age 4 years and much less remodelling after age 8 years]

2.1.2.10.4 Chronic Hip Dislocation with No Pain

- If chronic and no pain, and does not interfere with transfers, etc. – can be observed (especially if bilateral)

2.1.2.10.5 Painful Hip Dislocation with Symptomatic OA of Femoral Head

- Open capsule and look at head
- If good – reconstruction of hip on both sides
- If bad – resect femoral head, can consider a hypervalgus osteotomy (the previous Shanz operation described by Rang is less used nowadays)
- Other options for late OA. Not with good results and seldom recommended (hip arthroplasty unlikely to be good with this osteoporotic bone in wheelchair bound patients and uneven muscle pull; resection arthroplasty causes much post-op pain and proximal migration, even if post-op traction given.)

2.1.2.10.6   Avoid the Use of Triple Innominate Osteotomy in Hip Reconstruction

- Tend to retrovert the acetabulum and may dislocate, since these kids are chronically sitting in wheelchair

2.1.2.11   Two Major Neurosurgical Interventions For Significant Spasticity And Increased Tone

- Intrathecal Baclofen: Use intrathecal since Baclofen does *not* cross blood–brain barrier; hence, this method improves its effect with fewer side effects
- Selective posterior rhizotomy: not to be taken lightly as the operation is irreversible and involves painstaking severing of afferent rootlets. Needs careful patient selection, and should not be overdone, since it can produce too much weakness as well as iatrogenic spinal deformity

2.1.2.12   Treatment Goal in Non-Ambulators

- Balanced comfortable sitting by
  - Straight spine and level pelvis
  - Located mobile pain free hips
  - Mobile knees
  - Plantigrade feet
  - Appropriate adaptive equipment provided (e.g. wheelchair) plus supportive team

2.1.2.13   Wheelchair (Viewed as a Total Body Orthotic)

- Wheelchair hardware design
  Comfort, decreased pressure, stability
- Wheelchair hardware positioning components
  Headrest, trunk support, waist belt, may add spinal orthosis, etc.
- Wheelchair cushions
  Foam, gel-based, air-based, thermoplastic urethane
- Special custom designs
  Give fuller contact, optimise weight/pressure distribution, ?load sensor technology

2.1.2.14   Spine in Cerebral Palsy

2.1.2.14.1   Weinstein's Classification

It is assumed that the reader is acquainted with Weinstein's Classification for Scoliotic Deformity of Cerebral Palsy (CP)

2.1.2.14.2   Problems & Non-Op Problem

▨ (1) neuromuscular (NM) scoliosis, (2) unique problems – spasticity, seizure, etc.

▨ Non-operative treatment
  - Sitting support: good sitting aid hand function, sitting balance, aid feed/transport
  - Seating support: stabilise pelvis/trunk, choice depend on sitting balance, moulding
  - Curve control: sometimes brace
  - Delay surgery in some cases

2.1.2.14.3   Operative Principles

▨ The advantage of operation
  Sitting independent/endurance, better UL use, better lung function, better feeding and ease of nursing, pain control, ease of transport

▨ General surgery principle
  Fuse early, fuse long, pelvic level and balanced, stable internal fixation

▨ Indication of operation (OT)
  - Documented curve progression
  - Poor function (difficult sitting and balance)

2.1.2.14.4   Preop Assessment

Risk versus benefit

▨ Orthopaedic aspect: Also pay attention to the hip and pelvis

▨ Others:
  - Discuss with family
  - Nutrition (swallowing study, treat reflux, preop may need a jejunal tube)
  - Pulmonary function
  - Genitourinary Reflux
  - Neurology assess and fit control
  - Team assessment

2.1.2.14.5   Traction XR
▦ Help assess flexibility
▦ The pelvis level
▦ Spine/trunk
   – Level pelvis and balanced trunk: Posterior fuse
   – Tilted pelvis and unbalanced trunk: antero-posterior (AP) fuse

2.1.2.14.6   Surgical Tip
▦ Fuse long T2-S2
▦ Segmental fixation: flexible cable
▦ If fixation to pelvis planned → galverston/versus iliac bolts L5/S1/S2 screws
▦ Graft mainly cancellous and autograft
▦ Cell saver if expect blood loss of more than 2 l
   Postop → monitor lung function, nutrition, assess hips during follow-up to see any dislocation or contracture

2.1.2.15   Management of Upper Extremities Deformities in CP

2.1.2.15.1   General Comment
▦ Deformities in UL that may need surgery mainly in the hemiplegic CP children
▦ Surgery will not increase function in those with poor hand control and decreased sensation or stereognosis. Other children with mass or mirror movements as well as the athetoids are not good candidates for surgery

2.1.2.15.2   Clinical Assessment
▦ Examine the child for ability to grasp and release, reach or transfer objects. Ask the child to throw a soft object at the examiner, which gives a good assessment of the whole limb. Weak release will be obvious. Dynamic EMG has a place
▦ Check the resting hand position; look for contractures and instability
▦ Test hand placement by asking the child to put the hand on the head and then the knee. If the child can do this in 5 s, it carries a better prognosis if surgery contemplated for the child
▦ Test hand/finger control by asking the patient to play the piano. Look for independent movement of the fingers

2.1.2.15.3   Common Deformities and Management

- Thumb-in-palm deformity:
  - Common but difficult to treat, side pinch is impossible, and the child may use the tenodesis effect to get the thumb out of the palm by flexing the wrist
  - Four types according to House. Type 1 involved contracted AP, 1st dorsal interosseus; type 2 with added metacarpal-phalangeal joint (MCPJ) flexion from flexor pollicis brevis involvement, Type 3 also has MCPJ instability from overpull of extensor pollicis longus (EPL)/extensor pollicis brevis (EPB), Type 4 also has inter-phalangeal joint flexion from involved flexor pollicis longus
  - Type 1 involved soft tissue release, type 2 may need augment the weak EPL/EPB/abductor pollicis longus with palmaris longus/flexor carpi radialis/brachioradialis etc., and type 3 may need skeletal stabilisation
- Wrist and finger deformity:
  - Most with contracted pronator teres, flexor pollicis ulnaris (FCU) and finger flexors, resulting in forearm pronation with wrist flexion and ulna deviation
  - Children with tight finger flexors frequently depend on a mobile wrist and tenodesis effect for grasp and release. Wrist fusion alone in such cases can diminish function
  - Most hemiplegics have more problem with release than grasp; in these cases, FCU transfer to extensor digitorum communis (EDC) can work. For those with FCU active in grasp, FCU to extensor carpi radialis longus may be indicated. Wrist fusion is a salvage procedure. Finger flexion deformity requires release either as proximal slide procedure or functional lengthening at musculotendinous unit

2.1.2.16 Surgery for Lower Extremities in the Ambulatory CP patients

2.1.2.16.1   Principle

- Always assess the joint above and below a contracture and view the limb as a whole
- The same contracted posture can be caused by spastic muscle on one side or co-spasticity of both the agonist and antagonist, etc. The treatment is very different

▨ Gait analysis and dynamic EMG important if only to investigate more fully the frequently complicated problems of altered gait or postures such as crouching. It is also important to differentiate whether there is tonic spasticity or spasticity only in certain phases of the gait cycle

2.1.2.16.2 The Hip

▨ Loss of hip extension is a frequent cause of intervention, as it may produce secondary flexion of the knee and the ankle

▨ Commonly involves iliopsoas recession at the level of the pelvic brim to preserve some hip flexion power for gait; tenotomy is only reserved for the non-walker. Severe adduction contracture can lead to scissoring, and adductor longus intramuscular tenotomy together with gracilis myotomy can be performed. Anterior branch obturator neurectomy is obsolete and contraindicated, since the adductor brevis (a hip stabiliser) will also be taken out of action

▨ An occasional patient with significant IR deformity may need derotation

2.1.2.16.3 The Knee

▨ The same deformity of flexed knee posture can be caused by spastic hamstrings, weakened quadriceps or is secondary to hip flexion contracture. Careful assessment is required

▨ If hamstrings are the culprit, fractional lengthening can be performed

▨ Lack of swing phase knee flexion is frequently caused by rectus femoris, and transfer to semitendinosus can be useful to regain swing phase leg clearance

▨ An occasional patient may have knee hyperextension from spastic quadriceps, in which case one may need a distal rectus transfer

2.1.2.16.4 Foot and Ankle

▨ The same equinus deformity may be due to a contracture of the gastrocnemius or soleus or may be due to hip/knee flexion contractures. Also, careful clinical checking to differentiate whether only the gastrocnemius is tight or both gastrocnemius and soleus are tight is important

▨ Mild contracture of the calf muscles can respond to serial casting and ankle–foot orthosis (AFO). In diplegics, most opt for gastrocnemius recession nowadays if indicated to tackle the ankle equinus in favour of TAL to not overly weaken the power source of gait. It should be realised that excessive weakening of the triceps surae affects its control of standing posture, and normal/near normal strength is needed in running, jumping, etc. TAL only without tackling the joints above may also worsen a patient with a crouch gait

- Besides the equinus, the pes varus (as seen in hemiplegics) can be from spasticity of the tibialis anterior, TP or even gastrocnemius-soleus spasticiy, which can cause inversion of the ankle. Inversion of the ankle may need TAL. Inversion at the hind-foot may be corrected by either TP lengthening or split transfer. Inversion of the mid-foot caused by tibialis anterior can be treated by split transfer or total transfer

- Pes valgus can be due to spastic peronei, or triceps surae, and torsional moments during gait. Secondary hallux valgus (HV) is common. If AFO cannot adequately control the deformity, may need Evans calcaneal lengthening, or an extra-articular Grice subtalar arthrodesis. HV can be treated by a metatarsal osteotomy or metatarsal–phalangeal joint fusion

2.1.3   Poliomyelitis

2.1.3.1 Polio Virus
- Waterbourne, three types: If infected immune to one type
- Sabin vaccine effective
- Affinity to the CNS, especially the anterior horn cells (and cranial nerve nucleus)
- Three phases → acute, convalescent, chronic
- LL more affected, sometimes the trunk
- Severity increased by physical activity
- Differential diagnosis (DDx): encephalitis, meningitis, malaria
- Acute phase: treatment supportive
- Occasional death from respiratory complication (Cx)

2.1.3.2 Convalescence Phase
- Returnable power in 18 months
- Prevent deformity
- Physiotherapy: Motion, hydrotherapy, walking and ADL aids, splints, etc.

2.1.3.3 Cause of Deformity
- Muscle imbalance
- Example: Quadriceps weakness, the antagonists hamstring also slowed growth since intermittent stretching is the stimulus by opposition to growth
- As the femur grows, the relatively short hamstring causes a contracture
- It follows that deformities are less commonly seen in polio adults whose paralysis increased in adulthood (e.g. post-polio syndrome)
- The child frequently ambulates by crawling
- Scoliosis is common (sometimes no intercostal muscles to even hold the rib cage)
- Deformities usually do not occur in the totally paralysed
- Careful document with muscle charts [Medical Research Council (MRC) grading] of each and every muscle group

2.1.3.4 Key to Testing Different Muscle Groups
- Against gravity if weak
- If not that weak, against resistance
- Beware of trick movements (e.g. weak TA power with some plantar flexion still made possible by toe flexors)

2.1.3.5 Chronic Phase
- This is the phase that may need surgery
- Greater than 18 months
- Earlier neglect is a frequent cause that makes later repeated surgeries necessary
- XR: Osteoporosis and thinned cortices common

2.1.3.6 Options of Treatment
- Physiotherapy
- Casting: Milder ones ± wedging
- Surgery → e.g. TAL, or lengthen hamstrings, knee extension osteotomy (In more supple cases, tendon transfers may be considered)
- All three methods combined to treat severe deformities

2.1.3.7   Regional Tendon Transfers
- Power needs to be greater than grade 4
- Like excursion
- Synergistic
- Tension correct
- Straight line of pull preferably
- Glide on smooth surfaces
- No contractures
- Nerve and blood supply adequate

2.1.3.8   Role of Fusion
- When growth has ceased
- LL usually
- Usually fusion used in the deformed foot
- Triple arthrodesis commonly used in polio
- Age 14–16 years

2.1.3.9   Instruments/Orthotics Commonly Used
- Long leg calipers
- Below knees to control the foot

2.1.3.10   UL Management in Polio

2.1.3.10.1   Common Problems Encountered
- Flexion contracture elbow
- Sometimes uneven growth
- Supination contracture
- Variable hand deformity

Shoulder
- Shoulder: deltoid, loss of abduction, scapula control
- If there is still scapula control, sometimes need fusion after 15
- Never bilateral fusion, IR needed for toileting and propelling a wheelchair
- With scapular control for both sides, one fused shoulder still allowed, to have limited abduction
- 25° Abduction/forward flexion/IR is the usual position of fusion (to facilitate bringing the hand to the mouth)

Elbow [Biceps Paralysis]

- Biceps if paralysed are disabling, cannot bring food to mouth
- Three options:
  - Steindler flexorplasty (transfer origin of forearm flexors)
  - Pectoralis major transfer to the biceps
  - If deltoid also paralysed, may need fusion if scapular muscles functional (But avoid surgery if no hand function present)

Elbow (Triceps Paralysis)

- Cannot extend elbow with triceps paralysed
- Triceps is needed for Calipers walking
- No tendon transfer for triceps
- But not too disabling if the LL are functioning well, however

Forearm Contractures

- May need tendon transfers to restore muscle balance
- Pronation/supination contracture: may need to release the interosseous membrane (IOM), sometimes reattach site of insertion of biceps

Hand Problems

- Intrinsic hand muscle
- Extrinsic flexors and extensors
  - Differentiate between intrinsic versus extrinsic weakness or both and treat accordingly

Thumb Opposition Weakness

- Difficult to pick up objects
- May be forced to use the clumsy key pinch
- Example of operation: Camitz, flexor digitorum superficialis 4th; but test the extrinsics first

Interossei Weakness

- Clawing results (intrinsic minus hand)
- But much lesser than, say, leprosy or the usual ulna nerve palsy
- EPB → 1st dorsal plus tendon transfers as in ulna nerve palsy (to correct the MCPJ hyperextension)

Finger and Thumb Flexors Weakness
    Only if all long flexors lost is disabling (like a Volkmann)
    May spare the brachioradialis, flexor carpi radialis, FCU
    If no donors, thumb fusion and tenodesis of the flexors at the wrist

Finger and Thumb Extensors Affected
    FCU to EDC
    Palmaris longus → EPL
    PT → wrist extensors
    Can consider the above tendon transfers

Both Wrist Flexors and Extensors Are Affected
    May need fusion of wrist

2.1.3.11   LL Management in Polio

2.1.3.11.1   Hip in Poliomyelitis

- Gluteus maximus is a powerful hip extensor, is essential in walking (tested prone with knee flexed to relax hamstrings)
- Bilateral gluteus maximus paralysis cause the standing patient to flex uncontrolled at the hips, jack-knifing forwards: need stick or other aids
- Gluteus medius: Tested by lying on one side then abduct, but do not allow patient to flex the hip and abduct to prevent effect of tensor fascia lata (TFL). Gluteus medius if out of action causes the Trendelenberg sign: DDx of Trendelenberg sign includes short leg gait and unstable hip from other causes
- Hip internal or external rotators, e.g. walk with foot ER crablike
- ? Paralysed adductors less clinical significance if incomplete

2.1.3.11.2   Soft Tissue Contractures About the Hip

TFL Contracture
    TFL contracture: (the TFL is a small muscle with a very long tendon – the fascia lata; both fail to grow from a lack of stretching, as only the short muscle is elastic. The inelastic long tendon causes the deformity)
    – The deformity involves a flexion and abductor contracture of the hip: may later cause genu valgum and knee flexion deformity

– Sign: To show the ease with which the hip extends fully after relaxing the TFL to show no true hip flexion deformity from psoas/sartorius/gracilis. TFL tightens if ipsilateral leg adducted and IR, causes an apparent hip flexion deformity if other leg is flexed, as in the Thomas position. If the ipsilateral leg is later abducted and ER, which relaxes the TFL, the apparent hip flexion contracture will disappear

True Hip Flexion Contracture

More in a neglected case with an unopposed psoas pull

Not common

Some tried extension osteotomy

Many of these patients were unsuited for surgery and could not be made to walk from associated trunk paralysis

Hip Subluxation and Dislocation

Total paralysis will not dislocate the hip, but those still with powerful adductors and psoas do. Posterior capsule stretches and will not resist dislocation

Coxa valga per se does not usually need treatment

Hip on elevated side on a pelvic obliquity can be at risk, and pelvic obliquity in polio is common to be from a suprapelvic cause (that may need treatment)

2.1.3.11.3   Knee in Poliomyelitis

Quadriceps: An important muscle that keeps the knee stable in extension. Loss of power allows knee to collapse on walking and falls. Compensate by using the hand to straighten the knee; or use gluteus maximus to extend the leg

If quadriceps and gluteus maximus weak, can sometimes still extend by strong gastrocnemius via its origin of attachment at the popliteal surface

2.1.3.11.4   Ankle and Foot in Poliomyelitis

Learn to grade the power of triceps surae, sometimes the long toe flexors can take on the role of plantarflexion; loss of plantarflexion power causes poor push-off and slow gait

▨ Care to grade the power of tibialis anterior, make sure not confuse with action of the toe extensors; must be seen and felt before it is graded

2.1.4   Spina Bifida versus Spinal Dysraphism

2.1.4.1 Definition

▨ Spina bifida represents a group of disturbances of development of the vertebral arches, associated with abnormalities of structures derived from the neural tube and the meninges sometimes with cyst formation

▨ Spinal dysraphism involves a variety of hidden abnormalities that affect the spinal cord or cauda equina, which can produce either occult/ overt neurological disturbance

2.1.4.2 Spina Bifida

▨ Types
  – Myelocele
  – Myelomeningocele
  – Meningocele
  – Spina bifida occulta with a localised defect of the vertebral arches

▨ Associations: Arnold-Chiari malformation, hydrocephalus, hydromyelia, syringomyelia, diastematomyelia

2.1.4.2.1 Epidemiology, Aetiology and Recurrence Risk

▨ Incidence varies 1–5/1000 live births

▨ Possible causation involves a combination of genetic factors (probably polygenic) and environmental factors (folate/nutrition deficiency, drugs such as valproic acid, maternal diabetes, etc.)

▨ Likelihood of second child with the condition 1 in 5, but if already has two affected children, the risk increases to 1 in 10

▨ Prevention by prenatal USS, amniocentesis and folate supplements

2.1.4.2.2 Clinical Types

▨ Clinical presentation (and hence type of deformity) depends on lowest level of the lesion

▨ Three possible types of muscle imbalances around joints
  – One side normal, antagonist flaccid

- One side spastic, normal antagonist
- One side spastic, antagonist flaccid
  Situation in (c) produces greatest deformity

2.1.4.2.3 Pathogenesis of Deformities
▦ Muscle imbalance: Just described
▦ Intrauterine posture
▦ Posture assumed after birth
▦ Traction of nerve roots with later growth
▦ Others, e.g. any associated congenital malformation or arthrogryposis-like features

2.1.4.2.4 Goals of Management
▦ For those in whom standing is possible, try to obtain a stable extension posture by correction of fixed deformity. The extension posture helps maintain the centre of gravity directly over the feet with no/minimal hip/knee flexion. This should not only avoid flexion posture in the untreated child, but help free both upper extremities for other tasks
▦ The exact surgery, if any, needed depends on the exact neurological level

2.1.4.2.5 Neurological Levels in Relation to Treatment
▦ Thoracic level: will not be able to walk since both LL flaccid; this does not mean joint deformities of the LL will not occur. In fact, hip fixed flexion deformity can occur occasionally
▦ Lumbar lesions: If the lesion is L3 or below, i.e. reasonable quadriceps power, they may walk with the help of orthosis (those with strong quadriceps only require below-knee prosthesis); more affected cases may need hip-knee-ankle-foot orthosis (HKAFO)
▦ Sacral lesions: are useful walkers even into adulthood

2.1.4.2.6 Managing Deformities by the Region
▦ Foot: varus feet need early correction by plaster, although soft tissue release may be required near age 1 year; recurrence of deformity may require repeat release and/or ilizarov correction. Bony surgery reserved for later childhood (e.g. lateral column surgery) and triple arthrodesis for resistant cases after skeletal maturity. Valgus feet require

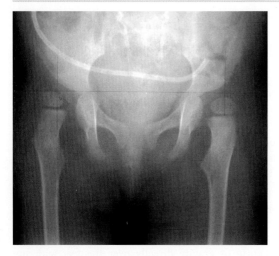

Fig. 2.9. Spina bifida affecting the hip

careful identification of the level of valgus. Correction will fail if there is unrecognised valgus at the ankle. Valgus ankle may need epiphysiodesis of the lower tibial growth plate. Subtalar valgus if not easily correctible by orthosis may need Grice subtalar fusion, or other bony surgery such as calcaneal osteotomy, or even triple if severe at maturity. Calcaneus deformity is not treated until age 3–5, when transfer of tibialis anterior may be considered

- Knee: fixed flexion deformities greater than 20° may need plastering, ± soft tissue release of the hamstrings and posterior capsule. Supracondylar femoral osteotomy is rarely required

- Hip (Fig. 2.9): soft tissue release sometimes required if there is fixed flexion deformity of the hip. For hip dislocations: in high lesions where gait analysis indicated an abnormally wide range of hip abduction is required for walking, surgery for a dislocated hip may result in stiffness and decreased walking ability, be it unilateral or bilateral. In low lesions with strong quadriceps, always reduce a unilateral dislocation; but whether to reduce a bilateral hip dislocation depends on individual cases, not always mandatory

- Spine: management of scoliosis will be discussed in the spine section. Kyphus is especially common in more severe cases, and these children are frequently born with a lumbar kyphus. If resistant and if recurrent skin ulceration, may need anterior and posterior surgery with kyphectomy to correct. In every patient, also look for occult lesions such as spondylolisthesis, diastematomyelia, partial absence of sacrum, etc.

2.1.4.3 Spinal Dysraphism
▦ It is believed by some that up to 10–20% of the population may have a degree of this abnormality, although clinically significant ones are rare
▦ May affect all or some of the primary embryonic layers to a varying degree

2.1.4.3.1 Common Clinical Presentations
▦ Trophic ulcers (e.g. of the foot)
▦ Short leg with wasting
▦ Small foot
▦ Cavus feet

2.1.4.3.2 Common Varieties
▦ Diastematomyelia (where the cord or filum is being split sagitally by bony septum)
▦ Lumbosacral lipoma
▦ Tethered filum terminale
▦ Other forms: dermoid cyst, hydromyelia, arachnoid cyst
  Dx by a combination of clinical features (e.g. hairy patch) and XR and magnetic resonance imaging (MRI) ± CT

2.1.4.3.3 Principles of Management
▦ Index of suspicion is needed to diagnose these conditions, since 20% of these lack cutaneous features
▦ Careful neurological work-up and definition of the anatomy
▦ Details of management depend on individual lesion; associated deformities (usually the feet) may need correction

2.1.4.3.4 Other Disorders
▦ Example: Charchot Marie tooth disease, etc., will be discussed elsewhere in the book

2.1.5   Malformations

2.1.5.1 Malformations with Chromosomal Abnormalities

▓ Examples include Turner's and Klinefelter's syndrome, which will not be discussed in this book

2.1.5.2 Malformations without Chromosomal Abnormalities

[Only neurofibromatosis (NF) will be discussed]

2.1.5.2.1 Introduction

▓ Multisystem
▓ Affects cell growth of neural tissue
▓ AD for types 1 and 2, 50% as new mutants in NF 1: Identification of mutation by the "protein truncation test". Detects a shortened p product; this test only can detect 70% of NF 1 mutations
▓ Not rare – 1 in 4000, NF 2 very rare
▓ Protein product of NF 1 is neurofibromin, of NF 2 is schwannomin
▓ Two peaks for severe clinical problems, age 5–10 years and age 35–50 years, the latter peak related to CA

2.1.5.2.2 Types

▓ NF 1: Protean manifestations, every patient with NF 1 will *eventually* show some features of the disease (sometimes more prominent after adolescence); categories include neurocutaneous stigmata, eyes, tumours, tibia dysplasia and orthopaedic problems – scoliosis, kyphoscoliosis, lordoscoliosis, etc.
▓ NF 2: not important orthopaedically, associated with acoustic neuroma, gene on long arm of chromosome 22

2.1.5.2.3 Dx Criteria (NIH Consensus Development Conference)

▓ Greater than six café au lait (5 mm diameter in child, and 15 mm diameter in adults)
▓ Greater than two neurofibromata (or 1 plexiform)
▓ Freckling axilla/groin
▓ Optic glioma
▓ Greater than two iris hamatomata (Lisch nodules)
▓ First degree relative (e.g. parent, sibling)
▓ Characteristic bone lesion, e.g. thinned long bone cortex ± pseudoarthrosis or spenoid dysplasia

2.1.5.2.4 Details of Neurocutaneous Stigmata

- Café Au Lait: most common; in 90% in NF, are hyperpigmented macules. Melanotic origin dispersed both in basal and upper layers. Most in areas not exposed to sun. Infants with spots alone not confirmatory of Dx; other features will occur later, usually by age 10 years
- Cutaneous neurofibromata: mixture of cells besides Schwann cell → also has fibroblasts, endothelial cells and glandular elements. Increase in numbers after adolescence ± pregnancy often seen
- Plexiforms: bag of worms feeling at subcutaneous plane, mostly under an area of pigmentation. When the pigmentation nears/crosses the midline, it is likely the tumour originates from the spinal canal and will be aggressive. Plexiforms have the potential for CA change
- Elephantiasis: rough, villous skin, not always successful in attempts to re-sect it (if occurs over long bones, can have dysplasia of nearby bones)
- Verrucous hyperplasia: thick, velvety skin. Crevice may form and break down. Most are unilateral
- Freckles: small 2–3 mm pigmented spots, second most common feature in child. By age 6 years, 80%
- Optic gliomas: most are static in size, occasionally enlarge and can cause exopthalmos and impair vision
- Lisch nodules – most will appear in adolescence or adulthood, well-circumscribed harmatoma in the iris

2.1.5.2.5 Spinal Manifestations

- Rule out C1–2 subluxation by cervical spine. XR a must prior to operation
- Scoliosis: dystrophic and the more common, non-dystrophic curves possible
- Kyphoscoliosis and lordoscoliosis
- Spondylolisthesis (rare)

Cervical Spine

- Rule out C 1–2 instability before operations
- Paraplegia from cervical-spine instability reported, as well as anterior dislocation of upper and lower cervical-spine, sometimes iatrogenic after tumour excision with kyphosis

Check for cervical-spine problems also before any halo-traction in those with neck pain and torticollis; may also see widened foramen in oblique views

Scoliosis

Most common osseous defect in NF 1

Scoliosis in 10–30%

Pathogenesis unknown but may be from: osteomalacia, localised neurofibromata that erodes bone, endocrine or mesodermal dysplasia

Most are non-dystrophic, but Crawford reminds us the possibility of a change to the dystrophic type especially in young age

Pathogenesis of dystrophic type may be from intraspinal lesions, e.g. meningoceles, and dural ectasia, but dystrophic change can also occur with normal spinal contents, here perhaps due to bone dysplasia

What Are the Dystrophic Changes

Scalloped posterior vertebral margin

Severe apical vertebral rotation

Vertebral wedging

Widened spinal canal and inter-pedicular distance

Enlarged neuroforamina

Defective pedicles

Pencil ribs: like twisted ribbon/diagnostic when a rib is smaller than midportion of second rib

Paraspinal mass

Spindling of the transverse process

Dystrophic Scoliosis

Short segment: Usually greater than six spinal segments

Sharp angulation, severe apical rotation

Other features, e.g. scalloping of vertebral, etc.

Dystrophic type can progress to severe, even sometimes subluxation or dislocation of vertebral body

Dystrophic Scoliosis Treatment

Less than 20°: Observe

If 20–40°: PSF & instrumentation – unlike in non-dystrophic cases for fear of curve progression and pseudoarthrosis

Greater than 50°: A+P Surgery

Importance of Dural Ectasia

- Note that dural ectasia, meningoceles, pseudomeningoceles and dumb-bell lesions are all related to presence of neurofibroma or abnormal pressure in and about the spinal canal neuraxis
- Dural ectasia is a circumferential dilatation of the dural sac; mechanics behind uncertain, the neural elements are not abnormal or enlarged and the expanded area contains increased cerebrospinal fluid and protein-like material
- The expanding dura erodes the bony structure, widens the canal, thins the lamina and destabilises the vertebral elements
- Its expansion outwards through the neural foramina causes meningoceles and gives the dumbbell appearance
- The spinal canal gross widening explains why paraplegia is rare despite marked angular deformity in dystrophic curves
- Others: destabilised costo-vertebral junction with rib penetration reported and even sometimes dislocation of the spinal column
- Most enlarged neuroforamen are due to neurofibroma rather than dural ectasia

Non-Dystrophic Curves

- Similar to AIS – curve to right
- Segments 8–10
- Treatment:
  - Less than 20°: Observe
  - 20–35°: Brace
  - Greater than 35°: Fuse
- (Close monitor needed lest change to dystrophic type)

Workup

- Tc 99 bone scan
- Tomogram
- Explore
- (MRI)

Kyphoscoliosis

- When scoliosis with Kyphus >50°
- Paraplegia rare since dura much dilated
- Sometimes caused by weakened stabilisers → e.g. facet, pedicles, ligament

Treatment: < 50°: brace, traction danger of neural loss

50°: A+P surgery, not posterior alone

(Some give a course of halo-traction if neurological deficit found at presentation)

Lordoscoliosis

- More likely pulmonary dysfunction (and mitral valve prolapse)
- Rarer
- May need long fusion well above cervicothoracic junction to prevent subsequent junctional kyphosis

Spondylolisthesis

- Very rare
- Erosion of pedicle or pas by lumbosacral neurofibromata or ductal ectasia
- Progressive cases may need A+P surgery

Fusion Levels for NM Scoliosis in General

- Non-ambulatory patients: most need fusion to pelvis, except:
  - Those who still walk and need to preserve the lower lumbar motion
  - Those (especially Duchenne cases) when we fuse early before lung function is less than 40%; hence, these curves are smaller and no pelvic obliquity
- Rigid criteria to fuse short of sacrum: Must be neither: fixed pelvic obliquity or oblique take-off at L5/S; the lowest instrumented level remains horizontal

Instrumentation for NM Scoliosis

- Most use Luque-Galverston technique. Advantage: has segmental spinal correction
- Construct: made of two contoured rods at either side of midline, fixed intimately to each laminar surface with sublaminar wires, now the rigid crosslink provides an even stronger rectilinear rigid construct restores near normal alignment in both the coronal and sagittal planes

The Galverston Technique

- Developed by Ferguson (and Allen): implanting the pelvic portion of rods into the posterior column or traverse bar of the ilium, which has the greatest bone mass and least likely to fail, maybe superior to hook/rod fixation devices
- After this single contoured rod inserted to transverse iliac bar, the resultant long lever arm used to correct the spine by progressive tightening of the sublaminar wires, provides much corrective forces and decrease pelvic obliquity

Pros and Cons of the Galverston Technique

- Disadvantage: crosses the SIJ (pain/OA), lucencies around rod of questionable significance
- Advantage:
  - Less fatigue failure as with screws
  - The multiplanar configuration of the rod provides an excellent triangulation fixation to the pelvis
    (P.S.: In difficult cases, sometimes use 'hybrid' constructs & anterior instrumentation to reduce a large lordotic deformity)

2.1.5.2.6 Congenital Tibial Dysplasia

- Will be discussed in the regional section

2.1.6   Metabolic Disorders (Discussed in Chap. 1)

2.1.7   Disorders of Joints and Soft Tissues

2.1.7.1   Marfan's Syndrome (Fig. 2.10)

2.1.7.1.1 Aetiology

- Autosomal dominant with variable expression
- An abnormal fibrillin gene was identified encoding a microfibrillar protein that is found in various tissues
- Most individuals are tall; long slender limbs arachnodactyly with decreased upper to lower segment ratio

2.1.7.1.2 Clinical Features

- Face: long and narrow with high arched palate
- Eye: upward lens subluxation is common as well as myopia and retinal detachment

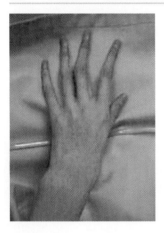

Fig. 2.10. Hand in a woman with Marfan's syndrome

- Chest: pectus carinatum or excavatum
- Upper to lower segment ratio: decreased
- Hands: arachnodactyly
- LL: protrusio acetabuli and developmental dysplasia of the hip (DDH) may occur; HV and long big toe common
- Spine: scoliosis common, kyphosis in infant common but may improve with time; flat-back may occur

2.1.7.1.3 DDx
- Homecystinuria: urine diagnostic, lens with downward dislocation, prone to thrombosis if surgery performed in these individuals
- Congenital contractural arachnodactyly: large joints stiff, not lax
- Others, e.g. Stickler's syndrome, Klinefelter's syndrome, may sometimes have the marfanoid habitus

2.1.7.1.4 Management
- AFO in infancy to provide better stance
- Scoliosis if progressive may need non-fusion rods during growth followed by fusion later
- Genu Valgum: if progressive may need hemi-epiphyseal stapling
- Pes Planovalgus: may need fusion if severe near maturity
- Most need a cardiovascular assessment to look for aortic arch anomalies and mitral valve problems

2.1.7.2 Ehlers–Danlos Syndrome

2.1.7.2.1 Nature

- AD disorder with hyperextensible skin, joint hypermobility (and proneness to dislocation) with fragile soft tissue/bone (sometimes calcification)
- Heterogeneous in pathogenesis: some are from mutations in genes for type 1 and 3 (Pro)collagen, others due to enzyme defects (lysine hydroxylase) in processing of procollagen

2.1.7.2.2 More Common Types

- Type 2: most common and least disabling
- Type 4: featured by vascular and bowel ruptures, and die earlier (middle age)

2.1.7.2.3 History

- Family
- Easy bruising, joint dislocations (sometimes recurrent), and bone fragility/severe forms may have history of bowel rupture

2.1.7.2.4 Physical Assessment

- Orthopaedic: paper-thin skin (cigarette paper); skin is soft, velvety and feels abundant over the hands and feet. Hyper-extensible but returns to normal shape on release, can be very fragile – split after minor trauma; wounds more likely dehiscence, sutures can pull out of surgical wound
- Other areas: scoliosis, history of joint dislocation (or currently dislocated) e.g. patella dislocation, past fracture or bony deformity
  - Other areas of interest: bowel, arteries, etc.

2.1.7.2.5 Orthopaedic Principles

- Wound: beware dehiscence and suture pull out
- Soft tissue orthopaedic procedures commonly fail
- Bony procedure sometimes needed (such as arthrodesis in some selected cases)
- Adjuncts: physiotherapy, orthotics, etc.

2.1.7.3 Arthrogryposis

2.1.7.3.1 Clinical Features
- The syndrome involves non-progressive, multiple congenitally rigid joints
- Joints did develop, but the periarticular soft tissues get fibrotic: incomplete fibrous ankylosis
- Mostly involve all four limbs, extent of involvement increases from proximal to distal, tend to be symmetric

2.1.7.3.2 Pathology
- Involved muscles marked decrease in muscle fibres, with fibrous replacement. Look pale pink and shrunken. Partially affected muscles have a mixture of normal and atrophic fibres
- In the spinal cord, there may be diminished number of anterior horn cells, but no inflammatory response. Posterior roots intact
- Fibrillation potentials detected in EMG, but nerve conduction velocity normal and muscle enzymes normal

2.1.7.3.3 Aetiology
- Unknown
- Theories include infection, abnormalities in the nervous system, muscles and joints

2.1.7.3.4 Physical Assessment
- Marked limited range of motion (ROM) of joints (active and passive)
- Motion limited by a firm inelastic block; joints can be fixed in flexion or extension
- Diminished muscle bulk make the joints look large, skin creases absent (can even be tense and glossy with or without webbing at knee and elbow)
- Reflexes: absent, sensation intact
- Common deformities at birth (if severe):
  - IR/adducted shoulder, elbow flexed/extended, wrist flexed/ulna deviated, ER/flexed/abducted Hip, knees flexed/hyper-extended, clubfeet common
- Common associated changes or deformities:
  - DDH, dislocated patella, scoliosis, low set ears, short neck, high arch palate, etc.

2.1.7.3.5 Management
- Early passive stretching should begin in newborn
- Goal of treatment to correct all LL abnormalities that may delay walking less than 2. Soft tissue surgery mostly in young child until age 6 years
- The combined use of physiotherapy and splintage is required to maintain correction
- Minimum functional requirement for functional ambulation is hip motion within 30° that of full extension, knee motion within 20° that of full extension, hip extensor strength of grade 4 and quadriceps strength of grade 3. The upper extremities should in addition be crutchable, and careful functional assessment is important

2.1.7.3.6 Management by Regions
- Foot: conservative usually fails, aim of treatment to convert the stiff deformed foot into a stiff plantigrade foot. Serial manipulation and casting are followed by full surgical release. Maintain with AFO until skeletal maturity. Surgical failures may need talectomy. But triple arthrodesis can be an option if near skeletal maturity
- Knee:
  - Most surgeries are part of overall treatment (Rn) plan, including correction of foot and hip deformities
  - Flexion contractures require serial stretching and casting. Severe cases may require posterior capsulotomy, even release of hamstring and collateral ligaments
  - The option of supracondylar osteotomy mainly reserved for those near skeletal maturity, not in the young child
- Hips:
  - Flexion contracture if significant, need operative release and hip spica: if severe, a total capsulectomy may be required, though there is risk of avascular necrosis (AVN; fixed flexion contracture greater than 35° causes increased lumbar lordosis, difficult in ambulation)
  - Dislocation is suggested by flexion, ER/abduction. treatment similar to DDH if mobile. If the hip is not reduced by age 2 years, sometimes left alone, especially if bilateral
  - However, a high dislocation can cause severe pelvic obliquity and need more aggressive treatment

▓ The upper extremity:
  – Goal is to increase function. In severe cases, have one extremity for mouth feeding and hygiene, the other used to push up from the sitting position or use the crutch.
    Thumb-in-palm deformity: needs Z-plasty and release of adductor
    Fixed flexion deformity of wrist needs release and splinting, with possible later fusion
    For fixed bilateral elbow extension, a unilateral posterior elbow capsulotomy combined with elongation of the fibrotic triceps can be attempted

2.1.7.3.7 Causes of Recurrence
▓ Recurrence of the corrected deformity is common as the limb grows, but the inelastic periarticular structures fail to stretch. Hence, the possible need of long-term orthotic control in selected cases to maintain correction

2.2   General Topics of Interest

2.2.1   Torsional Deformities of the LL

2.2.1.1   Terminology
▓ Version: normal variations in limb rotation
▓ Torsion: version beyond $\pm$ 2 SD from the mean considered as abnormal and described as deformity

2.2.1.2   Version
▓ Tibial: angular difference between the axis of the knee and the transmalleolar axis (do not be misled by any foot anomalies)
▓ Femoral: angular difference between the femoral neck axis and transcondylar axes at the distal femur

2.2.1.3   Normal LL Rotation
▓ The LL rotates medially during the seventh fetal week to bring the great toe to the midline
▓ Femoral anteversion declines from 30° at birth to about 10–15° at maturity
▓ Tibia rotates laterally from 5° at birth to 15° at maturity

2.2.1.4 Effect of Growth
▧ Growth is associated with lateral rotation in both femoral and tibial segments
▧ Medial tibial torsion and femoral antetorsion can improve with time
▧ Lateral tibial torsion usually gets worse with growth

2.2.1.5 Torsional Deformity
▧ Simple: Involving one level
▧ Complex: Multiple segments, additive or compensatory

2.2.1.6 Work-up
▧ History: onset and how discovered, severity, disability whether gait affected, any previous treatment
▧ Physical assessment:
  – The rotational profile: observe the foot progression angle = angular difference between the axis of the foot and the line of progression. In-toeing: $-5°$ to $-10°$ = mild; $-10°$ to $-15°$ = moderate; greater than $-15°$ = severe
  – In excessive femoral antetorsion, "egg beater" running pattern of the legs may be seen
  – Assess femoral version: measuring hip rotation with the child prone, knee flexed to right angle and the pelvis level. Normal degree of IR $<67–70°$
  – Assess tibial version: check the thigh foot angle. Measure with patient prone and knee flexed to right angle; check angular difference between the axes of the foot and thigh. This assesses the tibial and hind-foot rotational status (TFA)
  – TMA (transmalleolar axis) equals angular difference between the transmalleolar axis and the thigh. A measure of tibial rotation that will not be affected by foot deformity. (Note: difference between TFA and TMA equals hind-foot rotation. Normal range of both TMA and TFA is broad, mean value increases with age)
  – Assess any fore-foot adductus: the normal lateral border of the foot is straight. In metatarsus adductus, there is convex lateral border and adducted fore-foot

2.2.1.7   Management Principles

▨ Obtain correct Dx
▨ Adequate explanation to the family
▨ In-toeing spontaneously corrects in the vast majority
▨ Shoe wedges, inserts/night splints: ineffective
▨ Observational management the best: natural history less than 1% fail to resolve and need surgery

2.2.1.8   DDx in Infancy

▨ Out toeing: flatfeet with heel valgus, lateral rotation hip contracture
▨ In-toeing: adducted big toe, fore-foot adductus, internal tibial torsion
   Adducted great toe: involves a spastic abductor hallucis, occurs during stance phase, may associate with adduction of metatarsals, resolves spontaneously
▨ Fore-foot adductus
   – Metatatsus adductus: most resolve in first year
   – Metatarsus varus: rigid fore-foot adductus tends to persist, stiffness, most with rather incomplete resolution, cosmetic and shoe fitting problem. Treatment: long leg brace

2.2.1.9   DDx in Toddlers

▨ In-toeing: most common during the second year; usually noted when they begin to walk
▨ Due to: internal tibial torsion, metatarsus adductus and adducted great toe

2.2.1.9.1 Internal Tibial Torsion

▨ The most common cause of in-toeing in the toddler
▨ If unilateral: left side is more common
▨ Observation is best
▨ Dennis Browne night splints are commonly prescribed, but probably with limited long-term value
▨ Avoid daytime bracing and shoe modification: may slow running and influence self-image

2.2.1.10 DDx in Child

▨ In-toeing: commonly due to increased femoral antetorsion, rarely from persisting internal tibial torsion

- Out-toeing (late childhood): can be due to external femoral torsion and external tibial torsion

2.2.1.10.1   Influence of LL Rotational Growth with Age
- ER of LL with growth: (i). tends to correct any internal tibial torsion, (ii) tends to worsen any external tibial torsion

2.2.1.11   Clinical Scenarios
- Persistent internal tibial torsion in the older child
- Persistent external tibial torsion
- Excess femoral anteversion
- Effect of femoral retroversion on the hip

2.2.1.11.1   Persistent Internal Tibial Torsion
- Less common than external tibial torsion in older child
- May need operation if significant functional disability and cosmetic deformity in child greater than 8 years with TFA greater than 10 IR

2.2.1.11.2   Persistent External Tibial Torsion
- Worse with time, patello-femoral joint (PFJ) pain common
- Knee malalignment and the abnormality of the line of progression; more pronounced when combined with internal femoral torsion

2.2.1.11.3   Excessive Femoral Antetorsion
- More common in girls
- First seen mostly in age 3–5 years
- Mostly found to sit in "W" position
- Standing with the knees medially rotated (kissing patella)
- Runs like an egg beater if severe

2.2.1.11.4   Natural History of Increased Femoral Antetorsion
- Most severe around age 4–6 years
- Most do resolve with growth with decrease in femoral antetorsion
- Not usual to cause degenerative arthritis in adulthood and significant residual disability is rare
- Unaffected usually by non-operative treatment
- May need femoral rotational osteotomy if severe and when the child is greater than age 8 years

2.2.1.11.5   Effects of Femoral Retroversion
- More common in slipped capital femoral epiphysis
- Shear force on the physis increased
- Association with hip degenerative arthritis
- Out-toeing gait

2.2.1.12   General Operative Indications
- Rotational osteotomy usually effective in correcting torsional deformity
- Indications:
  - Age 8–10 years or more
  - Functional disability besides cosmetically unappealing
  - Single deformity three SD above the mean or combined deformity two SD above the mean
  - The child's problems should be severe enough to justify the risks
- Femoral rotational osteotomy
  - Most are performed at intertrochanteric level
  - Healing more rapid, fixation more rigid, scar less obvious, less noticeable if malunion occurs
  - Mostly considered if approximately 50° corrections needed
- Correcting the tibial side
  - At supramalleolar level
  - Bring the TFA to approximately 15°
  - Cxs: compartment syndrome, malrotation and non-union, which is most common in the fibula; avoid soft tissue interposition

2.2.1.13   "Rotational Malalignment Syndrome"
- External tibial and internal femoral torsion
- Axis of flexion of the knee not in line of progression
- PFJ problems common (pain, even dislocation)
- Most are treated conservatively
- Correction is a major undertaking as it will involve a four-level procedure

2.2.1.14   Prognosis of Rotational Malalignment
- Internal femoral torsion show little/no functional disability in adults
- Mild internal tibial torsion may even improves sprinting by improvement in push off

■ Knee degenerative arthritis may be associated with increased femoral anteversion

Hip degenerative arthritis may be associated with femoral retrotorsion

2.2.2   Leg Length Discrepancy

2.2.2.1   Introduction

■ Advantage about lengthening in adults: no worry of growth plates; disadvantage is slower healing (50–100% more time needed), not only of bone but soft tissues as well, especially if you do a diaphyseal corticotomy in a smoker

■ Advantage in children: no weak point as in adult, faster healing of bone and soft tissues. Disadvantage is need to worry about growth plates that sometimes behave unpredictably despite adequate protection (such as spanning circular frame across joint)

2.2.2.2   When to Lengthen

■ Depends on our calculation of expected LLD at maturity

- Earliest age is approximately 8–13 years of age when child can co-operate with this complex procedure
- Leg lengthening considered when greater than 5 cm, (if less than 5 cm, consider timed epiphysiodesis, unless short stature or refused surgery to good leg); if greater than 15 cm expected, possibility of prosthesis comes into consideration
- More leg lengthening required cases: can be divided into 2–3 stages. First stage around age 8, usually

2.2.2.3   Limb Length Discrepancy in General Population

■ Some discrepancy in 70%

■ Discrepancy of 1.0–1.5 cm in 30%

■ Discrepancy of 2–2.5 cm in 4%

2.2.2.4   Limb Length Discrepancy and Gait Analysis

■ Normal gait up to 3% with inequality of 2 cm

■ Variable compensatory methods start to occur with 3–5% inequality of leg length

2.2.2.5 Significance of Discrepancy
■ For 0–2 cm: no treatment usually
■ For 2–5 cm: shoe-lift ± shortening
■ For 2–5 cm: lengthening
■ For 15 cm: most need a prosthesis

2.2.2.5.1 Discrepancy of 2–5 cm
■ Shoe lift
■ Epiphysiodesis
■ Shortening after maturity

2.2.2.5.2 Role of Lengthening if 3–5 cm LLD?
■ If deformity correction is concomitantly needed
■ Err on side of correction if short stature
■ Especially if patient refuses surgery on good leg

2.2.2.5.3 Role of Lengthening if Greater Than 15 cm LLD?
■ Only very occasionally considered in acquired discrepancy
■ Otherwise good limb

2.2.2.6 Common Conditions for Leg Lengthening
■ Congenital group: main example FPFD and fibula hemimelia
■ Acquired/Developmental
  – Physeal plate related: trauma and other causes (tumour, sepsis, endocrine, vascular, idiopathic, e.g. hemihypertrophy)
  – Epiphyseal: e.g., bone dysplasia, achondroplasia
  – Not related to growth plates or epiphyses: e.g., anterolateral bowing and/or anteromedial bowing of the tibia. Positive constitutional delay

2.2.2.7 Basic Science of Limb Lengthening (Fig. 2.11)
■ Role of vascular endothelial growth factor under active investigation
■ Muscle: fibrosis, necrosis and element of inflammation, especially after 20% lengthened
■ Nerve: conduction changes after 20% lengthened, thereafter sometimes structural changes
■ Growth plate unpredictable: sometimes retarded after initial hyperaemia, sometimes increased because of better biomechanical alignments attained

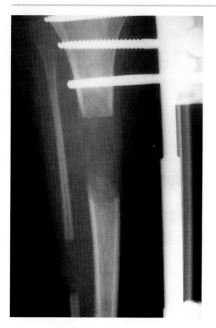

Fig. 2.11. Distraction osteogenesis

▨ Joint: danger of stiffness, subluxation and dislocation, e.g., in lengthening for congenital causes, e.g., knee stiff on lengthening congenital short femur, radial head dislocate on lengthening the radial club hand
▨ Articular cartilage: sometimes changes from nearby increased soft tissue pressure
▨ Vessels: changes begin also around 20% of lengthening

2.2.2.8 Calculating Expected LLD at Maturity
▨ Moseley graph: needs serial follow-up and plotting in order to make predictions
▨ Australian rule-of-thumb technique: can sometimes waive long serial follow-up if quite near maturity, mainly for less severe cases and useful in assessing the timing of epiphysiodesis
▨ Paley's "multiplier" method

2.2.2.9 Limb Lengthening Methods

- Principle
  - Distraction osteogenesis by corticotomy/osteotomy method that prevents injury to the blood supply. Based on Ilizarov experiments: need stable construct for bone formation by intramembranous ossification to occur
  - Lengthening near/spanning the growth plate: advantage no osteotomy, tackle right at the site of deformity, less counteracting muscle forces, e.g., distal to adductor tubercle in distal femur plate lengthening. Disadvantage risks of earlier growth plate closure

2.2.2.10 Which Fixator to Use

- Most common answer is the one most familiar to the surgeon, provided can do the job assigned
- Monolateral frame: less complex, more used in femur/humerus/fingers lengthening, more in straightforward deformities, less cost
- Circular frame: for more complex deformity, more used for the tibia, especially if rotation needs correction, more bulk and scar/pin tracks and less patient tolerance

2.2.2.11 Mode of Lengthening

- By EF, positive corticotomy
- Over IM nail: if straight, undeformed long bone with no deformity need be corrected
- Lengthen over IM nail, i.e. EF plus IM nail as internal splint (danger: high pressure to ream intact bone. Can do osteotomy first and cannulated reamer, more operative time and blood loss and IM sepsis. Advantage: less time for rehabilitation on EF, and less fracture of the regenerate)
- Acute correction: occasionally for mild rotation deformity on femur plus monolateral frame. Sometimes, acute correction after lengthening when there is some residual rotation element

2.2.2.12 Complications

- Neurovascular: intraoperative or developed during lengthening
- Fracture of regenerate: prevention important
- Stiffness, e.g., from muscle fibrosis, forgot for instance to splint knee in extension during say lengthening femur in congenitally short femur

and just ordering physiotherapy, likely in areas with thick muscles, sometimes from overtensioning

▦ Dislocation/subluxation of nearby joints: should check any dysplasia of nearby joints preoperatively especially in congenital cases; some experts like Paley do proactive surgeries

▦ Related to fixator: pins bent/break, loss of alignment, pin track sepsis

2.2.2.13 Ways to Avoid Cxs

▦ Avoiding fracture of regenerate: ensure good consolidate, selected cases lengthen over IM nail; avoid premature taking off external fixator

▦ Avoiding stiffness by prevention: need to allow, e.g. knee flexion despite use of extension splint at night or when not exercising; good therapists avoid overtensioning – experts like Paley stop whenever they encounter, for example, $40°$ knee motion loss during lengthening, and likelihood of stiffness more in areas with thick muscles, e.g. distal femur

▦ Avoiding dislocation: sometimes need to do surgery before lengthening/be proactive; e.g. Paley does a Dega pelvic osteotomy many a time if he finds a dysplastic acetabulum in his 1b class of PFFD (congenital short femur) prior to lengthening; other cases, if loose/dysplastic nearby joints are seen, close monitoring – if still subluxate, stop lengthening and assess need for soft tissue releases before recommence lengthening

▦ Neural Cx: most commonly encountered is the peroneal nerve, e.g. with pins near the proximal tibia; know your anatomy. Sometimes intraoperative nerve monitoring may be required

▦ Avoiding cartilage damage: not common but can occur even despite protecting joint by spanning it – manifested by loss of joint space and malalignment

▦ Avoid damage to growth plate: do not damage them but their behaviour is very difficult to predict

2.2.2.14 Special Cxs from Lengthening over IM Nails

▦ IM sepsis – 5% in one series

▦ Technique difficult: May need to use cannulated technique or AO miss-the-nail technique to place the large pins and avoid the IM nail

▦ Longer operative time

▦ More blood losses

2.2.2.15 Future

- Self-lengthening nail: driven either by electrical or magnetic forces under investigation

2.2.3 Angular Deformities About the Knee

2.2.3.1 DDx Bowed Legs

- Physiological bow legs
- Blount's disease (tibia vara)
- Rickets
- Trauma
- Dysplasias (e.g. metaphyseal chondrodysplasia, focal fibrocartilaginous dysplasia, Ollier's disease)
- Others, e.g. rarer metabolic disorders, old osteomyelitis

2.2.3.2 Physiological Changes in Angular Alignment about the Knee

- Growth around the knee accounts for up to two-thirds of LL growth
- Most normal children have Genu Varum less than 2 years old; and change to valgus by 4 years
- The knee is near neutral alignment at around 1.5–2 years of age. The adult anatomical tibio-femoral angle is reached by about 6–7 years old

2.2.3.3 Blount's Disease (Fig. 2.12)

- Involves a focal varus deformity of the proximal tibia from mechanical overload of the medial growth plate creating disordered growth
- The growth disorder resulted in abrupt medial angulation of proximal tibia distal to epiphysis, causing varus angulation of the proximal tibia and medial rotation of the tibia
- There are three types depending on age:
  - Infantile (age 0–3 years)
  - Juvenile (age 3–10 years)
  - Adolescent (age 11 years and above)

2.2.3.3.1 Microscopic Findings

- Islands of densely packed hypertrophied cartilage cells, not organised in the usual columnar fashion ± abnormal capillary loops

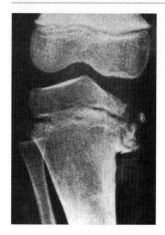

Fig. 2.12. Blount's disease

2.2.3.3.2 Predisposing Factors
- Obese children
- Early age of walking
- Female
- Afro-American lineage

2.2.3.3.3 Clinical Features
- Infantile: involves physeal lucency and depression and beaking of the corresponding epiphysis and metaphysis. Beak may be palpable, associated with feet pronation, medial tibial torsion and leg shortening. Tends to be bilateral and symmetric; may occasionally resolve by itself Drennan angle greater than 11°, tibio-femoral angle greater than 15°
- Juvenile/adolescent: abrupt medial angulation of the medial cortical wall of the proximal tibial metaphysis, narrowing of the medial half of the epiphyseal plate, Drennan angle greater than 11°, tibio-femoral angle greater than 15°. The proximal tibia is tender; there may be mild medial knee ligamentous laxity. More cases being unilateral, sometimes with a physeal bridge

2.2.3.3.4 Diagnosis
- Langenskiold described six progressive radiological stages from beaking to bone-bar formation. There is, however, low interobserver correlation. Resolution is possible with stage 4 or below

- Children age less than 2 years have inadequate ossification, Dx relies on the metaphyseal–diaphyseal angle (Drennan angle): the angle formed between a line through the medial and lateral beaks of the metaphysis and the line along the axis of the diaphysis. An angle greater than 11° is suggestive of Blount's disease
- To assess the extent of medial plateau depression, measure the angle between the medial and lateral portions of the tibial plateau
- Role of conservative treatment: not effective in adolescents. In infants, may try prosthesis like KAFO to be worn 23 h/day. Half still progresses. Assess effectiveness at the 1 year mark
- Operative:
  - Infantile: indicated if depressed tibial plateau and impending closure of the medial physis. May consider valgus derotation tibial osteotomy. Tomograms needed if bar suspected. If bar is found, either resect or close lateral side of physis. Tibial plateau need be elevated if depressed greater than 25°. Any residual LLD may need later correction
  - Juvenile/adolescent:
    Indications and management similar
    Consider lateral hemi-epiphysiodesis if deformity not severe and has greater than 2 years of growth remaining
    Selected cases require osteotomy of the proximal tibia ± distal femur
    LLD if greater than 2.5 cm will later need correction

2.3 Regional Problems

2.3.1 Longitudinal Deficiency of Proximal Femur in Children
(Fig. 2.13)

2.3.1.1 Myths
- Most people use the term PFFD to describe the congenital short femur (with a very different prognosis and functional potential), which may not always be appropriate
- It is now realised that PFFD is, in fact, strictly a misnomer, since anomalies are seldom really focal and many times the entire femur can be abnormal. The term FPFD is preferred

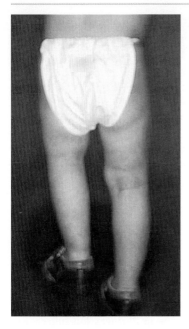

Fig. 2.13. Proximal focal femoral deficiency

2.3.1.2 Biomechanical Defects in PFFD (After Aitken)
- LLD
- Malrotated extremity
- Defect of proximal muscles
- Instability of the proximal joints

2.3.1.3 General Surgical Options
- Lengthening: if less than 15 cm LLD ± adjunct operations
- Amputations and prosthetics
- Rotationplasty: together with adjunct operations like knee arthrodesis sometimes
- Options in severe Aitken D deficiency
  - Iliofemoral fusion
  - Steel's, Brown's and Ilizarov's pelvic-support osteotomy

2.3.1.4   Technical Pearls if Limb Lengthening Planned

▦ If poor acetabular coverage and high chance of hip subluxation/dislocation on leg lengthening: operate to increase cover before leg lengthening commences

▦ Many suggest span the (frequently circular) fixator across the knee during lengthening. External splint sometimes for a 12 h a day, knee flexion exercises encouraged. Paley suggest to stop lengthening if knee flexion less than 40°

▦ Frequently quoted upper limit of lengthening is about 12–15 cm LLD; but this is a guide – depends on, for instance, whether there are Cxs during the lengthening process and status of nearby joints, e.g. deficiency of cruciates of the nearby knees

▦ Checking for the projected LLD prior to lengthening is important; these cases easy to calculate, e.g. if 40% at start, likely 40% at maturity

2.3.1.5   Pearls on Rotationplasty

Main risk/drawback:

▦ Psychiatric impact: can be serious on the child

▦ Timing: some perform at age 2 years as in Shriner's but others, e.g. Kostuik prefers the much later age 12 years, due to the problems associated with de-rotation

▦ Danger of de-twisting: most authors decrease this Cx by knee arthrodesis – by achieving most of the rotation at the knee, the muscles crossing the leg will be stretched to lesser degree; reduce de-rotation tendency over time. Will have to sacrifice the distal growth plate at time of knee fusion

2.3.1.6   Comparison:
Amputation and Prosthetics and Van Nees Rotationplasty

▦ Although Van Nees if properly done has an edge over amputation with prosthesis in terms of gait normality and oxygen consumption parameters; possible Cx must be bourn in mind

▦ Even discounting these Cx, Van Nees not always better in practice because these cases not that straightforward due to defective hip muscles; ER contractures, associated leg/foot anomalies

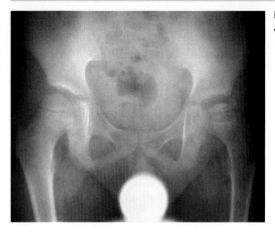

Fig. 2.14. Perthes disease affecting the left hip

2.3.2   Perthes Disease (Fig. 2.14)

2.3.2.1 Epidemiology
- 4–8 years
- Males more
- Bilateral 1/10: even if bilateral, occur in different stages
- Family Hx positive in 1/10
- DDx: MED, hypothyroidism and blood disorder/Gaucher's or septic arthritis

2.3.2.2 Natural History and Aetiology
- No true long-term natural history studies
- Real aetiology unknown; there is avascular necrosis of the femoral head going through the stages of necrosis, collapse and remodelling

2.3.2.3 Histopathology
- Primary vascular event
- Primary disorder of epiphyseal cartilage with collapse and necrosis as a result

2.3.2.4 Possible Aetiology
- Avascularity: interruption of blood supply
- Hyperviscosity states

- Venous hypertension
- Altered clotting (e.g. thrombophilia and hypofibrinogen states)
- Plus possible systemic disorder (delayed skeletal maturation, shorter, ± endocrine/IGF, ossification anomalies, cartilage changes on biopsy)

2.3.2.5 Classification
- Radiological staging: Waldenstrom's classification
- Severity: often use either the Herring Classification or others (Salter's or Caterrall's)
- Outcome: often use Stulberg's Classification

2.3.2.6 Waldenstrom Radiological Stages
- Initial: element of synovitis, increase in medial joint space, sometimes ↓ ROM
- Fragmentation: place where most classification refers to (e.g. Salter, Caterrall)
- Re-ossification: at which point treatment (even containment) may no longer be effective
- Re-model (healing)

2.3.2.7 Lateral Pillar (Herring) Classification
- Group A: no loss of height
- Group B: less than 50% loss of height at lateral pillar
- Group C: greater than 50% loss of height at lateral pillar

2.3.2.8 Head at Risk Signs (Catterall)
- Lateral subluxation
- Lateral calcification
- Lateral V-shape physeal defect (Gage sign)
- Metaphyseal: cystic changes
- Physis: horizontal
  Also check for:
  - Hinge abduction
  - Acetabular changes (on serial follow-up)

2.3.2.9 Stulberg (Outcome) Classification
- Spherical congruency: (1) if normal, (2) if big/small head
- Aspherical congruency: (3) if not flat, (4) if flat head + acetabular changes
- Spherical incongruency: (5) if flat head and spherical acetabulum

2.3.2.10 Alternative: Mose Circle Criteria
▦ Compares sphericity between AP and lateral views
▦ [good 0 mm, fair 1–2 mm, poor greater than 3 mm]

2.3.2.11 History and Examination
▦ Hx: painless/painful limp, acute onset rare, may have minor recent trauma
▦ P/E: limp, ↓ ROM (IR, abduction), thigh atrophy, (LLD)
(clinical at-risk signs → hip stiff, obese, ?female)

2.3.2.12 Investigation
▦ XR: classify into stages, check bone age
(Early stage XR: medial joint space widens, decreased size of ossific nucleus, subchondral fracture) (in fragmentation, area of radiodensity and lucency)
▦ Use of arthrogram: hinge abduction detection, check proper containment and head shape
▦ USS: synovitis, head shape
▦ Others, e.g. MRI

2.3.2.13 Factors Affecting the Development of Femoral Head Deformity
▦ Growth disturbance of epiphysis and physis
▦ Repair
▦ Disease process
▦ Type of treatment being given

2.3.2.14 Possible Residual Deformity
▦ Coxa Magna
▦ Premature physeal arrest
▦ Deformed femoral head
▦ Overgrowth of trochanter
▦ Osteochondritis dessicans

2.3.2.15 Prognostic Factors
▦ Age most important (cut off age 6 years): reflects remodel potential
▦ Other important areas:
  – Extent of involvement (Herring class)

- Head at risk signs (of Caterrall)
- Ratio of unaffected to affected femoral head size
- Stulberg class can help predict long-term outcome (type 1 good, type 2 intermediate, type 3 bad)

2.3.2.16   Management
▦ (Refer to multi-centre study headed by Herring)

2.3.2.17   Principle of Containment
▦ Prevent deformity
▦ Permit physiological motion
▦ Promote remodelling

2.3.2.18   Main Management Options (as Used in Different Treatment Arms in Recent Multicentre Trials)
▦ No treatment
▦ ROM only
▦ Bracing
▦ Femoral varus osteotomy
▦ Salter pelvic osteotomy

2.3.2.19   Preliminary Result (Recent Trials)
▦ Lateral pillar A: all do well, young and old
▦ Young lateral pillar B: many do well
▦ Old lateral pillar B: surgery better, femoral osteotomy seems better, brace intermediate
▦ Young lateral pillar C: as in (3) but brace less effective
▦ Older lateral pillar C – as in (4)

2.3.2.20   Appendix

2.3.2.20.1 Femoral Osteotomy
▦ Pre-requisite:
  - No hinge-abduction
  - Regained ROM possibly can be performed without perfect sphericity
▦ Advantage:
  - Load relieving effect on joint
  - Medialise femoral head
  - Reduce venous hypertension

- Disadvantage: (a) persistent varus; (b) trochanteric prominence; (c) LLD
- Pearls: avoid neck-shaft less than $105°$ (these cases need combined with pelvic osteotomy); do not derotate, prefer open wedge

2.3.2.20.2 Hinge Abduction
- Dx: (arthrogram/abduction X-ray)
  - Widened medial space greater than 2 mm with hip abducted
  - Lateral corner of head to rotate under lateral acetabulum
  - Lessened superolateral joint space with hip abducted
- Treatment: valgus extension osteotomy $\rightarrow$ allows remodel, correct deformity, more motion and less pain

2.3.2.20.3 Pelvic Osteotomy (Salter)
- Most result reported on Salter
- Salvage: Shelf and Chiari
- Success varied: 75–95%
- Advantage: better anterolateral cover, no coxa vara, improve leg length, no Trendelenberg gait, (no pathological fracture through screw holes)
- Disadvantage: technique demanding
- Rationale to perform Salter: more cover, possible more vascularity, lesser joint stress

2.3.2.20.4 Use of Braces as Method of Containment
- Abduction cast
- Abduction orthosis
  Examples of orthosis $\rightarrow$ Scottish Rite, Toronto, (Tachdjian, Newington)

2.3.2.20.5 The Scottish Rite Orthosis
- Permits near normal activity, avoid knee stiffness, contains the head
- Structure: pelvic band, thigh cuff, abduction bar, hinges – hip, abduction bar/thigh cuff

2.3.2.20.6 Other Methods to Regain Motion
- Home traction
- Non-steroidal anti-inflammatory drug (NSAID)
- PT, ROM exercise, Adductor tenotomy, brace wear 22 h/day

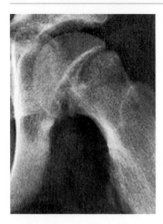

Fig. 2.15. Slipped capital femoral epiphysis

2.3.3   Slipped Capital Femoral Epiphysis (Fig. 2.15)

2.3.3.1 General Features
- Age 9–16 years (mostly 12–13 years)
- Males more
- Racial difference (Polynesian >Black >White >Chinese)
- Bilateral in 20–50% (becomes 60% in longer follow-up)

2.3.3.2 Traditional Classification
- Acute (>3 weeks)
- Chronic (<3 weeks)
- Acute-on-chronic (>3 weeks, recent more severe symptoms)
  Critics: the child may not remember and not always correlate with prognosis

2.3.3.3 Clinical Classification (Loder)
- Stable slip: can walk (with or without crutch)
- Unstable slip: cannot walk
  Prognosis: unstable slips 50% AVN rate (uncommon in stable cases)

2.3.3.4 XR Diagnostic Sign
- Klein sign
- Metaphyseal Blanche sign
- Posterior and inferior slip most common

2.3.3.5 XR Assessment of Severity
▨ Epiphyseal–metaphyseal displacement: less than one-third mild, greater than one-half severe (in between moderate)
▨ Lateral epiphyseal-shaft angle less than $30°$ as mild, greater than $50°$ as severe (in between moderate)

2.3.3.6 Aetiology (Biomechanical Versus Biochemical Theories)
▨ Mechanical theory
  – Obesity (greater than 95th percentile in more than half of the patients)
  – Femoral retroversion (more in obese)
  – Physeal obliquity
  – More acetabular coverage (from centre edge angle)
▨ Biochemical theory
  – Estrogens increase physis strength, androgens will decrease
  – Association with some endocrine disorders: ↓ Thyroid, ↓ gonads, growth hormone (GH) supplementation

2.3.3.7 Histology
▨ Slip at hypertrophic zone of the physis
▨ Ultra-structure → defective collagen fibrils and collagen binding

2.3.3.8 Management Principle
2.3.3.8.1 Treatment Goals
▨ Prevent further progression of slip
▨ Avoid Cxs:
  – AVN
  – Chondrolysis
  – Problems related to internal fixation devices

2.3.3.8.2 Main Treatment Options
▨ Conservative: casting – unpopular, many side effects
▨ Operative:
  – In-situ pinning (1 pin): smooth pin
  – Others:
    Open epiphysiodesis
    Percutaneous epiphysiodesis
    Osteotomies: (1) through physis (Cuneiform), (2) base of neck, (3) inter-trochanteric

2.3.3.8.3 Overall Trend

▨ Stable: in-situ pinning, perpendicular to physis in the AP/Lat projection – centre of physis

▨ Unstable: controversial. May consider doing gentle positioning by placing the foot in neutral position, screw fixation within less than 24 h, non-weight bearing ×6 weeks, then partial weight bearing ×6 weeks

2.3.3.8.4 In-situ Pinning (Details)

▨ Advantage: low progression, good remodelling, little blood loss

▨ Disadvantage: AVN, especially posterosuperior pin; chondrolysis, associated with pin protrusion

2.3.3.8.5 Surgical Principle of In-situ Pinning

▨ Some evidence to support use single screw: has 70% stiffness of two screws, avoids the higher Cx of two screws

▨ Screws positioning: things to avoid: (remember slipped capital femoral epiphysis causes a retroversion deformity of the femoral neck)
  – Avoid lateral shaft of femur: place the pin antersuperior
  – Never enter the epiphysis of the femoral head posterosuperiorly by exiting the posterior neck, ↑ AVN
    To minimise risk of injuring vessels, the ideal position for a screw is to aim at the centre of the femoral head

2.3.3.8.6 Surgical Technique

▨ Biplanar XR

▨ Make sure can see head and neck of femur before start

▨ Location of skin incision marked

▨ Lines drawn on the skin, skin incision at junction of the lines

▨ Guide pin advanced freehand parallel to skin lines

▨ Insert pin into epiphysis perpendicular to physis

▨ Some say that perhaps screw should "not" protrude laterally, as toggling by soft tissues can cause loosening. Advantage of leaving the screw head proud is possibly to allow easier removal later

▨ Outcome: 92% physis fusion and full activity, AVN around 2%

2.3.3.8.7 Casting

- Disadvantage: abandoned by many since progression of slip, chondrolysis, pressure sore, difficult in obese child
- Advantage: no operation, prophylactic protection to opposite hip

2.3.3.8.8 Options Other than Osteotomies: Epiphysiodesis

- Open epiphysiodesis:
  - Advantage: no pin Cx, lower AVN
  - Disadvantage: high risk of progression, invasive
  - Involves: window in anterior neck, tunnel across physis, pack iliac crest bone graft inside
- Percutaneous method reported but not widely used

2.3.3.8.9 Various Osteotomies

- Cuneiform: wedge excised from femoral neck metaphysis, reduce epiphysis and pinned. High AVN risks
- Base of neck: may cause shortening, LLD, corrects 35–55°, lower AVN
- Inter-trochanteric: low AVN but shortening occurs

2.3.3.8.10   Complications

AVN: causes

- Unstable hips/severe displacements
- Attempted reduction especially of chronic slips
- Pin in posterosuperior physis
- Cuneiform (neck) osteotomy
- Most develop in less than 1 year
- Clinical features: ↓ ROM, especially IR, irritable hip
- XR: early may not see changes; later on see collapse, cyst and sclerosis, etc.
- Bone scan: sometimes may predict its development but does not change management
- Treatment:
  - NWB status
  - ROM maintained
  - NSAID
  - Obviously, if protruding pin, should be removed or repositioned (CT may be used if really uncertain if pin protruding and whether physis is closed)

Possible salvage: later on, realignment osteotomy, fusion/trapdoor/ later plasty

Chondrolysis
  Pin protrusion
  Severe slip
  Occasionally reported caused by spica
  Occasionally reported association with inter-trochanteric osteotomy
  Clinical features and management such as AVN
  XR: less than half in affected side
  Bone scan: more periarticular uptake

Hardware Problem
  Poor fixation
  Pin breakage
  Pin protrude
  Less Cx if: (1) XR guidance, (2) use cannulated screws

2.3.4   Developmental Dysplasia of the Hip (Fig. 2.16)

2.3.4.1   Definition of Terms
■ Hip dislocation: no contact between femoral head and acetabulum
■ Dislocatable hip: hip dislocates with certain provocative manoeuvre and relocates with abduction and flexion

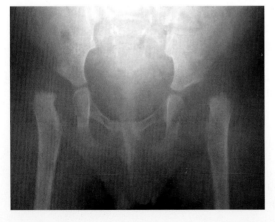

Fig. 2.16. Bilateral developmental hip dysplasia

- Hip subluxation: femoral head not articulate with the medial most portion of the acetabulum
- Hip dysplasia: includes all the spectrum of congenital hip anomalies from hip subluxation to dislocation
- Acetabular dysplasia: refer to abnormal development of the acetabulum, usually shallow and more vertical
- Teratological dislocation: most are high riding and irreducible, associated with abnormal anatomy and NM disorders (e.g. arthrogryposis)

2.3.4.2 Incidence and Screening
- 5–10/1000 live births
- Use of static and dynamic USS in neonatal screening: Not foolproof since some cases present later on (hence the more appropriate term developmental hip dysplasia rather than congenital hip dysplasia)

2.3.4.3 Indications for USS
- Positive physical examination
- Breech
- Oligohydramnios
- Strong family history
- Child with congenital torticollis

2.3.4.4 Physical Assessment
- Neonates:
  - Ortolani: check for reduction of a dislocated hip. Clunk felt upon hip abduction and 90° flexion with slight upward pressure over the greater trochanter
  - Barlow: a provocative test for a dislocatable hip. Done by applying outward and downward pressure on the adducted hip and the thumb on the inner thigh
- Infant
  - There may only be reduced abduction, with shortening of the femur (Galeazzi's sign Fig. 2.17) asymmetric skin fold

2.3.4.5 Aim of Management
- Aim at reduction of the femoral head into the true acetabulum by CR or OR at any age
- There is great remodelling power in young children and less need for concomitant procedures

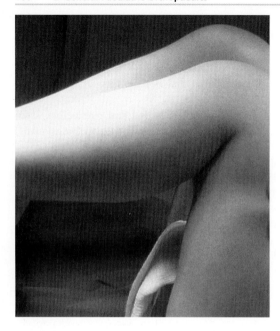

Fig. 2.17. Galeazzi sign

- Older children often need concomitant procedures like femoral or pelvic osteotomy
- Proper reduction of the femoral head is important for the proper development of the acetabulum and lower incidence of subsequent acetabular dysplasia

2.3.4.6 Treatment: Newborn to 6 Months of Age
- Pavlik Harness is most often used, with the hips flexed 100° and 30–60° abduction or the safe zone to prevent AVN
- Need to monitor the status of the hip by serial USS
- On day 1 30% of hips reduce, on day 2 65%, by first week 85–90%. In hips that do not reduce by 3–4 weeks the harness should be discontinued in favour of CR plus spica
- Those hips that reduce with the harness should be worn for 6 weeks, but up to 3 months in the older child at presentation or if the hip was dislocated at presentation

■ The harness is not recommended in a child greater than 6 months since it will no longer be useful to hold the older child in the correct reduced hip position

2.3.4.7 Cxs of the Pavlik Harness

■ AVN: if improperly applied and not keeping the hip within the safe zone
■ Persistently dislocated hip left undetected can wear away the acetabulum, so-called Pavlik Harness disease
■ Femoral nerve palsy

2.3.4.8 Role of CR in Children up to 12 Months

■ CR: must be gentle, hips flexed >90° abduction in the safe zone between 30°–60° abduction (human position). Mostly successful in children 12 months old or younger and can be performed for failed Harness cases
■ Role of traction: less used nowadays, employed in the past to "aid" reduction of the hip, with enough weight to lift the infant's buttock just off the mattress
■ Confirmation of concentric reduction by arthrogram: advocated, look for medial dye pooling less than or equal to 5 mm accepted but greater than 7-mm cases are associated with a poor outcome. Most also perform adductor tenotomy
■ Hip spica application: after successful CR, recommend CT to confirm reduction, change of cast every 6 weeks. (For children 1 year or younger, 3 of 12 casting mostly, after off cast, apply abduction splint until XR normal)

2.3.4.9 Use of Open Reduction in Children 12–18 months Old

■ As the child ages, there is higher chance that CR will fail and OR will be needed, e.g. from soft tissue contractures that hinder CR. Below 18 months, the good remodelling potential of the child's hip is such that concomitant procedures like femoral and/or pelvic osteotomy are seldom required

2.3.4.10 Open Reduction

■ Structural obstacles to CR are: hour-glass capsular contracture, ligamentum flavum, iliopsoas, pulvinar, transverse acetabular ligament

- OR should be performed by experienced surgeon. Repeat operation after failed OR only 1 of 3 satisfactory results
- Approaches to the hip:
  - Ludloff: medial approach, although has the advantage to tackle the structural obstacles directly, cannot perform capsulorraphy
  - Anteromedial approach of Weinstein, essentially a variant of the medial approach, 15% AVN chance
  - Anterolateral bikini incision: incise on the iliac apophysis, then using the interval between TFL and sartorius. Besides tackling the obstacles, perform iliopsoas recession and capsulorraphy. Immobilise in the most concentric position usually 30–40° abduction and IR, spica ×6 weeks

2.3.4.11 DDH Presenting at 18 Months

- Problems at this age:
  - Less remodelling potential: one-half of remodelling potential occurs by age 4 years; most of remodelling of the acetabulum by age 8 years
  - Progressive dysplasia: from deformed head and acetabulum, variable muscle contracture, hypertrophic ligamentum teres, redundant contracted capsule, labral deformity and thickened transverse acetabular ligament
- Principles of treatment:
  - Aim at stable, concentric reduction of the hip without too much pressure (may need shortening), followed by a period of post-operative immobilisation of 3 months
- Salter pelvic osteotomy:
  - The tendency is to perform the Salter at the time of OR rather than do it later on a pressing need basis, since the hip development may never catch up if delayed for around 2 years
- Femoral osteotomy:
  - May be required if shortening necessary to reduce the joint in proper tension
  - Derotate only if too much anteversion

2.3.4.12 Delayed Presentation (Fig. 2.18)

- The natural history of Bilateral neglected DDH is better than Unilateral DDH. By adulthood, most with reasonable ROM, some Trende-

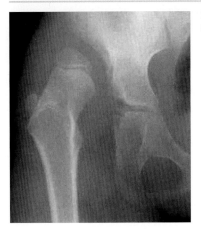

Fig. 2.18. Late presentation of developmental dysplasia of the hip (DDH)

lenberg lurch. Opinion differs as to the upper age limits for operative intervention but a reasonable age will be age 5 years
▪ As the natural history of unilateral dislocation is worse, the upper age limit that operation will be considered is higher, but one has to bear in mind that the potential for acetabular remodelling falls significantly after about age 8 years

2.3.4.13 Management of Late Presenters
▪ Will be covered by the section on management of hip dysplasia in young adults under adult orthopaedics

2.3.5   Problems Around the Paediatric Knee

2.3.5.1   Congenital Knee Dislocation

2.3.5.1.1 Clinical Features and Aetiology
▪ Rare, 2 per 100,000
▪ Female greater than male, 1/3 Bilateral
▪ Severity varies from subluxation to dislocation
▪ Associated with Larsen's syndrome
▪ Other associations:
  – DDH, clubfeet and others (e.g. cleft palate, spina bifida, arthrogryposis, etc.)

– Aetiology: packaging problems (associated with fetal positions, more in breech), possible hypoplastic cruciates, or fibrotic quadriceps

2.3.5.1.2 Pathological Findings
- Quadriceps fibrosis and contracture
- More anterior situated iliotibial band/hamstrings
- Absent suprapatella pouch
- Underdeveloped patella
- Hypoplastic cruciates

2.3.5.1.3 Physical Findings
- Hyperextended knee with anterior tibial subluxation with respect to femur
- Soft tissue contractures as mentioned
- Signs of associated conditions, e.g. Larsen's syndrome
- There may be delayed ossification of distal femur/proximal tibia

2.3.5.1.4 Management
- Conservative treatment like manipulation/splints usually not effective
- Operation near 6 months of age before weight-bearing. Involves soft tissue release and reconstruction and postoperative spica for 6 weeks

2.3.5.2 Congenital Patella Dislocation

2.3.5.2.1 Clinical Features and Aetiology
- Present at birth/within first few years of life
- Patella dislocated and permanently fixed to the lateral aspect of the femur
- Possibly due to failure of myotome (containing the quadriceps and patella) from internal rotating in the first trimester

2.3.5.2.2 Pathology
- Following may be present:
  - Shallow trochlea
  - Atrophic VMO
  - Contracted iliotibial band, vastus lateralis
  - Anterolateral abnormal insertion of the extensor mechanism
  - Genu valgum

2.3.5.2.3 Management
- Operation up to age 1 year
- Involves either Roux-Goldthwaite (distal realignment) or extensive lateral release and medial plications

2.3.5.3 Osgood–Schlatters Disease

2.3.5.3.1 Clinical Features and Aetiology
- Involves pain and swelling at the apophysis of the proximal tibial tubercle, likely caused by microavulsions caused by repeated traction on the ossification centre of tibial tuberosity
- Often referred to as an osteochondrosis, but AVN seems unlikely (and excellent blood supplies from the anterior, medial and lateral surfaces of the tibial tuberosity). Recent opinion is that patella tendinitis may be as important as apophysitis
- Normally ossification centres fuse with each other to coalesce with proximal tibial epiphysis around age 13 years
- Males greater than females, bilateral in nearly 50%

2.3.5.3.2 Work-up
- Clinical Dx
- Local heat, pain, swelling and increase of symptoms with resisted knee extension
- XR: fragmentation of the tibial tubercle may be seen, although Ddx from normal variation in ossification is needed
- MRI/USS: thickening and signal changes near patella tendon insertion

2.3.5.3.3 DDx
- Jumper's knee
- Sinding–Larsen
- Fracture of tibial tubercle
- Others, e.g. infection, tumours

2.3.5.3.4 Management
- Most respond to activity modification, ice, analgesics, infrapatella strapping. Although persistent pain on kneeling common
- Consider plaster if very symptomatic
- Surgery rarely needed since tend to resolve spontaneously with closure of physis

- A very occasional case may benefit from careful removal of still mobile not fused ossicles to prevent recurvatum
- More likely to have chronic symptoms if see fragmentation on X-ray or cases with persistent mobile ossicles

2.3.6   Lesions Around the Leg

2.3.6.1 Congenital Pseudarthrosis of the Tibia (Figs. 2.19, 2.20)

- Rare 1:150,000
- NF in 50%
- Involves anterolateral bowing of the tibia
- Numerous classifications (Boyd, Anderson, Crawford)
- Type may even change during treatment
- Results of treatment are better in older patients
- Early type, bowing present at birth; fracture before 5 years and poor prognosis
- Late type
  - Normal at birth; fracture after 5 years and good prognosis

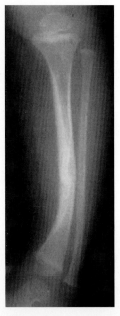

Fig. 2.19. Anterolateral bowing of the left leg

2.3.6.1.1 Special Characteristics

- Because of the possibility of non-union or pseudoarthrosis after osteotomy, an increase in angulation is not addressed surgically if the limb has no fracture and can be braced
- Always remember pseudoarthrosis can develop: (1) spontaneously; (2) after fracture; (3) after osteotomy of the involved bone

2.3.6.1.2 Pathology

- Fibromatosis-like
- Highly cellular, similar to other pseudoarthroses

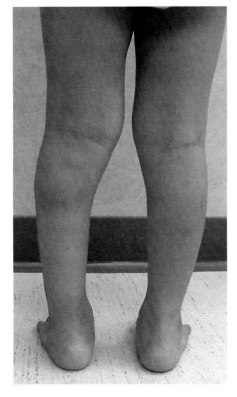

Fig. 2.20. Clinical picture of a child with anterolateral tibial bowing

2.3.6.1.3 "Rule of 2" to Ease Memorisation of Congenital Tibia Dysplasia

Two Causes of LLD
- Disuse atrophy
- Deficient of growth potential of the distal tibial physis

Two Causes of Ankle Valgus
- Sloping distal tibial epiphysis
- Deficient lateral buttress from fracture or pseudoarthrosis of lower fibula

Two Main Types
- Non-dysplastic: as radiological "sclerosis" of medullary canal and increased bone density and sometimes as "loss of tubulation" of long bone
- Dysplastic: with three subtypes
  - Failed tubulation
  - "Cystic" subtype radiologically
  - Severe type is like "sucked candies" appearance

Correlation Between Types 1 and 2
- Note possibility of conversion to dysplastic type after osteotomy to correct the angulation

Two Main types of Braces During Different Ages of Child
- Small: AFO (long); for the pre-walker
- Child walks → KAFO
  (The drop-lock type of knee joint hinges as child gets older, which allows sitting with knee flexed)

Two Main Uses of Braces
- Pre-fracture, i.e. prophylactic
- Therapeutic
- All cases need to be worn at least to skeletal maturity

2.3.6.1.4 Those Presenting as First Fracture
- Pseudarthrosis excision
- Iliac crest bone graft
- IM rod including ankle

2.3.6.1.5   Those Presenting as Second Fracture
- Repeat procedure
- Free vascularised fibula grafting can be considered
- Ilizarov transport is another option

2.3.6.1.6   Free Vascularised Fibula
- Technically demanding
- An option in recurrent fractures
- Persistent length discrepancy and donor morbidity

2.3.6.1.7   2 Main Drawbacks of Vascularised Fibula Grafts
- Potential to cause instability in the opposite leg syndesmosis; also check whether opposite side is dysplastic (harvest of ipsilateral dangerous, but reported; do not mention in examination setting, no large series supporting its use) and further pseudoarthrosis/angulation
- Not able to correct LLD and deformity well as does the Ilizarov and demanding technique

2.3.6.1.8   Ilizarov Procedure
- Resection
- Correction of deformity
- Bone grafting
- Compression at resection site
- Proximal lengthening

2.3.6.1.9   Advantage of Circular over Monolateral Transport
- More versatile
- Use for smaller fragments
- Adjustable during treatment

2.3.6.1.10   Pros and Cons of the Ilizarov Technique

Disadvantage
- High re-fracture rate despite good initial union
- Cumbersome for paediatric age group with psychological impact
- Others: pin tract problems, stiffness, non-union, neurovascular injury

Advantage
- Burns no bridges, not touch the opposite leg
- No need to sacrifice the opposite fibula and possibly sometimes less ankle stiffness than with William's rodding
- Many theoretical advantages: address LLD, angular deformity, fibular non-union, fibula migration, ankle valgus

2.3.6.1.11   Williams Rod and Graft (Fig. 2.21)
- An IM rod placed from proximal tibia across pseudoarthrosis site, incorporate the graft and extend through the ankle across the talus to calcaneus. Shriners' hospital uses rush rod for transankle stabilisation with good result

2.3.6.1.12   2 Main Drawbacks of William's Rodding positive bone graft (BG)
- Ankle stiffness almost the rule (and need to cross the physis; growth affected)

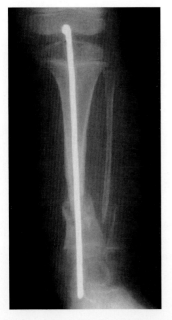

Fig. 2.21. William's Rodding procedure

▦ Changing of rod/rod migration due to growth usually required
▦ Others: ankle valgus, lateral planter nerve
▦ Advantage: (a) less technically demanding than Ilizarov or vascular fibulas, (b) reported results not bad, e.g. by Shoenecker or at Shriners' hospital

2.3.6.1.13 Amputation
▦ Some experts consider this option after three or more failed attempts
▦ Especially if the expected ultimate outcome expected is a short scarred limb with fibrotic ankle

2.3.6.1.14 Reasons for Boyd-Syme procedure
▦ Mid-leg amputation predispose to subsequent bone stump overgrowth
▦ Better length of stump adds biomechanical stability for prosthetic wear

(The new "Seattle foot" and runner's foot have made children's prosthetics much more functional, and team sports such as soccer are not out of the question)

2.3.6.1.15 Outcome
▦ Long-term results are guarded with any method
▦ Gait analysis of options mentioned versus Symes amputation were studied in the past
▦ Early onset of disease, early surgery and transankle fixation lead to a rather inefficient gait, comparable with that of amputees

2.3.6.2   Fibula Hemimelia (Fig. 2.22)

2.3.6.2.1   General Introduction
▦ As in "PFFD", it will be naive to think that fibula hemimelia only involves the fibula, for associated defects of the ipsilateral LL are quite common
▦ Many classifications exist, but none stresses the importance of whether there is an associated functional foot
▦ Check associated anomalies such as: Knee joint, tarsals, meta-tarsal (MT), phalanges, - that sometimes may be absent; tibia itself can be straight or bowed or shortened and the distal tibial epiphysis usually involved

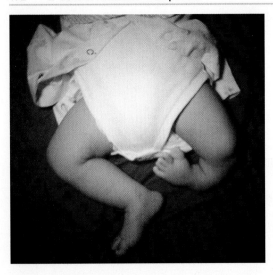

Fig. 2.22. A child with fibula hemimelia

2.3.6.2.2 Summary of Possible Associations

▓ Foot: equinovalgus, valgus hind-foot, sometimes absence of one or more lateral rays
▓ Ankle: absent lateral malleolus, or hypoplastic. Ball-and-socket ankle joint
▓ Fibula: hypoplastic or absent
▓ Tibia: can be shortened (proximal/mid/distal with valgus)
▓ Knee: ligament lax sometimes PFJ problem or foot instability
▓ Femur: acetabular dysplasia, femur varus/valgus, femur sometimes short, lateral femoral condyle hypoplastic

2.3.6.2.3 Kalamchi Classification

▓ Types IA, IB: hypoplasia with a portion of fibula present
▓ Type II: complete absence of the fibula → hip, knee anomalies common as are cruciates and knee valgus and maldeveloped lateral femoral condyle. The distal tibial plate/epiphysis can be abnormal. Sometimes tarsal bones anomalies
[More severe forms there can be ankle valgus (stable or unstable); tarsal coalition that will eventuate in a ball-and-socket ankle joint. Notice tibial bow uncommon with partial fibula deficiency]

2.3.6.2.4 Goal of Treatment
- Main goal of fibula deficiency treatment, whether partial or complete, is functional restoration
- This implies: a plantigrade functional foot and appropriate length equalisation. Cosmesis is only of secondary consideration

2.3.6.2.5 General Options
- Observe if minimal degree of length difference and normal foot
- Role of limb lengthening
- Amputation and prosthetics

2.3.6.2.6 Role of Limb Lengthening
- Staged lengthening sometimes in selected cases
- Lesser degrees consider merits of epiphysiodesis versus leg lengthening
- During lengthening: watch for progression in the knee valgus; may need excision of the lateral 'band' or Fibula Anlage plus supracondylar osteotomy for under-developed femoral lateral condyle and staple medial plate

2.3.6.2.7 Indications of Leg Lengthening
- Foot greater than or equal to 4 rays
- LLD projected less than or equal to 8 cm
- Stable mobile ankle
- Plantigrade foot
- Multi-disciplinary team

2.3.6.2.8 Amputation and Prosthetics Versus Limb Lengthening
- Treatment of choice especially with total deficiency, foot anomalies
- Experts like Paley think that planned repeat lengthenings with correction of foot to plantigrade may save some limbs
- Others argue that current Syme's prosthetic sockets are much improved and the cosmetic appearance of Syme or Boyd prosthesis are very acceptable

2.3.6.3 Longitudinal Deficiency of the Tibia

2.3.6.3.1 Classification of Tibia Hemimelia
- Type 1: distal femur hypoplastic, proximal tibia absent
- Type 2: two-thirds of distal tibia absent, distal femur fine

- Type 3: rare, amorphous segment of bone – appears like a "diaphysis" knee and ankle, both unstable
- Type 4: proximal end of tibia well developed

2.3.6.3.2 Work-up
- Associated anomalies → Hip, hand, spine in a large series by Shoenecker
- Short usually functionless leg with equino-varus posture in the ankle, there may be deficient/duplicated medial rays; knee joint is frequently also abnormal; shortened and anteriorly bowed leg

2.3.6.3.3 Management of Different Types in Lloyd-Roberts/Jones Classification
- Types 1 2 3: ablation usually involves knee disarticulation. (Not AKA as there will be bony stump overgrowth)
- Type 4: quite well-formed proximal tibia. May try reconstruction and limb lengthening
- Other main quoted treatment option – Brown's fibula-femur procedure for cases with reasonable fibula and retained quadriceps function

2.3.7   Lesions of the Foot

2.3.7.1   Clubfoot (Fig. 2.23)

2.3.7.1.1 Aetiological Classification
- Positional
- Congenital: common type
- Teratological: resistant
- Syndromal: spina bifida, arthrogryphosis, etc.

2.3.7.1.2 Functional Classification (Carroll and Dimeglio)
- Carroll 10 points (calf, posterior fibula, crease, lateral border curvature, cavus, navicular kissing medial malleolus, calcaneus fixation to fibula, equinus fixed, adductus fixed, fore-foot supination fixed)
- Dimeglio
  - Stiff-stiff = usually teratological 10%
  - Stiff>soft = resistant, but partial corrects in 60%
  - Soft>stiff = considerable reducibility 30%
  - Soft-soft = postural/mild no operation needed

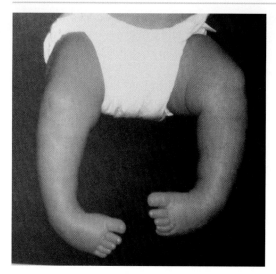

Fig. 2.23. A child with bilateral clubfeet

2.3.7.1.3 Physical Assessment
▪ General: shorter, wider, calf atrophic
▪ Crease: mid-foot and posterior ankle common
▪ Medial tibial torsion: assessment difficult since navicular adjacent to the medial malleolus
▪ Equinus: assess with knee F/E → true gastrosoleus contracture indicated by equinus with knee extended and may indicate amount of ankle stiffness. But feel posterior heel bone carefully, can be high away from heel pad
▪ Varus position and assess subtalar motion
▪ Talar head felt dorsilaterally
▪ Mid-foot stiffness indicated by amount of feeling the difficulty to reduce the fore-foot to the talar head
▪ Supination: check degree/extent
▪ (All deformities be assessed in relation to the next proximal segment, i.e. fore-foot on mid-foot, mid-foot on hind-foot)
▪ Check for mid-foot plantarflexion by feeling the medial column from the first MT to the talar head; plantarflexion at mid-foot can be caused by triangular navicular. If occurs postoperatively, can be due to dislocation of navicular relative to the talar head

- (Persistent varus after casting). Can be from varus deformity of the calcaneus and/or cuboid or varus of the MT

2.3.7.1.4 Differential Diagnosis
- MT adductus: lacks hind-foot varus and equinus
- Vertical talus: does have hind-foot equinus but with hind-foot valgus and fore-foot valgus

2.3.7.1.5 XR Assessment: Pearls and Pitfalls
- Feet held in position of best correction in weight-bearing or in infant, simulated standing
- Since the AP and lateral talocalcaneal (TC) angles are hind-foot angles, the XR beam be focused on the hind-foot (about 30° from the vertical for AP; the lateral can be transmalleolar, fibula overlapping the posterior half of the tibia, to avoid rotational distortion
- Sometimes lateral dorsiflexion/plantarflexion views assess ankle motion especially if flat topped talus, and assess mid-foot hypermobility. [In the older child → can also focus XR on mid-foot to assess the dorsaolateral subluxation of the talo-navicular joint (TNJ)]

2.3.7.1.6 Management: When Should It Start?
- From day 1 according to Ponseti
- Most need 4–8 casts, in fact seldom greater than 7
- Early recurrence needs a further 3–4 casts
- Later ones, TA transfer not to cuboid (valgus force), but to the third cuneiform

2.3.7.1.7 Conservative Treatment: Ponseti Versus Kite
- Main difference:
  - Kite not use tenotomy, sometimes feet kept in cast for 2 years
  - Kite uses calcaneo-cuboid joint (CCJ) as pivot instead of talar head, which Ponseti says is "wrong"

2.3.7.1.8 Possible Age Limit to Conservative Treatment
- Ponseti says not too rigid
- Others claim if present late at several months success rate low, but Ponseti thinks that several months old still possible to use his method

2.3.7.1.9 Pearls to Success in Ponseti Method and What to Do if Recurs

- Do not correct the equinus until the fore-foot adduction and hind-foot varus both have been corrected
- Tenotomy is percutaneous, done as outpatient procedure usually within few months
- Recurrence markedly reduced with postoperative compliant splintage with Dennis-Brown splint

2.3.7.1.10 Importance of Dennis-Brown Boots

- Key is holding both feet in abduction around 60–70°, (not more than in the cast); said to be the most effective splint by Ponseti to prevent recurrence – the child kicks both feet all the time

2.3.7.1.11 Role of Taping and Continuous Passive Motion (Dimeglio)

- Taping was tried but moderate effect
- Dimeglio's continuous passive motion machine is computer-controlled, allows dorsiflexion, eversion, etc.; connected 8 h a day. No long-term results

2.3.7.1.12 When to Do Surgery

- Failed Conservative
- Teratological type clubfeet
- Stiff-stiff variety to start with

2.3.7.1.13 Timing of Surgery Versus Attainment of Adequate Length (George Simon)

- George Simon is of the opinion that a foot of 8 cm or more is big enough for surgery
- Early school (surgery at 3–6 months): since much room for the bones to remodel especially in the first year of life (Carroll)
- Late school (surgery at 9–12 months), bigger and easier to see the culprit pathologies; postoperatively if weight-bear helps correct the deformity

2.3.7.1.14 Key Elements that May Need Correction in Open Surgery

- Posterior release
- Medial release

- Plantar release
- Posterolateral tether take down
- Lateral extended release

2.3.7.1.15 Surgical Approaches (Pros and Cons)

- Turco's posteromedial (not tackle posterolateral tether stressed by Carroll; some cases also need more extensive CCJ/lateral TNJ release)
- Carroll's two incision (main critic is residual varus danger since persistent posteromedial tether)
- Cicinati's cicumferential (difficult to deal with TA, but in practice no problem; sometimes difficult to do plantar release)

2.3.7.1.16   Elements of Release in Greater Details

During Posterior Release
- TA lengthened
- Posterior capsule need release [exposed by retracting peronei and flexor hallucis longus (FHL) and excise a piece of fat]

During Medial Release
- Keys are abductor hallucis and neurovascular bundle
- Abductor hallucis may need excision
- Part of posteromedial portion of deltoid ligament may need release
- TNJ capsule most require release

Plantar Release for Cavus
- Retract and protect medial/lateral plantar nerves
- Then eases release of plantar aponeurosis and short plantar muscles
- Sheaths of TP and FHL usually need releases
  [Avoid plantar release if already rocker buttom]

Posterolateral Tether Release
- TC and calcaneofibular ligaments released
- Peronei sheath released

During Extended Lateral Release
- May extend to the CCJ and the other side of the subtalar joint

2.3.7.1.17 Realignment on Table

▦ After all releases; finger at talar head dorsolaterally while the foot is laterally rotated in slight supination – similar in fact to Ponseti's manipulation

▦ This should correct the lateral border to straight, heel to slight valgus, reduce the talar head under the navicular (navicular be slightly proud as in normal feet) and no wedging open of subtalar joint

2.3.7.1.18 How Many K-wires

▦ Most authors use one or more, depends on what was done

▦ Do not over-reduce the talonavicular into valgus

2.3.7.1.19 Plaster Casting Post-op

Long leg plaster with knee flexed 90° for 6–8 weeks

2.3.7.1.20 Neglected Adult Club

▦ Not prevent standing and ambulation (some liken it to Syme's situation)

▦ Problems include: persistent deformity, abnormal gait, (and equilibrium), skin problems, and OA

(Even with the non-neglected ones, expect some residual calf atrophy, loss of ROM, and shape and size of foot, and talus vascularity sometimes affected)

2.3.7.1.21 Cxs of Plaster Casting Treatment

Spurious Correction (Transverse Breach of Mid-foot)
  Causes:
  – Dorsiflexion attempted with concomitant pressure wrongly under the MT heads rather than mid-part of the foot and with no correction of heel varus or fore-foot. XR: mid-foot equinus and fore-foot dorsiflexion with a break at the mid-tarsal joints
  – Premature hind-foot eversion before correcting the midtarsal varus. Abduction force transmitted to the hind-foot, which is rotated spuriously into lateral rotation (bean shape)
  Prevention: first, correct fore-foot adduction and supination, then correct the hind-foot varus and equinus (note: sometimes Bean shape not apparent until age 4–11 years; in this case, may need open wedge navicular osteotomy and close-wedge cuboid osteotomy)

Frank Inability to Correct

- Usually due to:
  - Faulty technique
  - Late age at first treatment
  - Severity of condition
  - Special conditions: arthrogryposis, spina bifida, Larsen's syndrome, diastrophic dwarfism

Flat-Topped Talus

- Here talus compressed by the nutcracker like effect in forced dorsi-flexion (sometimes compression fracture and ischaemia resulted)
- Prevention: less force, correct the posterior tight structures early

Fracture and Physeal Injury

- Metaphyseal compression of distal tibia/fibula
- Torus fracture distal tibia
- Fracture of distal fibula

Pressure Sore

- Injudicious moulding and lack of padding

2.3.7.1.22   Cx of Operative Treatment

Under Correction

- Inadequate post release (and TAL): equinus
- Inadequate palmaris longus tether release: persistent medial spin → with anterior calcaneus rotated beneath the talus
- TNJ plus first MT capsule plus abductor hallucis inadequate release → Fore-foot adduction
- Still subtalar rotation of the calcaneus → Heel varus
- TNJ inadequately tackled: Dorsal subluxed TNJ
- Inadequate/no release flexor digitorum longus/FHL: Claw toes

Over-correction

- Hind-foot valgus: at the level of ankle from dividing the deep deltoid, at the level of subtalar from excision of OI ligament and no fixation
- Fore-foot adduction: after TA transfer to fifth MT; prevent by split transfer with lateral limb to third cuneiform

- Pes planus: complete section TP+TC ligament ± section S Tali (or TP transferred with no subtalar stabilisation)
- Dorsiflexion/calcaneus deformity: overdone TAL plus casting in excessive dorsiflexion

Strange Correction (Some Over/Some Underdone)
- Skew foot: hind-foot valgus, fore-foot adducted

Correction Does Not Last
- No use of pin fixation
- Fixation time inadequate (recommend use 8 weeks)

Other Cxs
- Neurovascular
- Skin

Bone and Physeal Damage
- Bone damage to talus
- Physeal damage to distal tibial physis

Others
- Talus AVN: excess dissection at the Sinus Tarsi
- Possible aseptic necrosis with fragmentation of navicular reported

2.3.7.2 Pes Planus

2.3.7.2.1 Clinical Features
- Involves loss of the medial longitudinal arch of the foot
- Heel usually in valgus and fore-foot supinated the lateral column is short in relation to the medial column
- Can be rigid or flexible
- Biomechanical consequence of flat foot is talonavicular subluxation throughout stance phase of gait

2.3.7.2.2 Structures that Maintain the Normal Medial Arch
- Static structures
  - Bony structure (by virtue of the bony structure of the bony arch), plantar fascia (acting as a tie rod), spring and long plantar ligament
- Dynamic element
  - TP (works especially on weight bearing as medial stabiliser)

2.3.7.2.3 Classification

- Flexible:
  - Physiological: lax ligaments
  - Muscle imbalance (NM disease)
  - TP dysfunction (adults)
- Rigid:
  - Tarsal coalition: JRA/RA – trauma
  - Others
    Disorders that can resemble flat foot
    Congenital vertical talus: skew foot

2.3.7.2.4 History

- Duration of symptoms and location of pain if any
- Birth history, any trauma history, family history and previous treatment

2.3.7.2.5 Physical Assessment

- Look for the exact site of tenderness, uneven wear of shoes, any pressure points of the sole or mid-foot break, TA tightness, any general laxity
- Assess overall limb alignment
- Check the flexibility: tip toe test or jack test, on looking from behind, the heel valgus corrects on tip toeing if still flexible
- Assess the motion and flexibility of the ankle, subtalar and midtarsal joints
- Special test of TP in adults: single heel raise test, too many toes sign, inversion weakness

2.3.7.2.6 Investigations (Adults and in Older Child)

- Meary angle (in lateral view, line through talus, navicular and first metatarsal should normally be straight, in flat feet there is an apex plantarly)
- Standing hind-foot alignment XR to assess where the valgus is
- Others, e.g. Harris view and oblique XR of the foot useful to assess tarsal coalition; MRI useful in TP dysfunction

2.3.7.2.7   Natural History of the Normal Arch Development in Children
- Most cases the normal medial longitudinal arch will be formed in the first decade
- Refer to the landmark paper by Staheli on the development of the longitudinal arch in J Bone Joint Surg Am (1987)
- It is impossible to predict which planovalgus feet will become painful in adults

2.3.7.2.8   Management
- Physiological flat feet (majority of children's flat feet):
  - Most do not need surgery
  - Reassure parents; ± arch support if very symptomatic but will not correct the deformity
  - If really refractory, consider medial soft tissue reconstruction/bony surgery e.g., lateral column lengthening, calcaneal sliding osteotomy, extraarticular subtalar fusion, even triple arthrodesis if degeneration changes present near skeletal maturity
- Subgroup with hyperlaxity:
  - Severe cases may need subtalar fusion
- Subgroup with tight TA:
  - Will need TA stretching and/or lengthening
- NM flat feet
  - Orthosis may be useful, severe cases may need triple arthrodesis when skeletally mature

2.3.7.2.9   Metatarsus Adductus
- Involves fore-foot adduction at the tarso-metatarsal joint. Bilateral in 50%, present early at age 1–2 years
- Classification: mild/moderate/severe depending on whether the fore-foot can be abducted to the heel bisector or not
- Mild/moderate cases respond to conservative treatment by stretching/casting; only the occasional rare severe cases need metatarsal release and osteotomy

2.3.7.2.10   Skew Foot
- Involves fore-foot adductus and hind-foot valgus
- Can develop callosity over the plantar-flexed talar head ± tight TA
- XR: ↑ TC angle on AP and lateral view

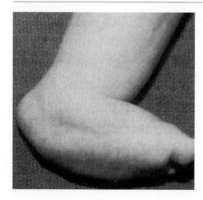

Fig. 2.24. A child with congenital vertical talus with rocker buttom foot

- Conservative treatment uncommonly successful, operation may need first metatarsal osteotomy, calcaneal osteotomy, and Achilles lengthening

2.3.7.2.11   Congenital Vertical Talus (Fig. 2.24)
- Aetiology: unknown, but look hard for associated conditions such as arthrogryposis, myelomeningocele, DDH, Marfan, Trisomy 13–15
- Pathology: hind-foot in valgus and equinus, talus is vertical, navicular articulates with dorsal cortex of talar neck. Talar head palpable on the medial plantar aspect of foot. Contracted posterior capsule and subtalar joint capsule. Contraction of nearby tendons: Achilles, extensor hallucis longus (EHL), extensor digitorum longus, peronei, TP, anterior tibial

2.3.7.2.12   Clinical Features
- Rigid flat foot
- Hind-foot valgus and equinus
- Fore-foot dorsiflexed and abducted
- Rocker-bottom deformity of sole
- Gait awkward with weak pushoff

2.3.7.2.13   Work-up
- XR: standing AP/lateral in plantarflexion and dorsiflexion. (assess the talar-metatarsal axis – a line bisecting the talus and the long axis of MT, Normal = 3°, ↑ in vertical talus)

▓ Usual anomalies: fore-foot abduction, ↑ TC angle calcaneum in equinus, talus vertical, fore-foot dorsally displaced on talus
▓ Lateral plantarflexion view to ddx congenital vertical talus and oblique talus (as in C.P.): only the latter condition aligns not the former

2.3.7.2.14   Management
▓ Goal: reduction and maintenance of the anatomic relationship of the navicular and calcaneum to the talus
▓ Serial casting: from birth to 3–4/12 stretches soft tissue
▓ Surgical: considered at 6–12/12, ST procedures – post capsulotomy, multiple tendon lengthening, reduce the TCJ and TNJ
Bony procedures in late presenters – Grice-Green subtalar fusion ± triple arthrodesis

2.3.7.3   Tarsal Coalition
▓ Involves connection between two or more tarsal bones. Most commonly TC and also calcaneonavicular. Bilateral in 50%
▓ Connection can be bony, cartilaginous or fibrous. Onset of symptoms usually associated with bar ossification
▓ Aetiology: possible defect of segmentation of the primitive mesenchyme. Thus, congenital rather than developmental

2.3.7.3.1   Clinical Features
▓ Age at presentation: TC bar at typically 12–16 years, and calcaneal-navicular bar at 8–12 years. Family history may be positive
▓ Can present as flat foot with hind-foot valgus
▓ Tender at site of coalition, e.g. sinus tarsi in the case of CN bar
▓ Peronei commonly shortened causing pain upon stretching with foot inversion. Frank spasm is rare
▓ Subtalar motion can be reduced in TC bar

2.3.7.3.2   Work-up
▓ XR: AP/lateral/oblique/and Harris view
   – CN bar can be easily seen in oblique view with the anteater nose appearance
   – TC bar sometimes seen in the Harris view, but may need CT to visualise

▪ CT: coronal cuts useful to assess TC bar and transverse cuts in assessing CN bar. Can also assess any degenerative changes and any associated coalitions

2.3.7.3.3 Management
▪ Conservative: activity modification and shoe-wear advice, period of casting ×4–6 weeks may help decrease pain and spasm if present
▪ Operative: CN bar: excision with muscle interposition. TC bar: Excision and fat interposition alone may fail and may require triple arthrodesis if near skeletal maturity especially if there is already degenerative changes

2.3.7.4 Pes Cavus
▪ High Arch foot (cavus) characterised by either mainly fore-foot plantarflexion (cavovarus) or hind-foot dorsiflexion (calcaneocavus)
▪ Always need to rule out underlying NM disorders frequently present
▪ Classification:
  – Acquired: neural disorders (Charchot Marie Tooth), muscular dystrophies, polio, spinal dysraphism
  – Traumatic: e.g. after leg compartment syndrome

2.3.7.4.1 Elements of the Deformity
▪ Fore-foot plantarflexion: from contracted plantar aponeurosis plus intrinsics and/or weak extensors
▪ First ray pronation: pull of peroneus longus
▪ Hind-foot calcaneus: weakened Achilles, normal or near normal tibialis anterior
▪ Hind-foot varus: adaptive in response to first ray pronation to get fore-foot on the ground
▪ Clawed toes: from weakened intrinsics. Big toe clawing can result from weak tibialis anterior and EHL overactivity

2.3.7.4.2 Clinical Features
▪ Look for deformities as mentioned and flexibility of hind-foot by Coleman block test
▪ Look at gait and pressure points/callosities
▪ Look at spine and neurological examination

2.3.7.4.3 Work-up

- XR: (1) Assess fore-foot deformity by angulation noted between line through the talus and 1st metatarsal. (2) Assess hind-foot calcaneus by calcaneal pitch (angle between line corresponding to the floor and calcaneus inferior border)
- MRI/radiology of the spine
- Nerve conduction testing/EMG and nerve or muscle biopsy

2.3.7.4.4 Management Principles

- Conservative: by heel and metatarsal pads, shoe-wear modification
- Operative: depends on flexibility of deformity, muscular imbalance, and any degenerative changes
- Soft tissue surgery: individualise, such as Jones procedure (EHL transfer to first metatarsal neck), standard procedure for claw toes, peroneus longus to brevis to prevent excessive first ray plantarflexion
- Bony surgery: e.g. Dwyer calcaneal osteotomy for hind-foot varus if rigid hind-foot and triple arthrodesis if degenerative sets in

2.3.7.5 Other Foot Disorders

- Hallus valgus: not uncommonly seen in patients with hind-foot valgus as in diplegics, and pes cavus. High recurrence rate in the youths. Better to wait till near skeletal maturity before operating. Growth plate damage should be avoided
- Hallux varus: can be iatrogenic after HV surgery (e.g. after excision of the lateral sesamoid) or from overactive abductor hallucis

2.3.8   Regional Problems Upper Extremities

2.3.8.1 Sprengel's Shoulder

2.3.8.1.1 Clinical Features

- Featured by small usually unilateral high riding scapula protruding into the base of the neck to a variable extent
- Accompanied by cervical or upper thoracic vertebral anomalies or abnormal ribs. An omovertebral bar may be present in the plane of levator scapulae and fixing the scapula to the cervical spine. Most cases have shoulder abduction range of $90°$ whether or not a bar is present

2.3.8.1.2 Management

▦ Mild cases with good function can be observed
▦ If surgery is indicated, the principle is attempt to reposition the scapula by either detaching the muscles from the scapula or secure/lower it down to a near normal position
▦ Management of associated spinal anomalies should be individualised

2.3.8.2 Congenital Dislocation of the Radial Head

▦ Clinically the radial head is palpable, movement is full or mild limitation
▦ Direction of dislocation can be anterior, posterior or lateral
▦ XR reveals a dysplastic capitellum due to the absence of the radial head, the radial head itself is usually conical
▦ Cases with little functional disability can be observed, as reduction of the radial head by shortening of the shaft and transfixation may still risk sacrificing some rotatory motion

2.3.8.3 Madelung's Deformity of the Forearm

▦ In this condition, there is subluxation/dislocation of the ulna with marked inclination of the distal radius articular surface towards the ulna side
▦ It is likely the deformity seems due to premature epiphyseal arrest of the anterior and medial quadrant of the radial plate that causes both forward and medial inclination and some shortening of the radius

2.3.8.3.1 Clinical Features

▦ Signs that may be present include a prominent ulna, wrist tenderness, weakness of grip and deformity. With time, there will be limitation of dorsiflexion and pronation

2.3.8.3.2 Management

▦ Many propose to intervene if there is presence of functional disability near skeletal maturity, with radial osteotomy and ulna shortening
▦ Conditions that may be associated include Turner's syndrome, diaphyseal aclasis and dyschondrosteosis, etc.

2.3.9   Regional Problems: Axial Skeleton

2.3.9.1   Congenital Muscular Torticollis

2.3.9.1.1 Clinical Features
- Painless condition usually discovered within first 2 months of life
- Involves tilting of the head from a contracted and fibrotic sternomastoid. Fibrosis of the sternal head may compromise a branch of the accessory nerve to the clavicular head, thus increasing the deformity

2.3.9.1.2 Aetiology
- Probably results from ischaemia of the sternomastoid muscle
- Cadaver dissections and injection studies defined the sternomastoid compartment
- Due to the association of congenital muscular torticollis with other intra-uterine positioning disorders, it is possible that head positioning in utero can selectively injure the sternomastoid muscle, leading to the development of a compartment syndrome (JPO Wenger 1993)

2.3.9.1.3 Physical Findings
- Non-tender enlargement in the body of the sternomastoid may be felt
- Contracture of sternomastoid muscle causes the head tilt to the side of contracture and the chin to rotate to the opposite side
- Most resolve within 1 year, persistent contractures if untreated can cause deformity of the skull or face (plagiocephaly) facial asymmetry can be caused by flattening of the face on the side of the contracted muscle
- Rule out associated disorders like DDH (occur in 20%)
- Check other areas: e.g. eyes, neck anomalies, neurological deficits

2.3.9.1.4 DDx
- In the newborn
  - Other tumours in the region of the sternomastoid (cystic hygroma, brachial cleft cysts, thyroid teratomas), ptergium colli, congenital anomalies of the cervical spine, posterior fossa tumours, eye disorders (e.g. superior oblique palsy of the ocular muscle)
- In the older child, torticollis may be due to
  - e.g. atlantoaxial rotatory subluxation (Fig. 2.25) which may be due to infection, trauma, etc.

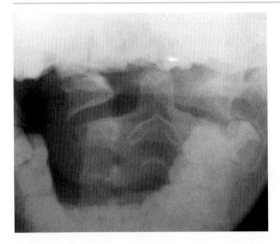

Fig. 2.25. Open mouth X-ray of a child with torticollis from rotatory subluxation of C1/2

2.3.9.1.5 Management

- Stretching exercises: 90% will respond to this simple regimen if started early, less than 1 years old
- Failure to respond to non-surgical measures by 1–2 years of age may need surgical intervention to prevent further facial deformity
- Surgery involves re-secting a portion of the distal sternomastoid muscle by transverse incision; avoid putting the incision immediately adjacent to the clavicle (incise transversely 1.5 cm proximal to the clavicle) More severe cases will need require proximal release as well (bipolar release)

2.3.9.2 Klippel-Feil Syndrome

2.3.9.2.1 Clinical Features (Figs. 2.26, 2.27)

- Includes all variants of failure of segmentation of the cervical spine, from failure of fusion of two segments to the entire cervical spine
- Segmentation occurs at 3–8 weeks of foetal life
- Frequent association with Sprengel's shoulder
- Other common associations include renal anomalies (Dx by USS) and anomalies in the cardiopulmonary or nervous systems

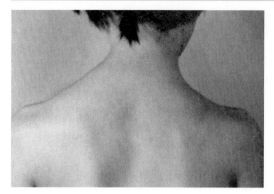

Fig. 2.26. Clinical picture of a child with Klippel-Feil syndrome. Note the low hair line and webbing

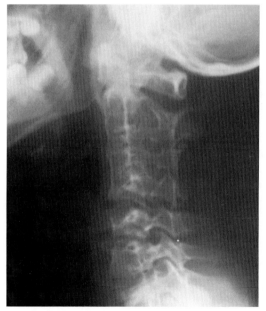

Fig. 2.27. Radiological appearance of a patient with Klippel-Feil syndrome

2.3.9.2.2 Physical Findings

- Many asymptomatic apart from variable loss of cervical spine motion especially lateral flexion
- The classic triad of low posterior hairline, short neck and decreased neck motion found in less than 50%
- Neurological deficit rather uncommon, more associated with higher cervical fusion (C2–C3) and those in whom most segments are fused except one or two segments, which then are more prone to instability

2.3.9.2.3 Treatment

- Asymptomatic patients only need observation
- With time, cervical spondylosis occur
- The proportion of patients requiring operative treatment is small

General Bibliography

Lyons Jones K (ed) (1997) Smith's recognizable patterns of human malformation, 5th edn. W.B. Saunders Company, Philadelphia

Benson M, Fixsen J, Macnicol M, Parsch K (eds) (2002) Children's orthopaedics and fractures, 2nd edn. Churchill Livingstone, Edinburgh

Selected Bibliography of Journal Articles

1. Leong JC, Wilding K et al (1981) Surgical treatment of scoliosis following poliomyelitis. A review of one hundred and ten cases. J Bone Joint Surg Am 63:726–740
2. Herzenberg JE, Paley D (1998) Leg lengthening in children. Curr Opin Paediatr 10:95–97
3. Ponseti IV (2002) The Ponseti technique for correction of congenital clubfoot. J Bone Joint Surg Am 84A:1889–1890
4. Sharrard WJ (1975) The orthopaedic management of spina bifida. Acta Orthop Scand 46:356–363
5. Herring JA (1996) Management of Perthes disease. JPO 16:1–2
6. Eyre-Brook AL, Price CH et al (1969) Infantile pseudoarthrosis of the tibia. J Bone Joint Surg Br 51: 604–613
7. Fong HC, Li YH et al (2000) Chiari osteotomy & shelf augmentation in the treatment of hip dysplasia. JPO 20:740–744
8. Ip D, Li YH et al (2003) Reconstruction of forearm deformities in multiple cartilaginous exostoses. JPO(B) 12:17–21

Contents

3.1   Congenital Hand Conditions

3.1.1   Introduction
- 1 in 600 live births
- 10% need surgery
- Associated anomalies: craniofacial, cardiovascular, neurological, musculoskeletal
- In half of the cases, aetiology is unknown; half occur from genetic (single/multi-genes, chromosome) anomalies and teratogens

3.1.2   Embryology
- Upper limb develops in a proximal → distal fashion
  - At 4 weeks, primitive limb buds are seen (undifferentiated mesenchyme): bulge at the lateral body wall and under control of apical ectodermal ridge
  - At 5 weeks, there is a hand paddle
  - At 8 weeks, fingers are separated (programmed cell death)
  - At 9 weeks movements begin to see joint creases

3.1.3   General Features and Operation Timing
- Child has exceptional ability to adapt
- Goal: improve and do not compromise function (cosmesis secondary consideration)
- Exact timing depends on the exact anomaly; usually takes place between 6 months and 18 months. Conditions that threaten limb viability – high risk of, for instance, deformity – should be treated earlier, e.g. constriction band syndrome

3.1.4   Classification According to the International Federation of Societies for Surgery of the Hand
- Failure to form: transverse versus longitudinal (e.g. radial club hand with frequent association with heart anomalies, Holt–Oram, blood anomalies, i.e. Fanconi's anaemia, etc.)
- Failure to differentiate, e.g. syndactyly
- Duplications, e.g. pre- and post-axial polydactyly. Thumb/pre-axial common in Asians; post-axial more common in blacks. Look for serious associated congenital anomalies if it occurs in the white population

- Overgrowth, e.g. macrodactyly (rare)
- Undergrowth, e.g. hypoplastic thumbs (five types/Blauth)
- Constriction band syndrome
- Generalised skeletal anomalies

3.1.4.1 Transverse Arrests
- Complete arm (amelia)
- Midarm
- Proximal forearm (most common)
- Wrist
- Midhand
- Fingers

3.1.4.1.1 Transverse Arrest
- Unilateral more, parts distal absent or rudimentary
- Forearm 1/20,000; arm 1/200,000
- Associated anomalies: club-hand, radial head dislocation, radio-ulna synostosis, meningocele

3.1.4.1.2 Treatment
- Infancy: passive prosthesis 3–6 months old
- Later: active terminal device, even myoelectric
- Role of Krukenberg operation:
  - Blind patients
  - Sometimes used in underdeveloped countries; if no prosthesis and unilateral amputees → involves separation of radius and ulna to function in a Pincer function

3.1.4.2 Phocomelia: A Form of Longitudinal Arrest
- Abnormal proximal → distal development. Three types:
  - Hand – trunk (complete)
  - Forearm – trunk (proximal)
  - Hand – arm (distal)
- Associated anomalies → cleft lip/palate; defective radial rays opposite side
- Most only treated with prosthesis and limb training
- ± A few – skeleton lengthening, tendon transfer
  1% all congenital anomalies, many from thalidomide

3.1.4.3 Cleft Hand Versus Symbrachydactyly

- Previously people separated cleft hand into typical (central V defect) and atypical
- Recent International Federation of Societies for Surgery of the Hand (IFSSH) meetings dropped the term atypical in favour of "symbrachydactyly"
- Severe cases of cleft hands still with fifth ray; severe symbrachydactyly usually still with first ray, a useful point in differential diagnosis (DDx). In symbrachydactyly, commonly see under-developed small hand bones, such as metacarpal (MC). Not usually seen in true cleft hands

3.1.4.3.1 DDx of "Symbrachydactyly"
- Cleft hand
- Constriction band syndrome
- Others

3.1.4.3.2 Central Ray Deficiency
- Also called split/cleft/sometimes lobster claw
- Two types: typical and atypical
    - Typical → V-shape from absent long ray. Two radial and two ulna rays; may have syndactyly
    - Atypical → three central rays absent
      X-ray: both types very variable; can have transversely oriented bones and split MCs

3.1.4.3.3 Cleft Hand: Features
- Associated anomalies: cleft lip/palate, cardiovascular anomalies, deaf, imperforate anus
- Typical more bilateral, atypical more unilateral
- Overall, many unilateral, most are sporadic
- Most do not need surgery as function is good

3.1.4.3.4 Any Role of Operation
- Reserved for more severe deformity when closure may be needed, e.g., suture fixation of the index finger (I/F) and ring finger (R/F) MC, ± MC osteotomy
- In cases where pinch and hand function compromised, correcting the thumb and index syndactyly may help
  (Flatt tackles the syndactyly first before attempting closure)

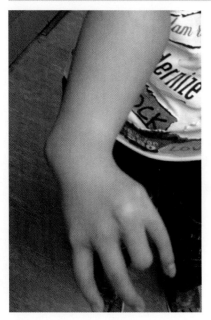

Fig. 3.1. A child with right radial club hand

3.1.4.4 Features of Radial Club Hand (Figs. 3.1, 3.2)

- Shortening and forearm bowing; can be both bones
- Radial angulation
- Radial displacements of the carpus with respect to the distal ulna
- Thumb never uninvolved, can be absent or hypoplastic. Decreased digital motion, I/F more
- Associated anomalies of other radial structures, e.g. radial carpal bones, such as scaphoid, articulation of the ulna and carpus not always present; always check for elbow stiffness as lack of flexion may contraindicate centralisation. Check any club of other side (bilateral clubs associated with TAR syndrome – thrombocytopenia absent radius syndrome); and/or other anomalies of tendons e.g., brachioradialis (BR), extensor carpi radialis longus (ECRL)/brevis (B), flexor carpi radialis (FCR), flexors/extensors. Radial nerve may terminate at elbow, even absent musculocutaneous nerve; radial artery sometimes also of small calibre, etc.

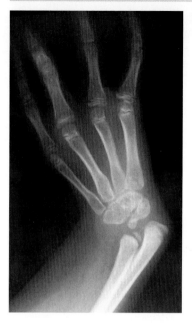

Fig. 3.2. The X-ray of the same child as in Fig.3.1 with radial club hand

- Systemic associations: Fanconi syndrome (pancytopenia), Holt–Oram (look for any atrial septal defect/ventricular septal defect). These are more often unilateral and if serious can limit the life expectancy
- Cause of deformity:
  - Ulna bow contributory
  - Tight radial soft tissue often known as the radial anlage, which, in fact, consists of either fibrous musculotendinous structures or even the median nerve
  - The carpus and hand are unsupported on the radial side, the mechanical advantage of the flexor mass is dissipated in increased radial deviation (RD) of the hand and palmar displacement of the carpus

    (Patients usually develop a side-to-side pinch in those with thumb aplasia; while this may be useful, it is restricted in the size of objects that can be grasped. An occasional neglected case adapts by using scissor-like action between the ulna two fingers and the radial two fingers)

3.1.4.4.1 Other Features of Radial Club Hand
▓ Half bilateral; most are sporadic
▓ Systemic association:
  – Aplastic anaemia (Fanconi Anaemia)
  – Heart (Holt–Oram)
  – Thrombocytopenia
  – Vater
▓ Local association → radial carpus/thumb with complete/partial absence; thenar muscle deficiency (ulna can be short and bowed)

3.1.4.4.2 Four Types (Bayne)
▓ Type 1: "Short" distal radius (may have delayed appearance of radial epiphysis) incidence 1/100,000
▓ Type 2: Defective proximal and distal epiphysis growth, radius rather hypoplastic
▓ Type 3: Partial (mid to distal third) absence
▓ Type 4: Complete absence of radius: most common

3.1.4.4.3 Treatment of the Different Types
▓ Types 3, 4 (and sometimes 2)
▓ Serial casting and stretching
▓ Check elbow: if poor elbow flexion, this contraindicates centralisation
▓ Centralisation at 6–12 months, adjunct operation, e.g. transfer ECRL to extensor carpi ulnaris (ECU) prevents recurrence, and/or distraction lengthening
▓ Pollicisation of I/F considered if severe thumb hypoplasia or absence → 6 months after centralisation (if only mild thumb hypoplasia, no need for pollicisation)

3.1.4.4.4 Treatment Principles
▓ Goal: Wrist stabilisation improves the mechanical advantage of the forearm flexor muscles by decreasing the abnormal radial movement of the flexor muscle mass; minimise power lost to increase the deformity
▓ The percentage of limb length discrepancy will be more apparent as the child grows; realignment helps physis plate growth and lengthening helps additionally, especially in activities that involve both hands
▓ Only by repositioning the hand out of the crouch of the forearm/elbow can we later do pollicisation procedures

3.1.4.4.5 Treatment for Different Grades of Severity

- Mild cases: 1–2 cm short, no instability, lengthening alone
- Severe: four basic components
  - Manipulation and casting: stretch early since pliable; change at weekly intervals
  - Realignment and stabilisation: several options are available – centralisation of the mainstay (into a notch created in the carpus by excising the lunate and capitate); radialisation (proposed by Gramcko; placing ulna radial to the central position to improve further the biomechanical wrist stability); soft tissue release alone quickly recurs; arthrodesis left for salvage and never for a bilateral deformity. The option to replace osseous support by free fibula is not good since no growth
  - Tendon transfer: especially of the ECU/flexor carpi ulnaris (FCU)
  - Correcting ulna bow as necessary: single/multiple closing wedges easier to perform paradoxically if radius is rudimentary – up to three osteotomies to straighten it. Better to perform at/around time of centralisation or the tightened radial structures will cause recurrence

3.1.4.4.6 Pollicisation Procedure

- To improve the function of prehension, especially precision pinch
- The procedure involves creating a new thumb from a digit, usually I/F, despite fact that it is usually rather stiff
- This procedure is complicated: involves reposition of I/F as thumb based on vascular pedicle; the MC is shortened and rotated
- The metacarpal phalangeal joint (MCPJ) becomes the new carpal-metacarpal joint (CMCJ). Tendon transfers are needed to produce a "balanced thumb" and create first web
- Always check angiogram and digital Allen before this operation – the former in severe cases, the latter in a child old enough. Doppler can also be used
- This procedure is always performed after centralisation, otherwise the tendon balance will be subsequently altered by the wrist procedure

3.1.4.5 Ulna Club Hand

3.1.4.5.1 Types
- Type 1: Ulna hypoplasia
- Type 2: Partly absent → most common
- Type 3: Completely absent
- Type 4: Associated radio-humeral synostosis. (50% radial head dislocation)
- In contrast to radial club hand; most ulna club hand with good hand/wrist function
- Associated anomaly: PFFD, club foot, spina bifida

3.1.4.5.2 Treatment Ulna Club Hand
- Mild: serial casts
- Radio-humeral synostosis: if severe internal rotation deformity → derotation osteotomy of the humerus
- Severe cases: associated radial head dislocation plus instability → may need to create one-bone forearm with excision of proximal radius and fusion of distal radius and proximal ulna (here, shoulder motion can compensate to some extent)

3.1.4.6 Syndactyly

3.1.4.6.1 Types of Syndactyly
- Complete versus incomplete (incomplete simply means joining of digits from web space to a point proximal to fingertip)
- Complex versus simple (simple means soft tissue bridge only; complex means both soft tissue and bony connections)
- Acrosyndactyly

3.1.4.6.2 More About Syndactyly
- A common anomaly
- Incidence: 1/2000, more in white male
- Half bilateral, many sporadic
- Most common site between middle finger (M/F) and R/F (50%); next common between ring and small (30%); least common between thumb and index (5%)
- Associated anomalies: i. component of syndrome; ii. polydactyly, constriction bands, toe webbing, brachydactyly, heart and spine anomalies

3.1.4.6.3 Poland Syndrome

The Four Main Features of Poland Syndrome

- Short or usually absent middle phalanx (M/P), mainly the I/F, M/F and R/F
- Syndactyly of the shortened digits
- Hand hypoplasia
- Absent sternocostal head of pectoralis major on same side, and sometimes no pectoralis minor, hypoplasia of breast/nipple or contracted axillary fold; sometimes no serratus anterior or latissimus dorsi, no deltoid; rib deficiency, even dextrocardia

Pulmonary Anomalies in Poland Syndrome

The letter "P" in Poland syndrome helps to remind the reader of the frequently associated pulmonary anomalies in this syndrome

3.1.4.6.4 Apert Syndrome (Fig. 3.3)

- Flat face, hypertelorism
- Mental retardation
- Craniosynostosis
- Ankylosed inter-phalangeal joints

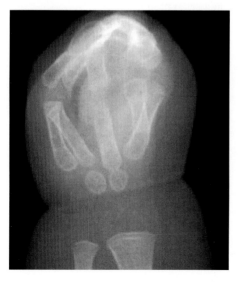

Fig. 3.3. X-ray of a patient's hand with Apert syndrome

■ Bilateral complex syndactyly with symphalangism: the digits are fused distally from the M/P onwards, triangular shaped bones, thumb if involved usually with delta phalanx; polydactyly rare. Vascular/tendon anomalies are common

The Three Types of Apert

■ The I/F, M/F and R/F as "Central Digital Mass", with thumb and little finger (L/F) free

■ Above and webbed fourth web, thumb free

■ Thumb and digital mass share a common nail
X-ray: Assess number of digits involved, number of MCs, number of phalanges, any cross-unions, any delta phalanx, sometimes joint surface configurations

Management of Apert

■ The aim of treatment: to achieve a functional hand in one or two stages, e.g.:
  – Thumb osteotomy to correct angulation, first web release, second/fourth web release
  – Central digital "mass" is divided to produce four digits and a thumb at around age 5 years of age
    (In type 3, a preliminary nail separation is needed)

3.1.4.6.5 Acrosyndactyly

■ Common association with constriction ring syndrome

■ Walsh classes:
  – Moderate: two phalanges [and one inter-phalangeal joint (IPJ) per digit]
  – Severe: one phalanx

■ Treatment: in general, release distal tethering bands early. This permits better growth; more proximal separation can be done later

3.1.4.6.6 Complex Syndactyly

■ In general, sometimes very tricky: accessory phalanges may be present between the skeletons of syndactyly digits either in organised form – "concealed central polydactyly" – or in an apparent jumble of bones lying transversely, obliquely and longitudinally

3.1.4.6.7 Pitfalls for Surgery in Complex Cases

- As the condition becomes more complex, the bifurcations of the common vessel become more distal and the arteries on the outer aspects become more rudimentary. Beware always of vascular compromise

3.1.4.6.8 Operation for Syndactyly

- Early surgery advised to prevent bone deformity and complete separation by school age
- Even earlier surgery is recommended for digits of unequal length to prevent flexion and rotation deformities

3.1.4.6.9 Timing of Surgery

- Thumb-index: 6 months
- R/F and L/F: 1 year
- Fingers of equal length: 1.5 year (Flatt)
  Multiple operations needed in severe complex types

3.1.4.6.10 Operative Pearls

- Beware of neurovascular (NV) anomalies in complex deformities
- One side corrected at a time in such cases (other side separated 3–6 months later)
- Zig-zag incision, with long volar or dorsal flap for web creation and separation: plus full-thickness skin graft
- Two major situations for early operation: (i) acrosyndactyly and (ii) syndactyly between rays of unequal lengths. If not, the longer ray will develop rotation and flexion deformity, which may not correct with later surgery. Thus, the rare thumb-index syndactyly mostly needs separation when first seen. Similarly, involved border digits in Poland and Apert syndromes require early release. Other cases can be left until 18 months

3.1.4.6.11 Other Technical Tips

- Where there are two digits with a common nail, precede with syndactyly separation by nail division and introduction of skin using a Thenar flap
- The sinus fenestration in acrosyndactyly is too far distal to form the new web and is excised during division
- Syndactyly release should not be performed simultaneously on adjacent webs, i.e. on both sides of single digit

▦ The shorter the digit, the more proximal be the new web: the limit being the MCPJ
▦ The new web should always be constructed with local skin
▦ Skin graft is required in nearly all cases, except those that are minor and incomplete
▦ When the thumb is involved, as in Apert, simultaneous rotation and angular osteotomy is required where all MCs are in the same plane and there is absence of thenar musculature
▦ Relatives of patients of Poland and Apert should be warned of a resultant smaller than normal hand and residual stiff fingers, which is common

3.1.4.7   Radio-Ulna Synostosis (Fig. 3.4)
▦ Two forms: (i) radial head not seen (absent) and (ii) radial head seen
▦ Treatment depends on the degree of forearm malrotation
▦ May sometimes need an osteotomy

3.1.4.8   Duplications

3.1.4.8.1 Thumb Duplication
▦ Mostly the radial duplicate more affected
▦ Mostly the ulna nerve-innervated intrinsics insert to ulna duplicate and median nerve-innervated intrinsics insert to the radial one
▦ Check joint stiffness and angulation
▦ Beware flexor and extensor can be duplicated, ±eccentric
▦ Nail – either shared or duplicated
▦ Wassel type 4 is the most common

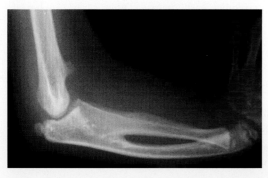

Fig. 3.4. Proximal radio-ulna synostosis

3.1.4.8.2 Other Features

- 1 in 10,000
- More in Asians, most being Unilateral
- Sporadic more common. ± AD (tri-phalangeal thumb)
- Timing of Operation: 6–9 months
  - If equal sized – can combine both – ensure articular congruent
  - If size unequal – excise smaller, reconstruct the collateral
  - If complex – add sometimes intrinsic/extrinsic tendon transfers, ± osteotomy and surgery on the plate

3.1.4.8.3 Post-axial Polydactyly

- Much more common in Blacks 1/300 versus 1/3000 in non-blacks
- Post-axial most common in Blacks
- Pre-axial most common in Asians and Whites
  (Post-axial most common overall)

3.1.4.8.4 Turek (and Stelling) Classification

- Type 1. Extra soft tissue mass, no bone
- Type 2. Normal-looking digit articulates with either phalanx or MC
- Type 3. With MC of its own
  'Central polydactyly' – involves either of the middle three digits; the extra digit mostly a Turek's type-2 anomaly [autosomal dominant (AD) and sometimes associated with foot polydactyly/syndactyly]

3.1.4.8.5 Treatment of the Turek's Types

- Type 1. Ligate; watch for bleeding (or by formal excision in theatre)
- Type 2. Preserve important structures such as the ulna collateral, of MCP of L/F and the abductor digiti quinti insertion
- Type 3. Excise extra digit
  (Type 1 with incomplete penetrance; types 2 and 3 AD with marked penetrance)

3.1.4.9 Macrodactyly (Figs. 3.5, 3.6)

- Pathomechanics: neural, vascular, and hormonal factors have all been implicated
- More than one digit not uncommon
- Two types – (1) starts in infancy and (2) starts in adolescence

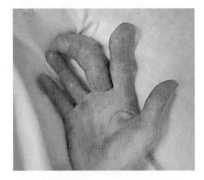

Fig. 3.5. Macrodactyly affecting the right middle finger

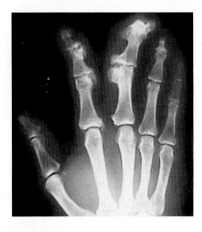

Fig. 3.6. X-ray of the same patient as in Fig. 3.5 with macrodactyly

3.1.4.9.1 Clinical Features

- Unlike the case for haemangiomas, AV-malformations, etc., all elements including bone, nerve, vessel and skin are involved
- Sometimes even hypertrophy of median/ulna nerve is involved
- Two forms exist: (1) noted at birth, growth rate same as fellow digits and (2) more common type, 'large' at birth, then grow out of its proportion to fellow digits
- Represents 1% all congenital anomalies
- Common site: I/F. Some authorities say multi-digit more common

3.1.4.9.2   Treatment

- Operation needed because function is compromised. The affected finger can also be stiff, and angulated
- Phased debulking each time on one side more prudent – remove excess skin and fat. Sometimes requires osteotomy to correct angulation. Sometimes epiphysiodesis (when size reaches that of the same digit) and/or bone shortening if digit is already too large, e.g. fusion of distal and M/P while part of M/P excised)
- Assess need of carpal tunnel syndrome (CTS) release and occasional case needs excision of the digital nerve. The areas supplied by the abnormal nerve are usually with abnormal sensation anyway
- Resistant cases result in amputation – especially when the rest of the digits are normal.

3.1.4.10   The Five Types of Hypoplastic Thumbs

- Absent – most need pollicisation (e.g. radial club hand) before prehensile function is fully developed in children less than 3 years old. In the case of radial club hand, centralisation ought to be done in 6–12 months, and pollicisation 6 months thereafter. If there is a delayed Dx of more than 3 years, the child with radial club hand sometimes would have adapted to the use of ulna 2 rays and there is a possibility that pollicisation might not be absolutely necessary. Also, never centralise in radial clubs if the elbow cannot be flexed
- Short thumbs [i.e. cannot reach level of proximal interphalangeal joint (PIPJ) of I/F]
- Adducted thumbs – associated 1st web contracture, needs opponensplasty
- Abducted thumbs – abnormal flexor pollicis longus (FPL) attachment
- Floating thumbs – possibility of reconstruction reported in some studies; others prefer pollicisation

3.1.4.10.1   Absent Thumb

- Many are associated with radial club hand
- Most will require pollicisation of the index

3.1.4.10.2   Floating Type

- Treatment: many favour amputation and pollicisation. In Japanese literature, there are attempts at reconstruction with variable success

- Most of these thumbs are connected by flimsy pedicle, and the two phalanges are hypoplastic. The MC may be rudimentary or absent
- The position of the floating thumb is usually more distal and radial than the normal thumb.

3.1.4.10.3   Short Thumb

- Most have little functional compromise
- Association with Holt-Oram Syndrome, and Fanconi's Anaemia; MC short and slender
- If there is short broad MC – think of myositis ossificans progressiva (dystrophic dwarfism)
- If there is short broad distal phalanx (D/P) – think of brachydactyly, Apert syndrome
- Operation: only if excess short: (i) deepen web space and (ii) distraction lengthening

3.1.4.10.4   Adducted Thumb

- Pathogenesis: web contracture, and poor thenar muscles
- Principle of treatment includes Z-plasties and/or fascial release (dorsal flap/SG), and opponensplasty
  [Opponenplasty options are transfer of abductor digiti minimi, flexor digitorum superficialis (FDS) and even the extensor digiti minimi]

3.1.4.10.5   Abducted Thumb

- Two main types according to Manske: (a) stable CMCJ – reconstruct; correct web release adduction, release abnormal slip, and provide stability and (b) unstable CMCJ – pollicise
- Pathogenesis – abnormal insertion of FPL (1 slip at volar D/P, 2nd slip passes dorsally and radially to join EPL); causes abduction with action of FPL

3.1.4.11   Constriction Band Syndrome (Fig. 3.7)

3.1.4.11.1   Introduction

- Definition: deep skin crease encircling a digit, thus causes varying degree of vascular or lymphatic compromise
- Four types (Patterson)
  - Mild groove
  - Deep groove, abnormal distal

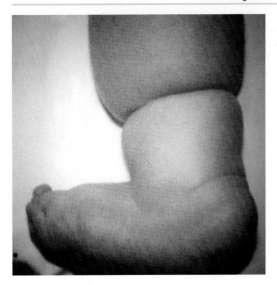

Fig. 3.7. An infant with constriction band syndrome

- Acro-syndactyly – incomplete or complete syndactyly of distal part
- Amputated

▦ 1/20,000

▦ Occurs more often in central digits; distal more common

▦ Associated anomalies → syndactyly, brachydactyly, and hypoplastic digits; sometimes also club feet, cleft palate, craniofacial.

3.1.4.11.2 Treatment

▦ Type 1 – observe

▦ Type 2 – release and z-plasty (depth of constriction determines whether complete or partial band release is indicated)

▦ If band is deep, only one side is released at a time to avoid vascular compromise. Second stage occurs 3 months later

▦ Type 3 – acrosyndactyly separation at 6 months; start early since multiple operations are required. Release border digits first, then central digits

3.1.4.12   Appendix

3.1.4.12.1   Symphalangism
- The affected finger is stiff, little/no skin creases
- X-ray: loss of joint space or no joint space
- Pathogenesis: failure of the finger IPJ to develop
- Represents only 1% of all congenital cases. AD most of the time
- Associations: syndactyly and foot anomalies
- Operation – not needed if adaptation is good; sometimes fuse in more functional position

3.1.4.12.2   Camptodactyly (Infancy and Beyond)
- Flexion deformity, usually of the L/F
- Mostly L/F. Deformity increases at growth spurts, but stops later
- Pathogenesis: e.g. flexor sheath contracture, FDS contracture, collateral contracture, volar plate contracture, lumbrical abnormal insertion, abnormal extensor, sometimes vascular/bone anomaly
- Treatment: try conservative splinting first
- Operation considered if progression was observed and flexion is greater than 60°
- Trick to operative treatment: operation involves release of all tight structures, e.g. lumbrical, skin, dermis, volar plate, etc., and sometimes even flexor to extensor transfer, phalangeal osteotomy

3.1.4.12.3   Congenital Clasped Thumb
- Can be normal in those up to 3 months old. Posture: thumb flexed and adducted posture
- Four types: (1) absent extensor, (2) hypoplastic extensor and strong flexor, (3) associated bony hypoplasia and (4) any other possibility
- Treatment: (1) try casting and stretching – may stimulate growth if hypoplastic and (2) if on table, absent extensor → EIP transfer considered and/or may treat any associated thumb hypoplasia

3.1.4.12.4   Delta Phalanx

Introduction
- J-shaped physis
- Associated with a C-shaped Epiphysis
- Usually as extra phalanx of the thumb or M/P of L/F → angulate towards the central axis of the hand

- Bilateral common
- Associated anomaly: polydactyly and syndactyly

Treatment Delta Phalanx
- Splints – no role
- Operate if severe angulation and/or for cosmesis
- Involves close wedge osteotomy

3.1.4.12.5   Clinodactyly

Introduction
- Deviation at M/P or at distal interphalangeal joint (DIPJ) causes lateral deviation especially of the L/F
- Incidence reported was 1–20%; much more in Down's Syndrome (30–50%)
- Sporadic or AD
- Associated anomalies → macrodactyly and brachydactyly
- DDx – delta phalanx

Natural History and Treatment
- Deviation towards radial side of the L/F usually
- Functionally, there is usually no/little impairment and operation is rarely indicated. Splintage not useful
- If operation is required, close wedge is usually used, but open wedge should be considered if phalanx is really short to start with

3.1.4.12.6   Kirner's Deformity
- Volar curvature of the D/P
- L/F common, most discovered at age 10 years
- Not rare – 1/400
- More bilaterals – sporadic or genetic
- DDx – trauma, infection, old frostbite
- Associated anomalies – Turner's, etc.
- Treatment – only if severe; consider osteotomy

3.1.4.12.7   Madelung Deformity
- Angulated and abnormal Ulna side and Volar aspect of the distal radial physis; the ulna half of the growth plate of the distal radius fuses early

- Bony changes – short bowed radius, short ulna, wedging of carpus between distal radius and ulna. Ulna head can be large and sub-luxated dosally
- Presents in late chilhood and adolescence
- Clinical features (C/Fs): can be stiff and there is ulna pain (impinged)
- Occurs more often in females; bilateral more common
- DDx: multiple exostosis, dyschondrosteosis, multiple epiphyseal dys-plasia, Ollier's disease
- Indication for operation: if persistent pain (splints may not work)
- Operation involves radial osteotomy, ulna shortening, and/or some-times can lengthen the radius

3.1.4.12.8 Mirror Hand

- Very rare, only 60 cases in three centuries
- In a true mirror hand, there are two mirror-image ulna bones, and no radius

3.1.4.12.9 Elbow Radial Head Dislocation

- Common congenital anomaly around the elbow
- Posterior dislocation most common; other possibilities include ante-rior and lateral dislocations
- Pathomechanics – abnormal development of the capitellum

Congenital Radial Head Dislocation

- Most common congenital elbow problem
- Check whether shaft of radius line bisects the capitellum
- Associated anomaly: nail-patella syndrome, etc.
- Cause – failure of development of the normal capitellum
- Direction: posterior>anterior/lateral; sometimes associated with radio-ulna synostosis

Treatment

- If there is no pain and patient is asymptomatic, continue to observe
- If there is pain (especially at the adolescence growth spurt), proceed with open reduction and/or radial head excision
  - Note: there is paucity of evidence to support the early open reduction

3.1.4.12.10 Congenital Trigger Thumb
- A1 constriction affects FPL gliding
- Bilateral >unilateral
- 25% of cases present at birth
- 30–40% of cases are resolved at age 1 year
- Operative timing therefore age 1 year or older

3.2   Brachial Plexus Injury

3.2.1   Causes
- Traumatic – open/closed; associated injuries – e.g. fractured clavicle, rib, cervical-spine, subclavian vessels
- Obstetric
- Pathological – radiotherapy, tumour, infected, cervical rib
- Iatrogenic – improper positioning in surgery
  - In adults, traumatic causes are most common – RTA, traction, open injury.
    Supraclavicular > infraclavicular (according to Naraka's large series); upper C5/6 more common if C8/T1 then more likely to be root avulsion since more tethering here. (Note that root avulsions type cannot be directly repaired or nerve grafted, may need to use such techniques as neurotisation)

3.2.2   Causes Secondary to Radiotherapy
- Much scarring
- Simple neurolysis may not work
- One way is to use free microvascular omentum transfer to give some padding sometimes providing pain relief

3.2.3   Causes in Children
- Causes include high birth weight, shoulder dystocia, etc.
- Most are Erb's palsy, Klumke's palsy occasional – mainly affects the hand
- Examination is not easy; need a calm child and serial assessment
- Good signs: lack of Horner's, presence of clavicle fracture, incomplete lesion, early recovery, not just of elbow flexion, but other aspects, for example, shoulder abduction

3.2.4   Lesion of the Child

■ Feature – most are neuropraxia or axonotmesis, but 5% need surgery
■ Usually should be observed for 3 months. Consider surgical intervention if biceps do not function by this time, or in fact muscles distal to it already regain function to repair the deficit

3.2.5   Assessment

■ History (Hx) – mechanism, position of body and arm during the accident, the magnitude of energy. In children, birth Hx and risk factors are important
■ Physical examination (P/E) – Horner's syndrome is suggestive of C8/ T1 lesion; proximal lesion indicated by rhomboid/ serratus anterior involvement, therefore look at type of breathing. Check motor power from proximal to distal. In total plexus injury, only most medial arm (T2) sensation remains

3.2.6   Clinical Types

■ Diffuse – all muscles paralyzed, sensory loss diffuse except for medial arm T2
■ Upper plexus – weak/absent abduction of shoulder and external rotation (ER); weak elbow flexion and supination; sensation loss in upper outer shoulder, lateral border arm, forearm; and I/F in thumb
■ Lower plexus – can affect shoulder adduction/IR, elbow extension, small muscles of hand (and forearm), sensation affected ulna side of the hand and forearm
■ Clinical signs of root avulsion – Horner's syndrome, dissociation of sweat and sensory function; affection of posterior neck muscles – supplied by the dorsal rami of the spinal nerves before the formation of the brachial plexus
■ Need to check each muscle of the upper limb to make a decision

3.2.7   Appendix

■ Sensory charting:
  – S0 = no sensation
  – S1 = deep pain only
  – S2 = superficial tactile and pain
  – S3 = recovery of tactile and pain in the autonomous area
  – S3+ = as above, two-point discrimination >1 cm
  – S4 = two-point discrimination <1 cm

- Motor charting:
  - M0 = no contraction
  - M1 = hint of contraction
  - M2 = movement with no gravity
  - M3 = move against gravity
  - M4 = move against some resistance
  - M5 = normal

3.2.8   Investigation

- Fluoroscopy – look at motion of diaphragm
- Computed tomography (CT) myelogram – still most accurate to detect root avulsions
- Magnetic resonance imaging (MRI) – can visualise root, present technology not yet too good to see the more peripheral nerve trunk
- Electrophysiology testing – electromyography (EMG) does not detect change immediately – needs 2–3 weeks; sensory nerve action potential still intact in root avulsions – beware. There is sometimes motor action potential testing and intra-operative nerve stimulation, favoured by Naraka
- X-ray – assess concomitant injuries, e.g. fractured clavicle, first rib (indicates high energy), etc.
- Intra-operative – ACh staining sometimes help identify the motor fibres but takes time (around 1 h)

3.2.9   Indications for Conservative Treatment

- Most are birth palsy, since 95% are neuropraxia or axonotmesis
- Non-root avulsion cases in adults, especially if we suspect neuropraxia/ axonotmesis – if unsure, a follow-up EMG, say in an interval of 1 month – in neuropraxia, there may be reinnervation of the more proximal muscles – if present one can wait for recovery of distal muscles; timing depends on distance from the site of nerve injury

3.2.10   Adjuncts to Conservative Treatment

- Splint – e.g. wrist extension to prevent flexion, shoulder abduction if deltoid affected
- Electrical stimulation – help prevent muscle atrophy
- Range of motion (ROM) should be maintained
- Active exercises – once the muscle groups begin to function
- Others? – gangliosides, etc.

3.2.11   Who Needs Urgent/Early Surgery

■ Open clean wound – do as emergency and it is easier than delayed surgery for a closed lesion
■ Closed wound but with vascular injury – sometimes the nerve can be tagged and repaired later
■ Gun shot/missile cases that are associated with vascular injury; many of these cases need to repair the subclavian vessels

3.2.12   Elective Surgery – Three Groups

■ Root multiple avulsions – no need to wait for long; go for early intervention (few weeks or less than 3 months) since root avulsion cases cannot direct repair or nerve graft, need neurotisation
■ Elective window lasts 3–6 months; results deteriorate if further delay and may not be useful after more than 12 months (wait at least 1–2 months; reason – time needed for nerve cells to activate the machinery for production of amino-acid needed for repair); period of observation is sometimes longer if there is a long distance between lesion and the nearest muscle – speed of axon advance 1 mm per day
■ Delayed referral – consider other strategies, e.g. muscle transfer and/or extraplexal neurotisation; tendon transfers, e.g. to restore trapezius/serratus anterior actions, to restore elbow flexion; occasional bony procedures, e.g. arthrodesis, and sometimes derotational osteotomy as in forearm pronation deformity

3.2.13   General Treatment Options

■ Direct repair – acute clean cut nerves
■ Observe – if only neuropraxia
■ Nerve graft – partial/complete ruptures of nerve trunks
■ Neurotisation – useful if root avulsions (either extraplexal source e.g. intercostal; or intra-plexal source, e.g. contralateral C7)
■ Late cases – tendon transfer, functional free muscle transfer and bony procedures

3.2.14   Comments on Neurotisation

■ Neurotisation of the avulsed plexus provides very few fibres in fact compared with the normal plexus; it will be a mistake to attempt to re-innervate too many muscles

- Functions that are vital need to be chosen, e.g. flexion of elbow, abduction of the arm with ER
- Restoring abduction of the arm with no ER is useless – since the forearm will drop onto the thorax

3.2.14.1 Choice for Neurotisation
- Intercostal nerves (usually take at least two, upper ones with more sensory fibres); most common connected to the nearby musculo-cutaneous nerve
- An alternative source to connect to musculo-cutaneous is the nearby ulna nerve (which sometimes can be vascularised)
- Spinal accessory nerve usually used to connect to the supra-scapular nerve
- Another possible choice to connect to the supra-scapular nerve is the phrenic nerve (but not if poor lung function or if patient is younger than 2 years)
- In last resort, with multiple root avulsions – contralateral C7
- Appendix – sometimes use stumps of C5, C6 but it is difficult to test their usefulness. This is another example of intraplexal neurotisation, e.g. if 1–2 of the upper roots avulsed, and 1–2 adjacent spinal nerves/trunks ruptured at the same time; then distribute the fibres of the available proximal stumps to all the distal stumps
- Some French authors also used the anterior cervical nerves

3.2.14.2 Use of Intercostals
- Two major problems with the use of intercostals, besides danger of decrease in lung function, contraindicated in patients under 2 years and in cases of Brown-Sequard since these are partially paralyzed: (1) mixed fibres (afferents and efferents) makes it difficult to identify and connect correctly; (2) motor fibres of all intercostal nerves receive their stimuli simultaneously – if an attempt is made to innervate more than one muscle, co-contractions occur, impair function, and fire only in deep inspiration

3.2.14.3 Use of Ulna Nerve
- Especially in cases where there is lower C8/T1 root avulsions and an upper trunk injury, some say neurotisation of these lower roots have a poor result; since the ulna nerve is unlikely to undergo spontaneous

re-innervation, it can thus be used as a free vascularised graft for repairing the higher part of the plexus

3.2.15 Prognosis – Adults
■ Type of nerve damage – root avulsion versus rupture versus clean cut
■ Site – more proximal is worse, and C5/6 better than C8/T1
■ Damage extent – diffuse worse than isolated cord/trunk/terminal branch
■ Surgeon factor – skill
■ Patient factor – age, smoke, etc.
■ Result of proximal C8/T1 usually not good and intrinsic hand function may not recover. The reason why fibres of upper C5/6 trunk recover more readily is not clear – probably because of the differing distance the axons have to cover to reach their destination
■ Root avulsions need be treated by neurotisation (of the distal stumps or better the terminal branches by means of transfer of other nerves). However, usually only a few functions can be restored – e.g. abduction/ER of the shoulder, elbow flexion. Notice restoration of shoulder abduction without ER restoration is useless
■ Proximal lesions usually fare worse, the reason being mingling of nerve fibres more proximally. The result of surgery is poorer in the spinal nerve and trunk lesions, while in the distal part of the plexus (cords and terminal branch) they fare better

3.2.16 Operative Pearls
■ Different types of nerve injury are frequently found in the same patient, and different surgical techniques may need to be combined
■ Necessary to confirm that lesions found correspond to clinical picture – if not may need more distal exploration. The reason is that injury at two sites is not rare (a sign of double level injury is a zigzag appearance of the suspected nerve)

3.2.17 Expected Time of Recovery
■ Proximal, e.g. suprascapular, in about 3 months
■ Very distal ones can take years

3.3   Tendon Injuries

3.3.1   Flexor Tendon Injuries

3.3.1.1 Vascular Supply of Flexor Tendons

▓ Longitudinal along musculotendinous units and along tendon-bone attachment areas

▓ Vinculae

▓ Diffusion – imbibition, more effective with finger motion

3.3.1.2 Healing of Flexor Tendon

▓ Extrinsic – previously thought to be the only healing mode, extrinsic healing may lead to adhesion formation

▓ Intrinsic healing – this form of healing proven in previous studies in which healing can occur inside the knee joint of experimental animals

– Our goal of repair is to encourage intrinsic healing and diminish adhesions. Although adhesions are almost inevitable, our protocol together with repair method should allow more friendly type of adhesions to form

– The epitenon is the active part of the healing tendon in the early phases of repair especially if there is some residual gap after repair. Intrinsic repair is more active if no gap remains

▓ Functional results of primary tendon repair are superior to results of tendon graft. This is because the revascularisation of the latter are at least 2–3 weeks behind that of primary tendon repairs

3.3.1.3 Goal of Flexor Tendon Repair

▓ Maximise excursion – the trend is to adopt the 'active extension passive flexion' programme which helps to reduce adhesions. Also, it is hoped that if adhesion does form, it will be of the more 'friendly' type

▓ Maximise strength – in order to prevent rupture of the flexor tendon with the above programme

3.3.1.4 Factors Determining the Success of Repairs

3.3.1.4.1 The Determining Factors

▓ Strength of repair

▓ Type of suture

- Prevention of adhesion
- Attention to the rehabilitation protocol
- Note: whether the sheath is repaired or not, no significant difference has been shown in previous papers

3.3.1.4.2 Strength of Repair
- Depends on the number of strands of the core suture
- Epitendinous suture augment the repair
- Dorsally placed sutures with 26% more strength than ventrally placed ones, though theoretically risk of impaired blood flow

3.3.1.4.3 Examples of Common Methods of Repair
- Standard modified Kessler with 4–0 monofilament core and 6–0 running epitendinous suture
- Silverskiold – uses the cross-stitch epitendinous suture and creates an external weave resembling a Chinese finger trap
- Strickland 4-strand suture – pairs a modified Kessler core stitch of 3–0 braided synthetic suture with a horizontal mattress stitch and a 6–0 epitendinous suture
- 6-strand suture method also reported

3.3.1.4.4 Epitendinous Suture
- Augment the repair
- Recent study showed deeper placement more effective
- Better contour, less bunching and overlapping

3.3.1.4.5 Methods to Prevent Adhesion Formation
- Active extension passive flexion programme by using suture methods with enough strength
- Prevent gap formation
- Use autogenous sources
- Role of tendon sheath repair controversial
- Use of synthetic materials (to surround the repair site), e.g. the polymer tetrafluoroethylene (PTFE)

3.3.1.4.6 Gap Formation
- Can occur with too aggressive rehabilitation protocol
- In vitro cyclic test shows that gapping is greatest at day 3 post-repair

▧ Tendon gapping is regarded as the hallmark of tendon failure – a gap of 2 mm or more is significant

3.3.1.5 Rationale of the Active Extension and Passive Flexion Programme

3.3.1.6 Basic Biomechanics

▧ Chicks tendon studies claim that motion and tension promote the greatest increase in cellular activity, but the absence of both components generates least activity

▧ Tensile strength of common repair technique may not be enough to reliably support active tendon mobilisation

▧ Too strong a repeated tensile stress too early will increase gap formation

▧ Tendons subjected to tensile stress in an active motion post-operative regimen maintained their strength to a far greater extent than immobile tendons

3.3.1.7 Partial Tendon Laceration

▧ Many recommend no repair if tendon is more than 70% intact, based on the reason that repair may delay healing

▧ Rehabilitation of these unrepaired tendons can follow Strickland's frayed tendon protocol

3.3.1.8 Zone 2 Flexor Tendon Injuries

▧ The reader is assumed to know the Kleinert zones

▧ Zone 2, or no man's land, has the special anatomy of Champer's chiasm as follows:
  – [Flexor digitorum profundus (FDP) travels through the decussation of FDS Champer's chiasm – during digit flexion, the two slips of FDS move forward toward the midline to compress the FDP, like a bat's tendon-locking mechanism]

▧ Although adhesion is more likely to form in zone-2 injuries, the modern trend is to repair both FDS and FDP in such injuries

3.3.1.9 Physical Assessment

▧ Resting posture sometimes typical, even diagnostic

▧ Proximal end of cut flexor tendon can retract to variable extent proximally. When the flexor tendon is under tension while being cut, it can retract significantly sometimes even to the carpal tunnel

▧ Also, for the above reason, depending on the posture of the finger during the time of the laceration, there can be great discrepancy between the site of the wound and the site of the tendon being cut

3.3.1.10 Timing of Acute Repair
▧ Best time for repair is within few hours
▧ Next best time is after day 10 and before 2 weeks
▧ Some studies found the worst result during days 4–7 after injury

3.3.2   Chronic Flexor Injury: Selection Between Tendon Graft and Staged Reconstruction
▧ Indications of staged reconstruction:
  - Badly scarred bed, previous multiple procedure
    Stage 1: clear the scar, preserve/reconstruct pulleys, implant silicon rod and establish gliding. Stage 2: graft attachment
▧ Indications of tendon graft:
  - Mature wound, full passive ROM, minimal scar
  - Donor: palmaris longus, plantaris, etc.
  - Preserve pulleys, attachment at D/P via drill hole, or directly attach into stump. Proximal attachment using Pulvertuft technique. Final ROM expected at 6 months, assess need for tenolysis

3.3.2.1   Importance of Pulleys and Sources for Reconstruction
▧ Especially important if deficient A2 and A4 pulleys
▧ More with bare hand rock climbing
▧ Pulley's normal function → prevent bowstringing, the pulleys hold the flexors close to the phalanges; enhance the flexor's ability to translate excursion into angular motion across the IPJ
▧ Pulley reconstruction sources:
  - Native pulley
  - Palmer plate

3.3.2.2   Tenolysis Indications
▧ Adherent repaired tendon or tendon graft. In addition there is a requirement of:
  - Good passive ROM
  - Good skin and NV condition
  - Motivated patient

- Pearls:
  - Incision depends on previous surgery
  - Preserve pulley
  - Post-operative physiotherapy important
  - Compliance of patient is important

3.3.2.3 Risk Factors of Overall Outcome

- Pre-operative: injury mechanics, contamination, associated injuries, medical problems/diabetes mellitus (DM)
- Intra-operative: excess dissection, NV injury, technique of repair
- Post-operative: re-rupture, non-compliance, triggering, contractures, etc.

3.3.2.4 Complications of Repair of Flexor Tendons

- Infection
- Re-rupture
- Contracture
- Adhesion is the most common tendon healing complication (Cx)
  In addition, there is sometimes difficulty in differentiating restrictive adhesions from rupture – sometimes need MRI to tell

3.3.3   Extensor Tendon Injury

3.3.3.1 The Zones

- Easier to recall the zones if remember that: odd numbered zones are over the joints
- For the thumb: zone 1 is over IPJ, zone 3 over MCPJ, and zone 5 over CMCJ
- Like flexor tendon injuries, the skin wound may not correspond to injury zone

3.3.3.2 Relevant Anatomy

- Less excursion than the flexors, always avoid further shortening in repair
- Feature in anatomy – juncturae tendinum – inter-connected; injury at one portion can therefore affect entire function of digit
- Sagittal bands used to centralise the tendon over the MCPJ
- Lateral bands are tendinous confluence of the termination of lumbrical and interosseous muscle. [The lateral bands join the central ten-

don at the level of proximal phalanx (P/P), proceed down the digit and insert to the dorsum of D/P]
- The reader is assumed to know the different zones

3.3.3.3 General Comments
- Few studies on vascularity – (1) major = synovial diffusion and (2) muscle branches under the extensor retinaculum and distal to it
- Flat shape and varying thickness and contour – placement of sutures is determined more by anatomy than by its vascular supply
- All suture methods weaker then flexors; the Kleinert modification of the Bunnell technique is strongest, followed by Kessler; others include mattress, figure-of-8, etc.
- Because of the flat shape, there is marked propensity for them to bunch during tenorraphy; this shortening can restrict PIP/MCP motions, and result in more loss of flexion
- The ideal suture technique with maximum tensile strength and minimum shortening has not yet been devised
- It is important to note that it is the post-operative splinting or sometimes k-wire that may help prevent post-operative rupture
- Zone-8 cases – epimysial invagination should be performed without strangulation of muscles, which could cause further necrosis. Forearm fascia repair may prevent muscle herniation

3.3.3.4 Complex Injuries
- Bone grafts, flaps or skin grafts should preferably be done before extensor tendon reconstruction in complex injuries
- Tissue equilibrium and full mobility of joints achieved before tendon transfer and grafting
- Refer to the section on rheumatoid arthritis (RA) for treatment of rheumatoid related tendon ruptures

3.3.3.4.1 Zone 1
- Closed mallet – nonstop splint for 6–8 weeks (recognised alternative is trans-articular k-wire. Cx: breakage of wire, chondrolysis, sepsis, etc.). Open repair of extensor if failed closed splinting treatment
- Open mallet – open repair
- Closed mallet with fracture and/or DP subluxation – consider open if it involves 30–50% articular area or more. If less than 30% and no subluxation proceed with closed treatment

- Open mallet with fracture and/or DP subluxation; methods to fix fracture vary from *k*-wire, tension-band, screw, etc. Even with anatomic fixation, splinting or trans *k*-wire may still be needed
- Untreated natural Hx may sometimes develop swan-neck deformity, the reason being that if patient has lax ligaments, the combination of proximal migration of the extensor hood with increased extensor force at PIP and volar plate laxity causes the deformity
- Stiffness and osteoarthritis (OA) of DIPJ to start with – may need fusion
- Chronic mallet but at less than 3 months – closed treatment mostly
- Chronic mallet and swan neck – a more complex situation which needs oblique retinacular ligament reconstruction and superficialis tenodesis

3.3.3.4.2 Zone 2

- Commonly associated with bony fracture, late tenolysis, and capsulotomy may be needed
- Complete open lacerations just repair (if untreated also causes mallet)
- Partial cases especially if closed sometimes conservative, especially if no significant extensor lag and encourage early motion

3.3.3.4.3 Zone 3

- Central slip cut – volar displacement of lateral band – boutonniere deformity may ensue
  - Closed acute central slip – extension splint and trans-articular *k*-wire
  - Open repair – may protect with transarticular *k*-wire for 6 weeks
  - Associated fracture – options include fixation versus excision of fragment and reattachment central slip
  - Chronic rigid – splint it straight (dynamic or serial static), then reconstruct by scar excision, and reattach (ensure balance between lateral bands and the repaired central slip). Once balance was established between lateral bands and the repaired central slip, consider transarticular *k*-wire spanning the PIPJ, and mobilise the DIPJ and MCPJ. (More difficult are cases in which PIPJ cannot be splinted straight – initial volar release to restore passive extension, then central-slip reconstruction)

Salvage operations include: (1) reconstruction with free tendon graft and dorsal suture of lateral bands and (2) tenotomy of tendon at D/P to restore D/P motion, while accepting a resistant PIP contracture sometimes for ulna fingers in labourers

3.3.3.4.4 Zone 4
- Complete cut uncommon since bone is wider
- Look for associated fracture

3.3.3.4.5 Zone 5
- Two common problems encountered: (1) bite wounds – never close, debride, antibiotics, early motion/prevent septic arthritis and osteomyelitis and (2) closed rupture of sagittal band results in subluxation into the (ulna) gutter, mostly
- In sagittal band ruptures, may need repair of torn sagittal band, augmented with tendon graft

3.3.3.4.6 Zone 6
- Two portions – at level of junctura versus proximal to junctura tendini
- More proximal cases more likely to retract; those at level of junctura can be missed
- If associated skin loss, may need grafting; beware of adhesions

3.3.3.4.7 Zone 7
- Worst prognosis – can produce mass healing of tendons adhering to underlying joint capsule, and nearby retinaculum
- This can cause limitation of finger flexion with wrist flexion – disability
- Technique: (1) try to retain some retinaculum to prevent bowstring and (2) protect dorsal radial/ulna sensory nerves and repair them if injured

3.3.3.4.8 Zone 8
- Two portions – proximal near posterior interosseous (PIN) or distally at musculotendinous units
- Feature – small skin wound, but injury can be extensive
  - Central core sutures for musculotendinous unit repair

– PIN branches may need repair

Appendix: (1) prognosis is reasonable since close to the motor units – reinnervation and (2) if beyond repair, some surgeons consider even primary tendon transfer

3.3.4   Tendon Transfer Principles

3.3.4.1 What Is Tendon Transfer

▓ Procedure by which a tendon insertion is moved from one location to another

3.3.4.2 Definition of Related Procedures

▓ Tendon graft – tendon moved without muscle, from one location to another; used to prolong/bridge gap. Sometimes also used to replace ligaments

▓ Free muscle transfer – a muscle with tendon transected both proximal and distal to its normal location; moved to different location. The NV bundle divided and reattached to NV bundle at its new location, vascularity restored at time of operation. Also, muscle is reinnervated gradually as the axons regrow from recipient nerve to the nerve of transferred muscle

▓ Other reconstruction procedures – e.g. nerve repair/grafts; tenodesis, arthrodesis, etc.

3.3.4.3 Other Options to Be Considered before Proceeding with Transfer

▓ Neurorrhaphy

▓ Intercalary grafting

▓ Tenodesis, tendon lengthening and arthrodesis

(If the proposed tendon transfer is likely to give better result than the above options, then proceed)

3.3.4.4 Summary of Pearls for Tendon Transfer

▓ Consider Options available, and pros and cons of transfer

▓ Discussion with patient and relatives about proposed treatment and post-operative therapy; assess whether can follow rehabilitation

▓ Prepare hand for transfer, which involves: reduce oedema, reduce joint contractures, prepare good tendon bed; reconstruct soft tissue cover, prepare the path of proposed transfer

▓ Select tendon: based on pathology, our treatment goal, motors available (position, synergy)
▓ Good post-operative care

3.3.4.5 Indications of Transfer
▓ Substitute the function of a paralyzed or weakened muscles
▓ Replace a ruptured avulsed or aplastic tendon
▓ Correct muscle imbalance caused by central nervous system disorders

3.3.4.6 Important Principles
▓ Use expendable tendon as donor if possible
▓ Donor of sufficient strength (since decrease one grade in power after transfer)
▓ Consider the needed excursion (amplitude) – the amplitude is the amount a muscle can be stretched from its resting position, plus the amount it contracts – this will be the main determinant of ROM
▓ Preferable to have a straight line of pull to optimise working of the transfer – not always possible and some transfers need to go through pulley or interosseous membrane. Significant altered line of pull weakens the action in general
▓ Tension needs to be correct – this is a critical step in order to provide useful function, though minor adjustments can be made by the patient, for example, with wrist motion
▓ Joints must be supple – need good ROM and any contractures released
▓ Avoid a scarred bed; preferable to go through fatty subcutaneous tissue to decrease adhesions
▓ One transfer for one function – do not expect a transfer to carry out two functions simultaneously
▓ As far as possible, synergistic muscles should be used; muscles work in groups and patterns are controlled at a subconscious level, e.g. finger flexors tend to work at same time as wrist extensors; while finger extensors work with wrist flexors
  – Synergy is preferred rather than essential – the transfer is more easily integrated into normal hand use if a synergistic muscle is used. If not, the new function will be more difficult to incorporate and result in a longer period of rehabilitation

3.3.4.7 What Things to Tell Patient before Operation

- Reason to perform the transfer
- Never 'normal' and realistic expectations
- Pre- and post-operative rehabilitation important to relearn the control of this transferred motor

3.3.4.8 Timing of Tendon Transfer

- Never if oedema still present
- Never do in scarred/grafted bed; will need a flap first
- Sometimes need to insert silicon rod to create tunnel, e.g. at time of flap to ease later transfer
- Some surgeons suggest to wait until the hand sensate before transfer. However, experts such as Pulvertuft think this is not an absolute necessity because restoration of useful motion will render the affected numb hand to many a helpful assistive function

3.4   Carpal Instability

3.4.1   Definition of Carpal Instability

- Carpal injury in which a loss of normal alignment of the carpal bones develops early or late
- It represents a disturbance of the normal balance of the carpal joints caused by fracture or ligament damage

3.4.2   Incidence

- 10% of all carpal injuries resulted in instability
- 5% of non-fracture wrist injuries had scapholunate (SL) instability

3.4.3   General Comment

- All wrist dislocations/subluxations, etc. are examples of carpal instability
- Not all imply joint laxity – some are very stiff
- Not all unstable wrists are painful

3.4.4   Kinematics of the Proximal Carpal Row

- In moving from radial to ulnar deviation, the whole proximal row moves from flexion to extension.

3.4.5   Carpal Instability – Pathomechanics

- The proximal row of the carpus is an intercalated segment with no muscle attachments
- Its stability depends on the capsular and interosseous ligaments
  - According to Gilford, a link joint, as between proximal and distal carpal rows, should be stable in compression and will crumple in compression unless prevented by a stop mechanism
  - The scaphoid may act as a stop mechanism

3.4.6   Aetiology

- Traumatic
- Inflammatory
- Congenital

3.4.7   Traumatic Aetiology

Fall on outstretched extended wrist

- If thenar first → supination → dorsal intercalated segment instability (DISI)
- If hypothenar first → pronation → volar intercalated segment instability (VISI)

3.4.8   Symptomatology

- Pain
- Weakness
- Giving way
- Clunk/snap/click during use

3.4.9   Carpal Instability – Classifications

Dobyns

- DISI
- VISI
- Ulnar translocation (rheumatoid)
- Dorsal subluxation (after fracture radius)

3.4.10 Carpal Instability – Classifications

Taleisnik: concepts of

- Dynamic instability – partial ligament injuries with pain but minimal X-ray change

- Static instability – end state; SL dissociation, fixed flexion of scaphoid, fixed extension of lunate

3.4.11 Other Carpal Instability Classification
- Carpal instability dissociative (CID) – interosseous ligament damage
- Carpal instability non-dissociative (CIND) – capsular ligament damage
- Carpal instability complex (CIC) – CID + CIND
- Carpal instability adaptive (CIA) – adaption to extracarpal cause

3.4.12 Carpal Instability – Common Clinical Scenarios
- Perilunate dislocation
- SL dissociation and lunotriquetral (LT) dissociation
- Unstable scaphoid non-union
- Extrinsic radiocarpal ligament insufficiency (inflammatory/traumatic/congenital)
- Distal radial malunion

3.4.12.1 Lunate and Perilunate Dislocations
- Lunate dislocation (Fig. 3.8) less common since bound by the stronger palmer capsular ligament
- Presence of chondral and osteochondral injury not uncommon and may not be seen on X-ray

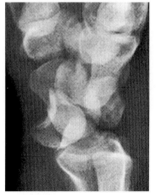

Fig. 3.8. Lunate dislocation of the right wrist, best seen in the lateral view. Notice the concomitant fracture of the distal radius, and look clinically for any median nerve palsy

3.4.12.1.1   Anatomy of Palmer Side Ligaments

▤ Two inverted 'V' structural constructs

- Centred on capitate = radioscaphocapitate (RSC) and ulnocapitate
- Centred on lunate = long and short radiolunate (RL) and lunolunate
  Note: (1) space of Poirier: weak point between capitate and lunate, through which Lunate dislocation occurs and (2) radioscapholunate ('RSL') – only a vestigial embryonic structure, though initially thought that this ligament of Testut was a key stabiliser

3.4.12.1.2   Dorsal Side Ligaments

▤ One inverted 'V' structure, centred on the triquetrum

- Intercarpal dorsal ligament
- Radiocarpal dorsal ligament

3.4.12.1.3   Mayfield Stages (Based on Cadavers)

▤ Based on wrist hyperextension and varying degrees of ulna deviation (UD) (and forearm supination)

▤ Postulate failure from the radial side/scapholunate interosseous ligament (SLIL) first

▤ Four stages – SLIL torn, followed by a sequence of ligament around the lunate in an ulna direction, with fracture of the carpal bone

▤ SLIL – c-shaped, intracapsular ligament, very important ligament of the wrist; controls the rotation of the scaphoid and the lunate without allowing gapping or translation between the two bones (the dorsal portion is the stronger part)

3.4.12.1.4   Mayfield Classes

▤ Stage 1: SLIL tear with DISI

- Class a. partial – positive scope
- Class b. partial – positive stress X-ray
- Class c. complete – gap seen and ↑ SL angle
- Class d. complete – complete and degenerative changes

▤ Stages 2–4: carpal dislocation with or without fracture

▤ Ulna, midcarpal or VISI patterns

▤ Vertical shear injury of the carpus

3.4.12.1.5   Investigation
- Plain X-ray
- Cineradiography
- Stress radiography
- Arthrography
- Arthroscopy

3.4.12.1.6   X-ray Interpretations
- Do not make final comments on AP X-ray alone
- Lateral important to ddx lunate vs perilunate dislocations
- Perilunate cases, look for fracture scaphoid or radial styloid/fracture capitate/ fracture triquetrum/fracture ulna styloid
- After reduction – still look for Gilula arc, carpal collapse and proximal migration of capitate through the SL interval

3.4.12.1.7   Treatment Principles
- Urgent reduction
- Most will need operation because 60% of cases with loss of reduction after initial reduction and casting is found in previous studies
- 65% of cases with open surgery give good results; most cases with no surgery give bad results. In summary, too unstable to be left unfixed

3.4.12.1.8   CR and OR
- Extending the wrist to recreate the deformity and apply dorsal pressure to reduce capitate into lunate fossa
- OR and repair of the SLIL and LT ligament is indicated in all perilunate and lunate dislocations

3.4.12.1.9   CR in Lunate Dislocations
- Flex wrist to remove tension from the palmer ligament
- Next, apply palmer pressure over lunate followed by wrist extension to reduce lunate to its fossa
- Flex the wrist to reduce the capitate to the lunate

3.4.12.1.10 Technical Tip
- A dorsal longitudinal incision, release 3rd extensor compartment and release EPL, elevate 4th compartment, longitudinal capsulotomy – exposes SLIL and LTIL and to reduce the scaphoid to the lunate and lunate to triquetrum

- Repair ligament avulsions with suture anchors, proceed with intra-operative X-ray to recheck alignment and place wire at scaphoid as joystick
- Additionally, need *k*-wires to pin scaphoid to lunate, pin triquetrum to lunate – but avoid pin from carpus to radius
- A separate palmer approach especially in lunate dislocations volarly and/or release median nerve
- Treatment of lunate dislocations similar to perilunate
- Whichever type, fix associated fracture, e.g. of styloid and scaphoid, etc.

3.4.12.1.11 Delayed Cases
- Long-term pain, weakness, stiffness, OA, CTS, attritional flexor injury
- Operation is still advised regardless of time lapse – but nature of operation options differ: open reduction, lunate excision, proximal row carpectomy (PRC), wrist fusion, etc. only proper reduction offers the greatest potential to normal wrist mechanics (PRC is a reasonable way to go if reduction cannot be achieved, provided head of capitate is not significantly injured – which alas may require fusion if the head of the capitate is abnormal)

3.4.12.1.12 Principle of Treating Chronic Injury
- Reducible: ligamentous repair
- Fixed – intercarpal fusion (also in athletes/manual workers)

3.4.12.1.13 Options in Late Static Chronic Instability
- Capsulodesis (may stretch out with time)
- Local fusion – adjacent OA
- Total fusion
- Proximal row carpectomy (salvage in SLAC wrist with old non-union)

3.4.12.1.14 Overall Management Depends on:
- Time of presentation
- Degree of pathology
- Associated carpal injuries

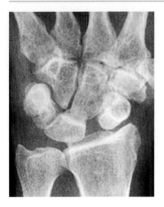

Fig. 3.9. A patient with scapholunate dissociation

3.4.12.2   SL Instability (Fig. 3.9)

3.4.12.2.1   Biomechanics of SL Instability
- Relative normal load distribution ratio of scaphoid:lunate is 60%:40%
- SL dissociation preferentially loads the scaphoid and unloads the lunate: scaphoid:lunate = 80%:20%
- SLAC – natural Hx – left untreated, DISI will progress to degenerative changes; however, timeline is still unclear

3.4.12.2.2   Pattern of Degenerative Changes
- Tip of radial styloid and scaphoid
- Remainder of scaphoid and scaphoid fossa
- Capitate/lunate joint

3.4.12.2.3   Anatomic Aspect
- Dorsal part stronger than ventral part (middle part membranous)
- Mayfield article on perilunate instability:
  - Stage 1: SL injury
  - Stage 2: SL and RSC affected
  - Stage 3: Above + LT ligament injury
  - Stage 4: Above + dorsal radiocapitate – palmer lunate dislocate

3.4.12.2.4   Clinical Exam
- Pain, snapping, weakness
- Pain at dorsal aspect of scapholunate joint, positive Scaphoid stress test

3.4.12.2.5   Radiological Assessment

- Terry Thomas sign
- DISI pattern
- Earliest cases may need arthroscopy to Dx
- Early cases may show up on stress X-ray
- Arthrogram: not all positive ones have symptomatic instabilities. Less used nowadays
- MRI – not yet very ideal
  (Arthroscopy is becoming the gold standard, but not needed if X-ray is diagnostic; however, it can offer a direct view and staging of chondral damage/wear)

3.4.12.2.6   Treatment Options

- Observe (in mildest of cases, one cadaver study claimed an incidence of 28%, i.e. many asymptomatic)
- Arthroscopic debridement – remember not all tears are part of a carpal instability (e.g. strong portion can be intact)
- Arthroscopic reduction and pinning – better if done in acute phase
- Blatt dorsal capsulodesis
- Tenodesis (by FCR)
- Limited carpal fusion – STT/SC fusions
- OR and repair ligament – still debated
- Bone-ligament-bone – no long-term result; many donors have been reported

3.4.12.3   LT Instability

3.4.12.3.1   Clinical Features

- Thought of as "reverse perilunate injury" pattern
- Pathomechanics – fall on a palmarflexed wrist
- VISI can develop
- No clear pattern of degeneration changes like the slack wrist counterpart

3.4.12.3.2   Goal of Treatment

- Less pain
- More strength
- Prevent static VISI

3.4.12.3.3   Anatomy of LT Ligament

- C-shaped like SL ligament
- Unlike SL, the dorsal part is thin and palmer is thick (just the opposite)
- Middle; membranous, consists of fibrocartilage and not true ligament

3.4.12.3.4   Physical Examination

- LT articulation tender
- Click on radial and UD
- Less grip strength
- Tests include:
  - LT allotment test – thumb and finger of one hand grasp pisotriquetral complex and use the other hand's thumb and finger to grasp the lunate – estimate AP translation of triquetrum relative to lunate
  - LT shear test – one thumb at dorsal lunate and the other thumb on palmer surface of pisiform – then RD/UD check for click
  - LT compression test – apply converging load to scaphoid and triquetrum, with pain in LT area

3.4.12.3.5   Radiological Assessment

- Look for VISI
- Assess Gilula arcs
- Check ulna variance
- Arthrogram – sometimes false and from ulna impaction
- Tc bone scan – non-specific
- MRI – not too easy to see the lesion
- Arthroscopy – new gold standard; refer to the different Geissler stages

3.4.12.3.6   Treatment Options

- Arthrodesis – not advised
- Ligament reconstruction – technique demanding
- Direct repair – reattach and k-wires
- Percutaneous k-wires
- Isolate injury can try conservative
- Goal – realign lunocapitate axis and establish LT stability

3.4.12.4   Ulna Translocation (of the Carpus)

3.4.12.4.1   Aetiology, Diagnosis and Treatment

▨ (1) RA – common, (2) from trauma – very rare

▨ Need global laxity (probably including RSC and long RL) to occur

▨ X-ray: assess – by degree of overhang by Gilula method (grip and stress view)

▨ Treatment:
  – Acute – ligament repair and fix
  – Chronic – Chamay procedure (radiolunate fusion) in RA cases. RSL fusion if the radioscaphoid joint is osteoarthritic.

3.4.12.5   Axial Instabilities

3.4.12.5.1   Types

▨ Radial column stays behind, ulna side displaced

▨ Ulna portion stays behind, radial side displaced

▨ Very rare

3.4.12.5.2   Clinical Feature

▨ Uncommon

▨ Most are crush injuries, e.g. printing presses of industrial type

▨ Cxs – skin, tendon, soft tissue loss, associated carpal fracture

▨ Treatment: open reduction and internal fixation (ORIF) with *k*-wires

▨ Stiffness common and less than 50% show a good result

3.5   Injuries and Instability of the Distal Radioulna Joint

3.5.1   Introduction

▨ The term triangular fibrocartilage complex (TFCC) was coined by Palmer in 1987

▨ Function – cushion, gliding, helps connect ulna axis to volar carpus

▨ Normally 80% load is carried at distal radius; can change a lot with differing ulna variance

3.5.2   Evolution

▨ One of the three most important advances after assumption of the bipedal gait

- The other two are higher brain centres and prehensile function
- Forearm rotation allows one to better manipulate the environment, handle tools and help in defence (after Lindshield)

3.5.3   Anatomy

- The reader is referred to the works of Palmer concerning load transmission across the wrist
- Correlation of the shape of the distal radioulna joint (DRUJ) articulation with the ulna variance
- Element of incongruity from differences in radii of curvatures of the two surfaces of the DRUJ – to allow not only rotation but translation with pronation or supination motions – the tradeoff is less stability

3.5.4   Primary and Secondary Stabilisers

- Primary stabilisers: especially the dorsal and palmer radioulnar ligament – they insert not only at ulna styloid, but also fovea of the ulna head (they are the dorsal and volar extents of the TFCC)
  (Implication – their avulsion from the ulna fovea may occur without ulna styloid fracture. However, basal ulna styloid fracture is suggestive of injury to these stabilisers; check DRUJ instability)
- Secondary stabilisers – ulno-carpal ligaments, sheath of the ECU, (articular disc)

3.5.5   Classes of TFCC Injury by Palmer

- Traumatic
- Degenerative

3.5.5.1 Natural Hx

- 50–70% of this structure damaged with age, according to cadaveric wrists studies

3.5.5.2 Common Clinical Scenarios

- TFCC/DRUJ instability – think of possible TFCC injury
- Patients with significant positive or negative ulna variance may predispose to TFCC injury
- One of the DDxs of ulna wrist pain – 'low back pain' of the wrist

3.5.5.3   Physical Assessment
- Area of tenderness at TFCC
- Test ROM of DRUJ and any subluxation
- Stress test
- Degree and direction of laxity
- ECU checked

3.5.5.4   Radiological Assessment
- Ulna variance and any ulna impingement – always check the elbow – can be cause of radial shortening
- Normality of form and tilting of distal radius
- Congruency of the sigmoid notch
- Subluxation/dislocate of distal ulna best seen in true lateral X-ray of the wrist
- Carpal height ratio and Gilula lines
- Look for degenerative changes

3.5.5.5   Role of Arthrogram versus Scope versus MRI/CT
- Arthrogram still has a role in judging the direction of dye leakage – but caution, the pores may fill up with fibrous tissue with time – less accurate for delayed cases
- Arthroscope – good to see lesions sometimes less well seen by MRI, such as in cartilage, and can probe joint and test for TFCC tension, can be therapeutic at the same time
- CT – good to assess congruency of the sigmoid notch and cases with bony deformity
- MRI – can assess soft tissue, non-invasive, but less good for cartilage

3.5.5.5.1 Scenario 1: Acute TFCC Injury and DRUJ Unstable
- If fractured, fix ulna styloid, and retest stability of DRUJ
- Try either (1) conservative (POP in supination) or (2) scope/open repair

3.5.5.5.2 Scenario 2: TFC isolated tear with Stable DRUJ
- Central lesion – debridement
- Peripheral lesion – repair (blood supply is from peripheral just like menisci)

3.5.5.5.3 Scenario 3: Ulna Styloid Fracture
- Need to treat any nonunion or malunion

3.5.5.5.4 Scenario 4: Chronic TFCC Injury
- Some study showed that one can still intervene with reasonable results up to 3–4 months
- DRUJ can be made unstable due to malunited distal radius. These cases may need osteotomy, especially if the distal radius is shortened with ulna impaction. In these situations, can consider a joint levelling procedure, which frequently involves osteotomy of the distal radius
- If Sigmoid notch area is degenerated, may need to salvage, e.g. Sauve-Kapanji

3.5.6   Example of DRUJ Reconstruction [Linshield Procedure]
- Use half of FCU as a sling
- Make in a strip
- Sling ulna head back

3.5.7   Examples of Procedures to Tackle Length Discrepancies
- Ulna alone – shortening, wafer operation, and Sauve-Kapanji
- Radius alone – osteotomy
- Both – rarely mentioned in the literature

3.5.8   Role of Joint Levelling
- Reconstruction procedure alone in the presence of significant length differences (between distal radius and ulna) with no joint levelling may not work
- Restoration of joint congruency is important

3.5.9   In the Setting of Distal Radius Injury
- Checking for clinical DRUJ instability is most important, since relying on X-ray assessment of ulna styloid is not good enough

3.5.9.1 Category I: Acute Situations
- Associated fractured distal radius: assessing integrity of the sigmoid notch, good restoration of radial shortening and prevention of the dorsal tilt are all very important. Hence, first ensure the adequate anatomical restoration of distal radius anatomy, then check DRUJ insta-

bility; if fracture base of styloid is found, fix it and recheck DRUJ instability even if there is no associated ulna styloid fracture

3.5.9.2 Management of Acute Instability
▓ Repair of TFCC (if subacute, avoid scope since may need open debridement of the granulation tissue)
▓ If still unstable, repair the secondary stabilisers
▓ If irreparable – extrinsic methods, like tenodesis

3.5.9.3 Category II: Chronic Instability
▓ Key: check whether there is OA
 – No OA: reconstruct the soft tissue – intrinsic versus extrinsic methods — extrinsic runs the risk of being not anatomical and more of a ROM limitation
 – With OA: severe; needs salvage (Sauve-Kapanji). Darrach tries to retain some ulna soft tissue; excision arthroplasty alone risks further de-stabilisation; Cooney suggests some role of DRUJ arthroplasty

3.6   Scaphoid Injuries

3.6.1   Features Peculiar to Scaphoid
▓ Most of its surface is intra-articular
▓ Tenous blood supply, main one from the dorsal ridge
▓ Twisted peanut shape, fracture can sometimes be visualised only by seeing multiple X-ray views

3.6.2   Scaphoid Fracture – Definition of 'Displaced' Fracture
▓ Definition of 'displaced'/unstable fracture → fracture gap more than 1 mm on any X-ray projection
▓ Extra evidence may be provided by: SL angle greater than 60°, RL angle greater than 15°; also intrascaphoid angle greater than 35°

3.6.3   Presentation of Acute Fracture
▓ Acute fracture – tender can be at anatomic snuffbox or distal tubercle
▓ Mostly after a wrist dorsiflexion injury

▨ Some cases are missed Dx, or else no fracture can be seen on initial X-ray or there is delayed presentation because the patient cannot recall any injury

3.6.4   Radiological Assessment
▨ X-ray:
  - Posteroanterior (PA) – distorted by flexion and normal curvature of the scaphoid
  - PA in UD better but does not completely solve the above
  - 45° pronated PA
  - Lateral – can see waist fracture better
  - Others – the distal third is best seen on semi-pronated oblique view; the dorsal ridge best seen on semisupinated oblique

3.6.5   Other Investigations
▨ CT – in the plane of the scaphoid, especially 1-mm cut; good for checking whether there is fracture; whether fracture is displaced; and in pre-operative assessment, for say malunion, etc., to check the intrascaphoid angle
▨ MRI – good to identify fracture, even within 48 h; Dx of occult fracture; and help check vascularity. Expensive

3.6.6   Different Clinical Scenarios
▨ Undisplaced fracture
▨ Looks like 'undisplaced' fracture – but in fact is displaced
▨ Displaced fracture – definition and implications
▨ Delayed presentation cases (over 4 weeks)
▨ Scaphoid non-union with advanced carpal collapse (SNAC) wrist
▨ Avascular necrosis (AVN) of scaphoid
▨ Unsure of Dx – what to do
▨ Malunited fracture

3.6.6.1 Really Undisplaced Fracture
▨ Refer to definition of undisplaced
▨ Treatment – many studies indicate only 4–5% nonunion even with simple casting
▨ Methods of casting – long versus short arm reported in literature with no statistical difference, some experts like Barton had suggested can

do away with thumb spica part – however, most surgeons still use the traditional teaching of Bohler, i.e. immobilise the thumb as well during casting

▣ Duration of casting – proximal pole needs too prolonged casting and chance of AVN/nonunion high (90%) that many choose primary (open or percutaneous) fixation via dorsal approach

▣ For the common mid-third waist fracture, there is a recent trend towards percutaneous screw fixation. There is as yet no long-term result but should be appealing for patients who have to return to their work early (sometimes for financial reasons) or are involved in competitive sports, such as athletes

3.6.6.2 Percutaneous Cannulated Screw Fixation

▣ Advantages:
  – Earlier return to work
  – No need for prolonged immobilisation
▣ Disadvantages:
  – Not yet very sure whether nonunion rate lower, no long-term study
  – Cx such as sepsis and trapezial erosion have been reported
  – Some recent arthroscopic studies show that passage of screw may cause fracture site distraction
  – Technically demanding

3.6.6.3 Labelled 'Undisplaced' Fracture
but in Fact Fracture Is Displaced

▣ Fracture displacement not easy to detect if hand casted
▣ Fracture displacement can be subtle and sometimes seen only in CT
▣ This difference is important since nonunion rate increases from 5% to 50% with fracture displacement
▣ Ease of fracture displacement also depends on fracture configuration, e.g. more likely with vertical oblique orientation

3.6.6.4 Acute Displaced Fracture

▣ Most use ORIF or percutaneous cannulated screw fixation if reducible
▣ Any suspicion intra-operatively of avascularity can check for punctate bleeding during open reduction (especially for cases with somewhat delayed presentation)

■ Screw used mostly of differential threads; most use headless screws, and screw head if present needs be countersunk. Placement of screw in the central third is essential

3.6.6.5 Summary of Operative Indications for Acute Scaphoid Fracture

■ Displaced fracture
■ Proximal pole fracture
■ Delayed cases (especially over 4 months)
■ Perilunate dislocation with scaphoid fracture
■ Concomitant scaphoid fracture and fractured distal radius
■ Possible advantage of fixing acute undisplaced fracture has been mentioned

3.6.6.6 Delayed Presentation (Fig. 3.10)

■ Operate
■ Vascularised bone graft sometimes needed if avasculasrity sets in
■ Mostly volar approach, but dorsal for proximal pole fracture (since not much more to loose with respect to vascularity). Preserve RSC during volar approach in open reduction

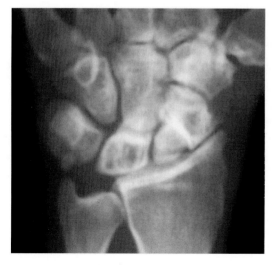

Fig. 3.10. X-ray of a patient with previously fractured scaphoid, the joint space of the radio-scaphoid joint is narrowed

3.6.6.7 Assessment of any AVN

- Increased radiological density not always indicative of avascularity of the proximal fragment (two factors new bone forming proximal fragment and porosis because of increased vascularity of distal fragment; these are only tentative explanations)
- Gelberman favours intra-operative punctate bleeding as most reliable method to assess any AVN
- Recently, there has been a trend to adopt the use of Gadolinium MRI to determine any avascularity

3.6.6.8 SNAC Wrist

- Pattern of arthrosis similar to SLAC wrist. Natural Hx of scaphoid nonunion is that given time degenerative arthritis will set in although sometimes the time lapse can be as long as 10 years
- Operative method used depend on stage of disease
- Early nonunion cases especially if no avascularity. Screw fixation may need wedge graft to correct humpback
- Late nonunion cases probably select among options like limited carpal fusion, PRC, even wrist fusion

3.6.6.9 Unsure of Diagnosis

- For most cases, cast for 2–4 weeks and then repeat X-ray (out of cast)
- Some propose a CT if still not sure by then

3.6.6.10 Malunited Fracture

- If untreated, also influence carpal biomechanics
- Clinically, there is loss of extension
- Treatment – operative, frequently need wedge graft to correct humpback and screw fixation
- Malunion rather uncommon

3.7   Compression Neuropathy and Peripheral Nerve Injuries

3.7.1   Compressive Neuropathy

3.7.1.1   Pathophysiology
- Mild – ionic block (recovers in hours)
- Moderate – myelin back-flow/ myelin intussusception (usually recovers in 3 months or less)
- Severe – axonotmesis (with Waller degeneration) takes longer to recover. Recovery related to distance between site of injury and motor end organs

3.7.1.2   More on Pathophysiology
- The more central fibres spared until late in compression process
- Proximal fusiform swelling of the nerve
- The only case of neurotemesis is that associated with fractures

3.7.1.3   Other Possible Contributing Factors Besides Compression
- Traction
- Excursion
- Tethering
- Scarring
- Ischaemia
  (Do not forget the 'Double Crush' syndrome)

3.7.1.4   Physical Assessment
- Sensory symptoms are sometimes not well localised and can be confusing
- Use provocative test to reproduce clinical symptoms if possible
- Accurate motor testing
- Refer to the indications for nerve conduction testing (NCT)

3.7.1.5   Prognosis
- Age – for elderly, prognosis is worse
- Chronicity
- Completeness of paresis – less likely to recover if paresis is complete and chronic, such as more than 1.5–2 years

▦ Underlying pathology
▦ If there is associated dissociated loss of motor or sensory function, prognosis is sometimes better

3.7.1.6 Median Nerve

3.7.1.6.1 Carpal Tunnel Syndrome
▦ Symptom – numbness, but can be nonspecific
▦ Nocturnal symptom
▦ Reduced motor control of thumb [only hand muscle control by median – 'LOAF': radial two lumbricals, opponens pollicis, abductor pollicis brevis (APB), flexor pollicis brevis (FPB)]
▦ Precipitating factors – pregnancy, thyroid disorder, ↑ anatomic contents (fractured carpus, fractured hamate hook, lipoma, abnormal muscle, median artery, synovitis/RA)
▦ Association – perhaps Dupuytren
▦ Beware of acute CTS secondary to trauma and fracture dislocation
▦ DDx – cervical cause, thoracic outlet syndrome, peripheral neuropathy

3.7.1.6.2 Boundaries of Carpal Tunnel
▦ Floor – carpus
▦ Roof – transverse retinaculum
▦ Radial border – scaphoid tubercle and trapezium
▦ Ulna border – hook of hamate and pisiform
▦ Contents: nine flexor tendons (the FDS of 3rd/4th fingers more superficial) and median nerve

3.7.1.6.3 Diagnosis
▦ Clinical:
  – Phalen
  – (Reversed phalen) – 60% sensitive, 85% specific, numbness in 60 seconds
  – Tinel – 75% sensitive, 90% specific
  – Gelberman median nerve compression test – elbow extend, forearm supinate, wrist flex $60°$, then press on the nerve
▦ Investigation
▦ Exact role of NCT:
▦ Not needed if Dx certain

▦ Needed (1) when Dx equivocal, but some false-negative (10%) (reason – even when a few normally conducting axons remain, can cause normal result), (2) if normal and suspect disease; can repeat later (there is always a small group with negative NCT but who respond very well to decompression); sensory is affected before motor on NCT

3.7.1.6.4 Operative Options
▦ Open release
- Avoid palmer cutaneous nerve – median nerve can be directly inspected, some release tourniquet to check revascularisation
- Some do external neurolysis if pallor of nerve remains. Internal neurolysis felt by many surgeons to cause further damage
- If dissociate symptom with more motor than sensory – explore the recurrent motor branch
- Beware of the anatomical variations of the recurrent thenar and palmer cutaneous nerves
- Full power does not return until 8 weeks
- Side effects: scar, pillar pain, neuroma of palmer branch, tendon adhesions, tendon bowstringing
▦ Arthroscopic
- Advantages: less scarring and pillar pain
- Disadvantages: occasionally serious Cxs, e.g. nerve damage, vascular injuries, learning curve, and it is costly

3.7.1.7   Pronator Teres Syndrome

3.7.1.7.1 Introduction
▦ Symptom: fatique of forearm after heavy use; on/off paresthesia
▦ Signs: (1) test pronator – resisted pronation of forearm with elbow extended, (2) test lacertus fibrosis – resisted elbow flexion and supination; and (3) test for the FDS arch – resisted flexion of PIPJ M/F (Tinel is non-specific)
▦ Investigation: use EMG but not NCT
▦ Aetiology: pronator teres (PT)/FDS arch/lacertus fibrsis ligament of Struthers (and underlying pathology such as fracture dislocation of elbow, repeated elbow trauma and abnormal anatomy of the pronator muscle)

3.7.1.7.2 Treatment
▪ Conservative: avoid repeated elbow movements, splint in flexion/pronation
▪ Operative – decompress

3.7.1.8 Anterior Interosseous Palsy
▪ Anterior interosseous supplies: FPL, radial FDP, PQ (pure motor)
▪ Symptom: vague forearm pain, 'less dextrous'
▪ Signs: cannot make an 'o', make a rectangle instead (reason: lost FPL action and FDP I/F actions), and weaker pronation with extended elbow (mostly with negative tinel)
▪ NCT not advised
▪ (1) Conservative, (2) operation – usually compression is by deep head of PT (humeral part of PT)

3.7.1.9 Ulna Nerve

3.7.1.9.1 Cubital Tunnel Syndrome (Fig. 3.11)
▪ Symptom: numbness ulna two fingers; dull ache forearm
▪ Signs: Froment's sign, Wartenberg sign (i.e. weakness of abduction of L/F), degree of ulna claw (less/none if weakened FDP and intrinsics), Tinel behind elbow, numbness, sometimes wasting of ulna forearm border
▪ NCT/EMG – more useful in general for ulna nerve since sometimes there can be more than one site of compression
▪ Location of compression:
  – At the elbow – valgus, spurs, tumours
  – At arcade of Struthers 8 cm proximally
  – At FCU distally (hypertrophied)

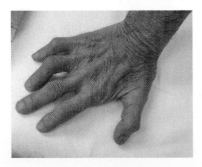

Fig. 3.11. Right ulna nerve palsy

▪ DDx: cervical causes, thoracic outlet, spinal cord pathology, pancoast tumour, (local peripheral neuropathy, motor neurone disease, etc.)
▪ Treatment:
  – Conservative: avoid elbow hyperflexion, extension block night splint,
  – Operative: some experts for nerve transposition, some are for decompression alone
▪ Cxs: scar, neuroma, regional pain syndrome, nerve dislocation, inadequate decompression, vascular supply affected
▪ Recovery: sensory symptoms improve better; can occur as late as after 3–5 years

3.7.1.9.2 Gyon Canal Boundaries
▪ Floor – transverse carpal ligament
▪ Roof – volar carpal ligament
▪ Radial side – hook of hamate
▪ Ulna side – pisiform
  Contents: ulna nerve and artery

3.7.1.9.3 Physical Assessment
▪ Sensation of ulna side of hand dorsum spared
▪ More severe ulna claw in distal ulna nerve lesions (ulna paradox)
▪ Others: numbness, tinel, swelling
  Investigation: NCT → delayed motor latency from wrist to 1st dorsal interosseous

3.7.1.9.4 DDx and Treatment
▪ Causes: any space-occupying lesion (SOL), fractured hamate, ulna artery thrombosis (by prolonged hammering), trauma and/or pisiform instability, pisotriquetral OA
▪ Treatment:
  – Conservative
    Splint
    Avoid trauma
  – Operative: decompression of motor/sensory branches and/or excision of pisiform/hamate hook

3.7.1.10   Radial Nerve

3.7.1.10.1   PIN Palsy

▪ Symptom: hand weakness and noted 'dropped fingers' – fingers in fact can still extend to some extent. Due to the intact intrinsics (interossei)
▪ Signs:
  – Can be wound in forearm
  – Drop fingers
  – Not frank drop wrist, – still intact BR/ECRL – but wrist deviates more to the radial side
▪ Pure motor loss

3.7.1.10.2   DDx of Causes

▪ Fibrous (arch) of the supinator
▪ Recurrent leash (Henry)
▪ Arcade of Frohse
▪ Carpi/brevis (ECRB)
▪ Supinator distal border

3.7.1.10.3   Investigation and Treatment

▪ Investigation: NCT – slowing across arcade of Frohse, EMG with evidence of denervation
▪ Treatment:
  – Conservative – 8–12 weeks if no masses
  – Operative – decompress

3.7.1.10.4   Radial Tunnel Syndrome

▪ Definition: a condition featured by minor compression of PIN without paresis
▪ Cause: PIN syndrome usually with no mass lesion
▪ C/Fs: ache in extensor muscle mass – more at end of day; tender 5 cm distal to lateral epicondyle
▪ Special test: M/F test (firm pressure applied by the examiner to the dorsum of P/P of the M/F) – reason: due to ECRB inserting into base of third MC. (The test is positive if it produces pain at edge of ECRB in the proximal forearm)
▪ DDx – tennis elbow

- Investigation:
  - NCT – more latency in active forced supination > (and/or injection test into the radial tunnel)
- Treatment:
  - Conservative
  - Operative: decompression, at the plane between ECRB/EDC interval, PIN found just proximal to arcade of Frohse

3.7.1.11   Wartenberg Syndrome
- Isolated neuritis of sensory branch of radial nerve
- Treatment: local steroid injection and/or release

3.7.1.12   Other Entrapments
3.7.1.12.1   Spinal Accessory Nerve
- Location: posterior triangle of neck
- Supply: sternomastoid, (superior) trapezius
- Aetiology: wound, after lymph node biopsy, radical neck
- P/E: shoulder girdle weakness (only abduct to 90°) → wasting trapezius, scapula rotates laterally and distally (flaring tends to disappear when arm is abducted, unlike long thoracic palsy)
- Treatment: primary/delay suture and/or nerve graft

3.7.1.12.2   Suprascapular Nerve
- Supplies: supraspinatus, infraspinatus
- Anatomy: upper plexus – post-neck – below transverse scapular ligament
- P/E: pain and weakness, wasted infraspinatus and/or supraspinatus
- Aetiology: trauma, cancer, fractured scapula, entrapment, SOL
- Investigation: EMG
- Treatment: no conclusive result of efficiency of direct repair
- Salvage: can transfer Teres Major, (Latisimus Dorsi)

3.7.1.12.3   Long Thoracic Nerve
- Supplies: serratus muscle (C567)
- P/E: winged scapula (cannot fully flex and abduct shoulder)
- Aetiology: trauma, traction (as when head forced acutely away from shoulder)

▨ Treatment: if stretched, conservative; if cut and paralysis, will need reconstruction

▨ Salvage: (1) pectoralis minor to distal scapula and (2) teres major transfer from humerus → Rib (5/6)

3.7.1.12.4   Axillary Nerve

▨ Supplies: deltoid and teres minor and sensation to regimen badge region

▨ Anatomy: from posterior cord, winds around at the quadrilateral space

▨ P/E: deltoid wasting/look at contraction (pitfall: but full abduction can sometimes be possible due to action of supraspinatus action and scapula rotation)

▨ Aetiology: fracture or fracture dislocation, etc.

▨ Treatment: closed cases, observe for 3–12 months (not many published results of nerve suturing)

3.7.1.12.5   Musculocutaneous Nerve

▨ Supplies: biceps, coracobrachialis, half brachialis, (exit as lateral cutaneous nerve of forearm)

▨ Anatomy: lateral cord plexus, (pierces coraco – brachialis)

▨ P/E: weaker elbow flexion (but partly compensates by BR) and/or sensory loss

▨ Aetiology: wound and/or shoulder dislocation

▨ Treatment: repair – good results

▨ Salvage: Steindler's flexorplasty, anterior transfer of triceps, transfer of pectoralis major and of pectoralis minor

3.7.2   Injuries of Upper Limb Peripheral Nerves

3.7.2.1   Radial Nerve Injury

3.7.2.1.1 General Features

▨ Causes of injury: fractured humeral shaft, cut wound, gunshot, pressure (Saturday night)

▨ Function: motor = triceps, supinator of forearm, extensors to wrist/fingers/thumb
Sensory = 1st web space of hand dorsally. Sometimes part of dorsum of radial three fingers)

- P/E:
  - Cut radial nerve – wrist-drop, check supinate forearm, cannot extend elbow
  - PIN – still able to supinate and extend wrist (with RD), since BR/ECRL intact
- Treatment:
  - Closed – observe, ± explore later
  - Open – explore and suture
- Results of suture: 90% good function to proximal muscle, 65% good function of all muscles (possible slightly less with extensors of finger/thumb). Never delay sutures more than 12–15 months
- Salvage – tendon transfer

3.7.2.1.2 Salvage of paralysis from Radial Nerve Injury

- Regain wrist extension → PT to ECRB
- Regain MCPJ extension → FCR (or FCU) to EDC, or FDS to EDC
- Regain thumb extension and abduction of thumb: PL to EPL
  (Note: try retain FCU which is important, as the wrist tends to work best in dorsiflexion and ulna palmarflexion)

3.7.2.2 Median Nerve Injury

3.7.2.2.1 General Features

- Causes: perilunate dislocation, fracture distal radius, open wounds
- P/E:
  - Low median: wasted thenar (APB sometimes FPB), numbness, and/or sometimes spare palmer cutaneous sensory distribution
  - High median: above, FPL + FDP (radial two fingers/Benediction sign)
- Treatment:
  - Closed observe
  - Open explore

3.7.2.2.2 Salvage of Paralysis from Median Nerve Injury

- Low median:
  (Notice thumb 'opposition'=a combinaton of flexion and adduction)
  - Restore thumb opposition, e.g. (i) Camitz operation, (ii) R/F FDS transfer to APB (via a pulley made in the FCU at level of pisiform)
  - Restore sensation → NV island graft from ulna side of R/F to thumb

- High median:
  - Restore flexion of I/F, M/F – side/side suture of their FDP to R/F and L/F (and/or strengthen by ECRL)
  - Restore IPJ thumb flexion – BR transfer to FPL
  - Restore thumb opposition – EIP more than APB, or Camitz
  - Restore sensation – same as low median lesion

3.7.2.3 Ulna Nerve Injury

3.7.2.3.1 General Features

- Cause: open cut wounds commonly
- P/E: Froment's sign (Wartenberg sign), weak abduct/adduct of fingers, hypothenar wasting, look at ulna border, clawing (beware ulna paradox) – hyperextension MCPJ flexed IPJ due to loss of function of interossei and lumbricals. High ulna nerve lesions do not spare dorsal sensation on ulna side of the hand and are less clawed
- Treatment:
  - Closed – splint, physiotherapy, observe – if not improve, then explore
  - Open – explore/ repair

3.7.2.3.2 Salvage of Paralysis from Ulna Nerve Injury

- Low ulna:
  - Tackle thumb opposition and adduction
    If FPB working and adductor not → EIP to adductor through interosseous membrane (but how do we know that FPB is working? – Jeannes sign and if there is thumb MCP hyper-extension on pinching; this means FPB is not working)
    If FPB is not working → R/F FDS to AP via pulley made at FCU tendon at level of pisiform
  - Lost interossei and ulna 2 lumbricals
    Tighten volar MCPJ capsule (Zancolli)
    Use tenodesis method: 'split tendon transfer of FDS and/or EIP to radial extensor apparatus'
- High ulna:
  As above and for lost FCU (can consider transfer ECRL)

3.7.2.4 Combined Median and Ulna Palsy

- With a low lesion one needs to face hand intrinsic problems (besides thumb):
    - Restore MCPJ flexion and IPJ extension: graft using ECRB/plantaris (to increase length) to intrinsics insertion
    - For thumb adduction: EIP to AP
    - For thumb opposition: FDS R/F to EPL (by pulley)
- High lesion:
    Thumb: consider arthrodesis, e.g. MCP
    Long flexor/intrinsics losses: ECRL–FDP; BR–FPL
    ECU (lengthened) – EPL; MCPJ volar capsulodesis

3.7.2.5 Digital Nerve Injury

- Most important digital nerves are: ulna digital nerve of thumb, radial digital nerve to 2nd, 3rd, 4th, and 5th fingers, and ulna digital nerve to 5th finger
- If both tendon and nerve are cut, repair tendon first (reason = avoid disruption of the delicate nerve repair) – use 8–9 0'nylon, epineurial repair/four sutures
- Post-operative splint ~ 2–3 weeks

3.8 Arthritis of the Hand

3.8.1 RA Hand Deformity

3.8.1.1 Presentations of RA

- Serositis – includes synovitis, tenosynovitis and bursitis
- Granulomas – vascular aetiology and fibrinoid necrosis, associated with more aggressive disease
- Vasculitis – PAN, Raynaud's, splinter haemorrhage, dry gangrene
- General body reaction

3.8.1.2 Stages of Synovitis

- Synovial reflection at joint margin
- Pannus invasion, loss of capsular and ligament support; periarticular porosis
- Fibrosis setting in
- Subluxation/dislocation versus ankylosis

3.8.1.3 Stages of Tenosynovitis
- Impaired nutrition
- Adhesion formation
- Ruptures from: ischaemia/bone spurs/direct invasion
  (In addition, tendon may enlarge from granuloma, sometimes triggering, entrapment, besides rupture)

3.8.1.4 Goal of Management
- Pain control
- Correct severe deformity
- Prevent early deformity
- Improve function/cosmesis
  (Note: always ensure adequate systemic control of the disease by physicians before surgery is contemplated)

3.8.1.5 Types of Operation
- Synovectomy/tenosynovectomy
- Soft tissue surgery (tendon surgery)
  Tendon repair – high failure rate
  Tendon – graft
  Tendon – transfer
  Tendon – rebalancing
- Bony surgery examples:
  - Arthrodesis
  - Arthroplasty (resection/hemiarthroplasty/total)
  - Osteotomy – mostly fail, hence avoid

3.8.1.6 Priority of Intervention
- Consider tackling the most painful joint first
- If disease is progressing, try to intervene early
- Some operations have higher priority
  - CTS release
  - C1/2 subluxation
  - Preventive dorsal wrist tenosynovitis to avoid extensor rupture
- Some operations have predictable outcome
  - Tenosynovectomy of hand
  - Arthrodesis of wrist and foot
  - Excision arthroplasty (DRUJ and forefoot)
  - Hip and knee arthroplasties

- Sometimes upper limb (UL) reconstruction undertaken before lower limb (LL) reconstruction if high demands are expected on the UL (for the use of walking aids) after LL reconstructive surgeries
- Souter's opinion of relative priority of reconstruction for the upper extremity:
  - Dorsal wrist tenosynovectomy
  - CTS release and flexor
  - MCPJ
  - PIPJ
  - Thumb
- In UL reconstruction, if proximal joints hinder accurate or functional positioning of hand for ADL, shoulder and elbow reconstruction, then they may take priority before hand surgery

3.8.1.7   Other Considerations on Priority
- Due to the linked nature of wrist and hand joints, it is advised to improve motion at one joint and stabilise the adjacent joint for surgery of RA hand deformity
- The 1st operation preferably has predictable outcome
- If bilateral hand involvement, the more severely disabled hand should be tackled first – other hand for ADL

3.8.1.8   Factors Causing RA Hand Deformity
- Attenuation of wrist ligaments and unbalanced wrist tendons:
  - RD of carpus and MCs
  - Carpal collapse and MC descent
  - Ulnar translation of carpus
- Bony erosion of MC head and P/P base
- Collateral ligament laxity allows unopposed pull of volar flexors
- Accessory ligament laxity allows ulnar and palmar displacement of volar plate and flexor sheath
- Flexor sheath stretching allows ulnar and volar displacement of flexor tendons
- Ulnar subluxation or dislocation of extensor due to radial sagittal band stretching
- Extensor rupture
- Intrinsic muscle contracture

3.8.1.9   Problems with Extensors in RA

- Sites of rupture and underlying aetiology
  - Ischaemic – typically distal edge of extensor retinaculum
  - Attrition – e.g. Caput ulnae syndrome; EPL at Lister's tubercle
  - Invasion – e.g. DIPJ mallet deformity; PIPJ synovitis and Buttonere deformity

3.8.1.9.1   DDx of Ruptured Extensor

- MCPJ dislocation with flexion contracture
- Extensor subluxating ulnarly – i.e. volar to axis of rotation – becomes flexors of MCPJ
- PIN palsy – motor compression at arcade of Frohse → C/F: elbow fullness, positive tenodesis present, RD of wrist due to ECU paralysis (retained ECRL)

3.8.1.9.2   Treatment of Ruptured Extensors

- Tenosynovitis – tenosynovectomy decompresses, prevents rupture
- Rupture may also need to treat associated DRUJ lesion
  - One tendon ruptured (extensor to L/F): L/F to R/F
  - Two tendons ruptured (extensors to L/F and R/F): EIP to L/F; R/F to M/F
  - Three tendons ruptured (extensors to M/F, R/F, L/F): M/F to I/F; EIP to ulna 2 fingers
  - All four extensor tendons: ECRL to I/F, M/F (with graft), EIP to ulna 2
  - EPL rupture – use EIP transfer

3.8.1.10   Problems with Flexors in RA

3.8.1.10.1   Clinical Problems

- Tenosynovitis – can cause trigger, swan neck, pinch test if positive indicative of associated synovitis
- Flexor tendon related problems
  - Thickened flexor sheath – may cause triggering
  - Distal nodule → finger may lock in flexion
  - More proximal nodule near A2 → lock in extension
  - Flexor ruptures → more at (1) palmer carpal bones, (2) trapezial ridge (FPL), (3) scaphoid tubercle and (4) edge of carpal ligament in carpal tunnel

3.8.1.10.2 Managing Flexor Tendon Problems

- Trigger/Tenosynovitis
    - Tenosynovectomy and/or excise RA nodule
- Flexor ruptures
    - FPL: if long stump, do tendon graft; if short, FDS transfer should be considered
    - FDP: if at digit, do tenosynovectomy, DIPJ fusion; if at wrist, do side–side repair and use mass action
    - FDS: if at digit, do tenosynovectomy, debridement; if at wrist, do side–side repair
    - Both FDS/FDP: if at digit, consider FDP/FDS tenodesis; if at wrist, do side–side repair and FDP graft

3.8.1.11   CTS and RA

- Synovitis causes pressure to increase and CTS
- DDx median nerve vasculitis (but lacks Tinel)

3.8.1.12   RA Wrist Problems

- Rotatory subluxation of scaphoid
- Scapholunate dissociation
- Attenuation of RSC ligament and deep ligament (RSL) of Testut
- Ulna translocation of the carpus

3.8.1.12.1 Result of Global Ligament Laxity

- Radiocarpal shortening (carpal collapse)
- Ulnar translation of carpus
- Failure of radial side structures (R-S-C volarly and dorsally)
- Sliding of carpus down the slope of distal radius ulnarward
- Impingement between TFCC and lunate

3.8.1.13   DRUJ Problem

3.8.1.13.1 General Features

- Destruction of ulno-carpal ligament complex, TFCC and ulnar disc
    - Volar displacement and collapse of lunate and triquetrum
    - Relative supination of carpus
    - Prominent distal ulna

3.8.1.13.2 Caput Ulnae Syndrome

Painful ulna head prominence and forearm rotation with unstable DRUJ

- Radio-ulna dissociation
- Dorsal displacement of distal ulna
- Volar subluxation of ECU

3.8.1.14   Treatment of RA Wrist (Fig. 3.12)

- Early stage
  - Synovectomy of radiocarpal joint and DRUJ
  - Wrist rebalancing
    If ECU dislocated – reposition with retinacular flap
    If ECU ruptured – do ECRL transfer
  - DRUJ arthroplasty
    For low demand – use Darrach procedure
  - Young, high demand
    DRUJ fusion and excision arthroplasty of distal ulna (Sauve Kapandji)

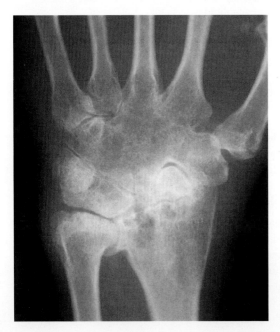

Fig. 3.12. Advanced rheumatoid arthritis affection of the wrist. Note the advanced bony erosion, spontaneous carpal fusion, and ulna head impingement, and loss of carpal height

3.8.1.15   Treatment of Ulna Translocation

▣ Radiolunate arthrodesis (Chamay)
  – Corrects RD of wrist
  – Prevents ulna translation
  – Cannot prevent deterioration of wrist
  Feature of Chamay operation:
  – Sparing of midcarpal joint for flex and extension
  – Sparing of the radioscaphoid joint for radial and UD
▣ RSL arthrodesis
  – Considered if radioscaphoid joint involved
  – Expect no radial or UD post-operatively
▣ Proximal row carpectomy
  – Destroyed RSL joints; retained intercarpal joint cartilage
  – Expect very good motion but reduced grip strength

3.8.1.16   Treatment of Advanced RA Wrist (Fig. 3.13)

▣ Indications of wrist arthrodesis:
  – Ankylosing or disintegrating wrist, or advanced OA type with pain, deformity and/or instability

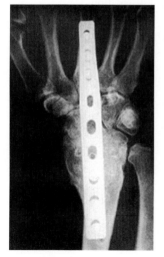

Fig. 3.13. Post-operative X-ray of a wrist after fusion of the right wrist with plating

3.8.1.16.1 Wrist Fusion
- Fusion usually in neutral position
- Requires reasonably good shoulder and elbow control
- Technique (inter or intra MC methods)

3.8.1.16.2 Role of Total Wrist Arthroplasty
- Pan-arthritis of wrist, bilateral involvement, bilateral UL multiple joint stiffness
- Low demand patient
- Sufficient bone stock
- Moderate residual ROM
- Reasonable extensor and flexor function

3.8.1.16.3 Contraindication to Wrist Arthroplasty
- High demand group – weight-bearing wrists
- Poor bone stock, poor range, rupture extensors
- Sepsis

3.8.1.17   MCPJ Disorder in RA

3.8.1.17.1 Contribution of Normal Anatomy Towards Tendency to MCPJ UD
- Smaller slope of ulnar condyle of MC heads
- Shorter ulna collateral ligament length and orientation
- Stronger hypothenar muscle than other interosseous muscles
- Flexion of 4th and 5th MC bases with grip
- Normal forces
  (e.g. lateral punch pressure and power grasp)

3.8.1.17.2 MCPJ Disease and UD
- Erosion starts at insertion of collateral ligament at MC heads with progressive cartilage and bone lost
- Resultant deformity:
  - UD of finger
  - Volar subluxation/dislocation of P/P

3.8.1.17.3 Treating MCPJ Disease
- Synovectomy:
  - Painful synovitis despite conservative treatment
  - Young patient associated with deformity

- Soft tissue reconstruction:
  - For UD: (a) intrinsic release: ulna side of I/F, M/F and R/F and ADQ of L/F; and (b) intrinsic transfer: transfer to radial side of M/F, R/F and L/F, at lateral band or radial collateral ligament

3.8.1.17.4 Operation for Volar Subluxation and Ulna Drift
- Extensor relocation: reefing of radial, release of ulna fibres
- Zancolli's procedure: extensor tenodesis to base of PP through drill holes

3.8.1.17.5 Role of MCPJ Resection Arthroplasty with Flexible Implant
- For deformed, destroyed and painful MCPJs
- For dislocated MCPJs
- Quite good result, arc of 40° and/or combined with intrinsic release, collateral ligament repair and extensor relocation

3.8.1.18   Finger Deformity and RA

3.8.1.18.1 Swan-Neck Deformity
- Pathology: volar synovitis and flexor tenosynovitis (DIP extensor lag, PIP hyperextend, MCP flex)
- Surgical options:
  - If DIPJ is the cause – arthrodesis of DIPJ
  - If PIPJ is the cause:
    PIPJ not fixed: do tenosynovectomy, sublimis sling and/or lateral band translocation
    Associated MCPJ disease: do MCPJ plasty
    PIPJ fixed: do extensor lysis and collateral release, mobilise lateral band, and do flexor tenosynovectomy
    PIPJ destroyed: arthrodesis of PIPJ

3.8.1.18.2 Boutonniere Deformity
- Pathology: dorsal synovitis produces DIP hyperextend, PIP flex, MCPJ hyperextend
  - PIP 10–15° extensor lag, dorsal synovitis, attenuated central tendon, volar subluxation of lateral band
    PIP synovectomy, reefing central slip, and/or extensor tenotomy over M/P

- PIP 30–40° extensor lag, intrinsic tight, oblique retinacular ligament shorten, volar lateral band
  Repair/reconstruct central-slip; centralise lateral band
- Fixed flexion and severe
  → Consider arthrodesis

3.8.1.19 Surgery for RA Thumb Deformity (Fig. 3.14)

▨ Game-keeper's: reconstruct UCL, release adductor fascia (and/or plasty/fusion if MCPJ destroyed)

▨ Swan-Neck (Fig. 3.15):
  - Early – splint
  - Subluxed CMC– CMCJ fascial hemiarthroplasty
  - Dislocated CMC – CMCJ plasty, MCPJ fuse

▨ Boutonniere (Fig. 3.16):
  - Mobile MCPJ subluxation: synovectomy MCPJ, transfer EPL
  - Fixed MCPJ: plasty versus fusion (depends on nearby IPJ/CMCJ)

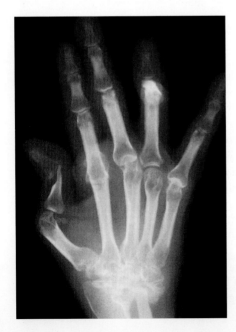

Fig. 3.14. X-ray of a patient with rheumatoid arthritis affecting especially the bones of the thumb

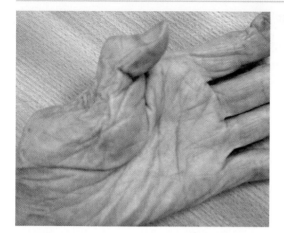

Fig. 3.15. Swan-neck type deformity of the left thumb from rheumatoid arthritis

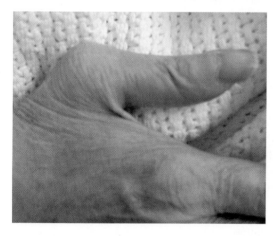

Fig. 3.16. Boutonniere type deformity of the right thumb from PA

- MCPJ destroyed and IPJ fixed: e.g. if CMCJ preserved, MCPJ plasty and IPJ arthrodesis, etc.
- Hyper-extended MCPJ
  - Either fusion or volar capsulodesis in flexion

3.8.1.20 Arthritis Mutilans

- Poor bone stock
- Grossly very unstable
- Many types of deformity are possible
- Example: lateral deformity at MCPJ; hyperextend deformity at IPJ, etc.
- Treatment: arthrodesis with BG (to maintain length)

3.8.2   Hand OA

3.8.2.1 Incidence of OA of the Hand

- Most common form of OA
- Younger than 40 years – 50 new cases per 1000 person – years at risk
- Older than 60 years – 110 new cases per 1000 person – years at risk

3.8.2.2 Pattern of Joint Involvement

Most commonly affected joints

- DIPJ
- 1st CMC
- PIPJ
- MCPJ
- Others – sesamoid, trapezial scaphoid/trapezoid, pisiform-triquetral OA

  Prevalent OA in one joint increased the incidence risk of OA in:
- Other joints in same row
- Other joints in same ray

  OA in DIPJ or PIPJ increased incidence risk of OA in any other hand joint. However, thumb CMC is not a strong predictor of generalised disease

3.8.2.3 Clinical Presentation

3.8.2.3.1 Fingers

- Swelling around joints
- Lateral deformity
- Osteophytes/exostoses
  - Heberdens nodes
  - Bouchards nodes
- Mallet finger
- Mucous cysts/ganglion – hyaluronic acid filled cysts

3.8.2.3.2 Thumb CMC
▦ Subluxation of the CMC – MC base prominence
▦ Z-deformity – bony collapse at the MC base leads to adduction of the
MC and hyperextension of the MCP

3.8.2.4   Physical Examination

3.8.2.4.1 PIPJ/DIPJ
▦ Tenderness at joint line
▦ Lateral instability
▦ Pain on axial compression
▦ Crepitus on axial compression
▦ Reduced ROM

3.8.2.4.2 Thumb CMC
▦ Tenderness over 1st CMC
▦ Pain and crepitus on axial compression – torque test
▦ Decreased pinch strength
▦ Subluxation – intermittent pressure to MC base while patient pinches

3.8.2.4.3 Sesamoid Arthritis
▦ Pain palmar plate at thumb MCP
▦ Good joint space
▦ Elicited by pressing on palmar plate

3.8.2.5   Radiological Features
▦ Joint space narrowing
▦ Osteophytes
▦ Subchondral sclerosis
▦ Bony cysts
▦ Joint deformity
▦ Cortical collapse
   X-ray classification: Kellgren scale

3.8.2.6   Treatment Options
▦ Conservative
   – Splints
   – Non-steroidal anti-inflammatory agents
   – Intra-articular injections

- Surgical
  - Stabilisation
  - Arthrodesis
  - Arthroplasty

3.8.2.6.1 Surgery for the 1st CMC

Anatomy
- Palmar/ulna collateral ligament
- Dorsal inter-MC ligament
  - Congenital laxity can lead to subluxation and OA, e.g. Erlers–Danlos Syndrome
  - Pattern of joint involvement influences choice of procedure

Indications for surgery
- Failure of non-surgical methods
- Pain
- Instability – weakness in grip

Arthrodesis of the 1st CMC
- Disease limited to CMC
- Positioned 45° palmar and radial abduction
- Cup and cone arthrodesis: 2–5% non-union

Arthroplasty of the 1st CMC
Trapezium excision arthroplasty
- With or without ligament reconstruction
- Possible role of silicon interposition arthroplasty; many side effects
- Fascia/tendon interposition
  Note: ligament. reconstruction and tendon interposition may improve grip strength and endurance; produce stronger hand than trapezial excision alone, although they have a slower recovery

3.8.2.6.2 Surgery for the DIPJ
Indications
- Pain
- Instability
- Mucous Cyst
- Deformity

- Options:
  - Arthrodesis (if significant destruction or instability)
  - Arthroplasty
  - Synovectomy and removal of osteophyte

3.8.2.6.3 Surgery for the PIPJ
Indications
- Pain
- Instability
- Deformity
- Options:
  - Arthrodesis
  - Arthroplasty
    Cemented
    Silicon interposition

3.8.2.6.4 Options for Thumb MCP/IPJ
- Arthrodesis – either IPJ or MCP
- Interpositional arthroplasty – MCP
  - Cemented prosthesis
  - Swanson silicon rubber
  - Soft tissue arthroplasty

3.9   Hand Infections and Tumours

3.9.1   Hand Infections

3.9.1.1   Relevant Anatomy
- The pulp
  Separated into many tiny compartments by strong septae from skin to bone
  Immediate pain with any swelling
- Web space
  Each hand with three webs between fingers; fat filled just proximal to the superficial transverse MC ligament at level of MCPJ
  Often these begin under palmer calloses/labourer often points dorsally since skin yielding – but it is the palmer extension into the deep palmer space that is dangerous

■ Deep palmer space (thenar and mid-palmer spaces)
Lies between: (1) fascia dorsal to flexors (roof) and (2) fascia that covers MC and its muscle (floor)
Radial border: fascia of adductor/thenar
Ulna border: hypothenar fascia
Separated into 'thenar' and 'mid-palmer' spaces via fascia plane that passes the 3rd MC shaft (and the fascia dorsal to the I/F)
Note: I/F and thumb infection can spread to thenar; and the other three fingers infection can spread to mid-palmer space
■ Flexor sheath
  – Thumb flexor sheath can spread to radial bursa
  – L/F flexor sheath can spread to ulna bursa
  – Occasional 'horseshoe' collection if the above bursae are connected

3.9.1.2 General Approach
■ Hx: systemic, e.g. DM
Mechanism, e.g. human bite
Organism, e.g. staphylococcus is three times as common as other microbes, such as streptococcus, enterobacteria, pseudomonas, enterococci and bacteroides
Rare microbes: TB, gonococcus, Pasteurella (cat/dogs), Eikenella (humans), aeromonas, haemophilus
■ P/E: check spreading of lymphangitis and check lymph node → 4th/5th fingers drain to epitrochea, while other fingers are more likely to drain to axilla nodes
  – Cellulitis only, treat with antibiotics (cloxacillin and benzyl penicillin and/or augmentin if the result of a bite)
  – If there is pus under pressure, always operate

3.9.1.2.1 Pulp (Felon)
■ Cx: osteomyelitis
■ Incision: lateral; avoid fishmouth
  – Deeper incisions partitioned by septae – dorsal to the tactile surface of the pulp and not more than 3 mm from free edge of nail; if not, digital nerve will be damaged
  – Superficial and pointing volar midline; possibly midline longitudinal. Never fishmouth, as this is slow to heal and leaves painful scars

3.9.1.2.2 Paronychia
- Nail fold infection
    - Drain by incision with blade angled away from nail bed to avoid damaging it
    - Alternative: wedge excision of nail
    - If it is a bilateral infection and it migrates under the nail, excision (proximal third) of the nail should be undertaken

3.9.1.2.3 Web Space
- Never incise on the web
- May need to use two incisions – one dorsal and one ventral
  Most point dorsally, but it is the palmar part which can spread deep that can be dangerous

3.9.1.2.4 Deep Palmar Spaces
- P/E:
    - Thenar space: systemic upset, I/F held flexed and ̄ROM for thumb and I/F
    - Mid palmer space: ̄ROM for M/F and R/F, and general hand swelling
- Drainage:
    - Thenar space: drain by curved incision in thumb web along the proximal side of thenar space; avoid recurrent branch
    - Mid palmer space: curved incision beginning at distal palmer crease, extending ulnarward to just inside the hypothenar eminence

3.9.1.2.5 Tenosynovitis
- Kanavel four signs:
    - Finger flexed
    - Sausage shaped
    - Tender at sheath
    - Pain on passive extension
- Cause spread from pulp space/punctures, etc.
- Treatment:
    - Intravenous antibiotics if < 48 h
    - Drain if: (a) not improved at 24 h and (b) late presentation after 48 h

- Two types of incisions:
  - Open
  - Incise at distal palmer crease and distal finger crease (or perhaps midlateral at M/P)

3.9.1.2.6 Radial and Ulna Bursa Sepsis
- Cause: from infected flexor sheath
- Treatment:
  - Drain radial bursa: make lateral incision over P/P of the thumb, enters sheath; insert probe and push towards wrist. Make 2nd incision at its end. Irrigate
  - Drain ulna bursa: open at ulna side of L/F, then proceed proximally at the wrist. Irrigate

3.9.1.2.7 Other Areas
- Osteomyelitis – similar to large bones, if amputation is needed, it is done at the joint proximal to the infected bone
  - D/P cases may improve after abscess drained
- Human bites: must be aggressive with intravenous cepalosporin and penicillin washout on any exposed joint (commonly MCP)
- TB: associated with fish tanks/pools. An atypical example is as persistent synovitis – culture can take weeks; treatment involves synovectomy /excision of lesion and anti-tuberculous medications by microbiologist
- Herpetic whitlow: pain swelling and vesicular rash – on thumb and I/Fs; – self-limiting, lasts 3 weeks; do not drain
- Sporotrichosis – from roses, lymphatic spread and lumps are seen. Treatment involves KI (potassium iodide)

3.9.1.3 Appendix: Atypical Mycobacteria

3.9.1.3.1 Introduction
- Majority of chronic hand infections
- Strive at lower temperature, hence involve upper or lower extremities, rather than the lung
- Treatment: debridement and anti-TB drugs according to suggestion of microbiologists
- Common examples:

- *Mycobacterium marinum* – fish tanks, pools, etc.
- *Mycobacterium kansaii*
- *Mycobacterium avium-intracellulare*

3.9.1.3.2 Mycobacterium Marinum
- Type I – self-limiting verrucal lesion observed; biopsy; minocycline ×1 month
- Type II – single or multiple subcutaneous granulomas and/or ulceration excision; minocycline ×3 months
- Type III – deep infection surgery; minocycline ×3 months
- Non-caseating granulomas

3.9.2   Hand Tumours Overview

3.9.2.1 Ganglion
- Most common
- Possible aetiology: trauma, mucoid degeneration, synovial hernation
- Location: dorsum of wrist more than volar wrist
- Need to identify the stalk to decrease recurrence
- Recurrence: 5–20% after surgery

3.9.2.2 Giant Cell Tumour of Tendon Sheath
- Second most common hand tumour
- Occurs in 40- to -60-year olds
- Finger volar/dorsal surface can be affected, with or without circumferential
- Can wrap around NV bundle; needs meticulous dissection
- Painless
- Pathology – foam cells, histiocytes, giant cells (resemble PVNS)
- May need to include joint capsule and tendon sheath during excision in difficult cases

3.9.2.3 Epidermal Cyst
- Trauma aetiology
- Volar aspect D/P typically
- Painless
- Histology – inclusion of squamous epithelium within fibrous capsule
- Treatment: complete excision including curettage of D/P in difficult cases

3.9.2.4 Glomus Tumour
- 1–5% of hand tumours
- More than 50% subungual in location
- Symptom: painful and tender, and cold sensitive; not usually relieved by aspirin
- Signs: ridged nail, blue spot
- X-ray: may see lucent, eccentric lesion
- Histology – polyhedral cells, fibrous stroma
- Treatment excision

3.9.2.5 Enchondroma
- Occurs during 2nd to 4th decades
- More in P/P
- Most present as pathological fracture or incidental finding
- Treatment curettage and bone graft may recur. If pathological fracture, let fracture heal then do BG and curettage
- May occasionally become malignant – chondrosarcoma

3.9.2.6 Osteochondroma
- Either solitary hand lesion or part of multiple osteochondromata
- Location: often at MCs or P/P
- Treatment: excision after skeletal maturity
- Malignant change 2–11% chance if multiple

3.9.2.7 Osteoid Osteoma
- Rare in the hand
- Pain typically relieved by aspirin
- X-ray – eccentric cortical sclerosis and lucent nidus
- Treatment curettage using image intensifier
- 10% recurrence

3.9.2.8 Malignant Hand Tumours
- Primary malignant tumours rare
- If older than 40 years of age these tumours are likely to be metastatic until proven otherwise
- Look for primary (e.g. commonly Ca lung)
- Enneking grading and staging plus incisional biopsy for primaries

3.9.2.9 Soft Tissue Malignancy
- Wide range of different pathologies, e.g. epitheloid sarcoma, synovial sarcomas
- Work-up as for sarcomas in general

3.10   Microvascular Replantation

3.10.1 Indication for Replantation
- Multiple digits
- Thumb
- Child
- At the level of MC/wrist/forearm
- For individual digit, if distal to FDS insertion – often results in reasonably satisfactory function

3.10.2 Contraindication to Replantation
- Local
    - Crushed – segmental; distal to DIPJ
- General
    - Serious disease – arteriosclerosis; mental disturbance

3.10.3 Relative Contraindication
Single digit replantation proximal to FDS insertion causes a digit with significant functional impairment – average PIPJ ROM 35, although cold intolerance and sensation are comparable to more distally amputated cases. For cases with concomitant PIPJ injury, amputation may also be considered

3.10.4 Ischaemia Time Allowed

	Warm	Cold
Digit	12	X 2
Proximal division	6	X 2

3.10.5 Initial Assessment
- Care of the amputated part:
    - Irrigate with Hartmann
    - Wrap in wet swab
    - Place in bag and place in ice

■ Associated injuries (e.g. mangled extremity score) if severe
■ General state of patient: save life, then save limb

3.10.6 Surgical Technique
■ Bilateral mid-lateral incision
■ Isolate vessels and nerves
■ Shorten and fix bone
■ Repair nerves
■ Repair arteries first, not the reverse, since toxins will enter the body if veins are repaired first
  – Regarding the repair of veins – two for each artery, more than three total
■ Repair flexor and extensor tendons (some prefer to repair tendons before NV)
■ Repair skin
  In the case of hand or forearm replantation, consider use of arterial shunt before the vascular anastomosis and give heparin

3.10.7 Post-operative Monitoring
■ Check any arterial insufficiency
■ Check any venous congestion
■ Keep warm
■ Anticoagulant
■ Rest and no smoking
■ Monitoring progress, e.g. temperature probe, clinical, Doppler sometimes for bigger vessels, etc.

3.10.8 Complication
■ Early
  – Arterial insufficiency: loosen dressing, change position, heparin bolus, – return to operation if no effect in 4–6 h
  – Venous congestion: medical leeches – need to give antibiotics to cover for *Aeromonas hydrophilia*
  – Sepsis: especially if some myonecrosis has set in
■ Late
  – Function impairment: e.g. Lost differential gliding, motion of digits also affected by the overall injury sustained
  – Cold intolerance: might sometimes improve over 2–3 years

3.10.9   Recovery

- Cold intolerance sometimes improves over the long term
- Neural recovery – depends on type and level of injury; fine tactile discrimination rarely ever returns

3.10.10   Ring Avulsion Injuries (Classification by Urbaniak)

- Class 1: satisfactory circulation → manage bone and soft tissue injury
- Class 2: inadequate circulation → repair vessel
- Class 3: completely degloved → many need amputation

3.10.11   Managing more Complicated Cases

3.10.11.1   Mangled Extremity Scores

- Bone and soft tissue injury: energy level involved – low E (1), medium E (2), high (3), very high E (4). Contamination/high speed injury
- Circulation: Normal (1), decreased (2), nil (3)
- Shock: BP over 90 mmHg (0), transient ↓ BP (1), persistent ↓ BP (2)
- Age: younger than 30 years (0), 30–50 years (1), over 50 years (2)
  If mangled extremity scores are over 7, it is nearly 100% predictive for amputation

3.10.12   Overall Results of Replantation

- 80% Success in adults, some quote slightly lower figures in children but this could be because of a more aggressive approach taken
- The outcome measure in replantation can be classified into the following classes:
  - Resume original work; MRC 4/5, ROM 60%
  - Some suitable work; MRC 3/5, ROM 40–60%
  - ADL ok; MRC 3/5, ROM 30–40%
  - No function remains

3.11   Miscellaneous Conditions

3.11.1   Kienbock's Disease (Fig. 3.17)

3.11.1.1   C/Fs and Management

- Clinical: asymptomatic, possible symptoms – grip weak, pain at wrist or proximal forearm, limited motion – especially extension – and sometimes discomfort on extending M/F

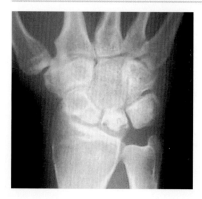

Fig. 3.17. X-ray of a hand with Kienbock's disease

- Goal – when OA absent, decrease the axial load on lunate, hope for spontaneous revascularisation. Options in this category:
  - Radial shortening, which is more popular (does not need BG). Usually only 2 mm needs be taken away to unload the lunate, quite regardless of the degree of ulna variance
  - Lunate revascularisation from 2nd to 3rd MC artery
  - Lunate excision with replacement by silicon spacer not popular since synovitis. Other options: STT fusion, capitate shortening, etc.
- When OA is present, needs salvage, e.g. PRC (if pristine proximal capitate and lunate fossa) or total wrist fusion

3.11.2 Dupuytren Disease

3.11.2.1 General Features
- Association – family Hx, race (more in UK/USA, while rare in China), males, epilepsy, DM
- 'Dupuytren diathesis' – strong heredity and family tendency (AD with varying penetrance)

3.11.2.2 Normal Anatomy
- Digit fascial layout: – three layers
  - Superficial to skin of distal palm
  - Middle to NV bundle as digital sheet
  - Deep passes around the flexor sheath lateral to MCP

▦ Palm
  – Long fibres of palmer fascia pass into each digit
  – There are two transverse systems:
    Natatory ligament at base of digital web
    Deep system as transverse fibres of the palmer aponeurosis

3.11.2.3 Pathoanatomy

▦ Cords follow the anatomical pathways
▦ Myofibroblasts form early. In later stages – mostly acellular and mature collagen bundles
▦ Ectopic deposits – knuckle pads produce local thickenings over the dorsum of PIP; plantar nodules – medial insole (Ledderhose); and Peyronie's disease – local thickening in dorsum of the penis, sometimes as concavity curving upwards

3.11.2.4 Aetiology

▦ Vascular theory – source of myofibroblast appears to be from perivascular
▦ Mechanical factors

3.11.2.5 Clinical Examination

▦ Nodule – forms early distal to the distal palmer crease
▦ Pit – at level of distal palmer crease
▦ Blanching sign – forced digit extension will blanch the skin distal to area of tethering
▦ R/F, L/F more than other fingers/thumb
▦ Test digital circulation
▦ Table top test
▦ Assess flexibility of PIP and MCP contractures
▦ Associations – knuckle pad, Peyronie's disease

3.11.2.6 Treatment Principles

▦ Tension has a key role in maintaining the tissue's abnormal response; considerable resolution of the process may occur with disappearance of nodules and softening of tissues if tension is successfully released. Permanent release of tension is preferred to using a radical excisional approach as in tumour surgery

- Fascial ends are prevented from re-uniting – interposition of normal tissue, such as fat, or excision of involved subcutaneous tissue and skin grafting
- Minimise cell reproliferation by means of dead space elimination, and hold out to length post-operatively (until collagen maturity is established)

3.11.2.7   Mainly Surgical Disease
- Little success with conservative treatment
- Operative options

3.11.2.8   Timing of Operation
- Rapid progression needs early surgery
- In the case of severe contracture, if it starts to become fixed, one needs no delay
- Table top test
  - Operation rarely needed for palmer nodules per se
  - PIP contracture, unlike MCP, is very difficult to release once contracted

3.11.2.9   Consent
- Warn of adherence to post-operative rehabilitation and sometimes splinting
- Warn of recurrence
- Warn of danger to NV injury in digit

3.11.2.10   Other factors in surgical decision making
- Age – most young individuals have more aggressive conditions – more radical
- Motivation – needs assessing
- Type of hand – the hands of a labourer tend to have a greater risk of post-operative stiffness. Also, elderly with pale cold hands have a poorer prognosis

3.11.2.11   Choice of Surgery

3.11.2.11.1 Option 1: Fasciotomy
- Open/closed
- More used in elderly
- Procedure initially described by Dupuytren

3.11.2.11.2 Option 2: Partial Fasciectomy
- Aim at excision of nodules and involved cords
- 'Selective' fasiectomy means retain the transverse fibres of the palmer aponeurosis

3.11.2.11.3 Option 3: Radical Fasiectomy With or Without Open Palm
- Diffuse severe disease and/or absence of fat
- Involves removal of all of palmer fascial structures, involved or not. However, extensive dissection has not been confirmed to lower the recurrence rate
- Open palm method not popular in USA and UK
- Advantage of open palm option: quick pain and complete relief; early mobilisation
- Disadvantage of open palm option: some patients are afraid of such big and open wounds

3.11.2.11.4 Role of Skin Graft
- Indications:
  - Skin involvement – dermis involved
  - Separate the ends of affected fascia
  - Skin deficient after release

3.11.2.11.5 Urgency of Tackling PIPJ More than MCPJ Disease
- Options for PIP disease
  - Release – tendon sheath, ligament release, volar capsulectomy
  - Arthrodesis
  - Arthroplasty
  - Osteotomy
  - Accept deformity
  - Amputation

3.11.2.11.6 Dermofasciectomy
- Considered when there is no clear plane of separation between fascia and dermis

3.11.2.11.7 Salvage Options
- Amputation – selected cases, L/F only not R/F
- PIPJ – arthrodesis, fusion, arthroplasty

3.11.2.11.8 Miscellaneous Surgical Tip

▪ PIP disease – use of excess force can cause vessel spasm, or even joint subluxation; be gentle

▪ Removal of dead space and prevention haematoma important

▪ Skin incision – use Brunner zig-zag, and z-plasties where indicated

3.11.3   Gamekeeper's Thumb (Fig. 3.18)

▪ Also called skier's thumb

▪ Caused by injury to the ulna collateral ligament of the first MCPJ, sometimes associated with fracture base of P/P

▪ Dx is usually obvious, but can resort to stress testing under X-ray control in case of doubt

▪ Conservative treatment may fail in the presence of a Stener lesion due to interposition by the aponeurosis of the adductor pollicis. In case of doubt, ultrasound or even MRI has been reported to confirm the presence of the Stener lesion

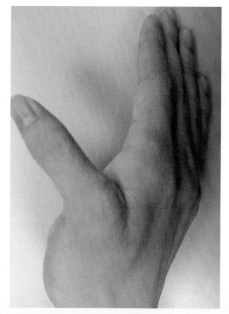

Fig. 3.18. Gamekeeper's thumb in a skier

▓ Open repair is necessary in many cases, if only to address the stener lesion. However, if the ligament is much attenuated in chronic or neglected tears, then bone–ligament–bone type of ligamentous reconstruction may be tried

General Bibliography

Smith P (ed) (2002) Lister's the hand (Diagnosis and Indications), 4th edn. Churchill Livingstone, Edinburgh
Weinzweig J (2001) The wrist, 2001 edn. Watson K (ed). Lippincott Williams and Wilkins, Philadelphia
Birch R, Bonney G, Parry CBW (eds) (1998) Surgical disorders of the peripheral nerves, 1998 edn. Churchill Livingstone, Edinburgh

Selected Bibliography of Journal Articles

1. Boyer MI, Strickland JW et al. (2003) Flexor tendon repair and rehabilitation, state of the art in 2002. Instructional Course Lectures 52:137–161
2. Ring D, Jupiter JB et al. (2000) Acute fractures of the scaphoid. J Am Acad Orthop Surg 8:225–231
3. Gelberman RH, Cooney WP et al. (2001) Carpal instability. Instructional Course Lectures 50:123–134

4 Principles of Foot and Ankle Surgery

Contents

4.1   Gait Analysis

4.1.1   The Gait Cycle
- Gait cycles from initial contact to subsequent contact of the same foot
- Two phases are included: stance (60%) and swing (40%)
- There are four sub-phases of stance; the first and fourth are double support
- There are three sub-phases of swing
- The position of the ground reaction force (GRF) with respect to the joint centre depends on two factors – muscle activity and posture (body segmental alignment)
- There must be an equilibrium between the externally applied forces and the internally applied forces
- External forces in stance include the GRF; external forces in swing include gravitational and inertial forces
- Internal forces include muscle, ligament, capsule and structural anatomy of the bone itself

4.1.2   The Different Phases
- Loading response: shock absorption and transfer of body load onto the limb; centre of motion (COM) is low
  - At the end, GRF is located relative to hip and knees such that muscular activity is needed to balance
- Mid-swing: climbs up an energy hill using the hamstring as hip extensor to pull the thigh segment back; COM is at its highest, but only one muscle group is active – ankle plantar flexors. The body is aligned so that the GRF falls through the joint centres
- Terminal stance: COM falls down an energy hill, but only one muscle group is active – the ankle plantar-flexors. With respect to the joint centre, the GRF is such that internal and external forces tend to balance out with little muscle activity (large moments by ankle PF)
- Pre-swing: COM is low and moving quickly; the body is preparing for phase shift and load transfer to the other leg. Hip flexors (second most important) are active
- Initial swing: shortens the limb to achieve clearance; thigh segment accelerates from hip flexors
  - The knee flexes, but there is no active hip flexor firing. As the limb leaves the floor, the GRF disappears and gravitational and inertial

forces now become significant; the shank segment lags behind and the knee bends (shortens the leg functionally, cleared by a mild action of pre-tibial muscles)

■ Mid-swing: shift from flexion to extension; eventually the shank segment comes forward, with or without rectus assistance
  – The knee extends and the ankle dorsiflexes to achieve clearance

■ Terminal swing involves deceleration. Hamstrings are active (hip extensor), stopping the thigh segment from moving forward; the knee extends as a result of inertia from the shank segment. By the end, activity occurs on both sides (dorsiflexion to pre-position the foot)

4.1.3   Running
■ Only two sub-phases in stance
■ Still a heel contact
■ Two periods of double support replaced by double float

4.1.4   Sprinting
■ Feature: toe strike, not heel strike, at initial contact
■ In general, velocity = cadence × stride length

4.1.5   Key to an Effective Gait
■ Stability in stance and pre-positioning of the foot prior to heel strike
■ Clearance in swing
■ Effective phase shift
■ Energy-efficient fashion

4.1.6   Oxygen Consumption
■ Walking is less than twice that for standing and sitting
■ Very efficient
■ Any deviation of normal gait is costly in terms of oxygen and energy consumption
■ Fast walking and below knee amputation – 60% more consumption
■ Above knee amputation – 100% more consumption
■ Crutches walking – 300% more consumption

4.2   Acute Ankle Ligament Injuries

4.2.1   Acute Injuries

■ Possible predisposing factors to ankle sprain:
- Pes cavovarus
- History of previous injury
- Fore-foot valgus or dropping of first ray with compensation through the hind-foot
- Altered proprioception

■ Common injury pattern: plantar-flexion inversion injury

4.2.1.1   Usual Sequence of Events

■ Injury to anterior talofibular ligament (ATFL)
■ Followed by a varying degree of calcaneofibular ligament (CFL) injury
■ Can classify injuries as stable or unstable according to the degree of talar tilt and anterior drawer sign upon stressing
■ Besides clinical testing, stress testing under X-ray (XR) can be performed, but always compare with the opposite normal ankle. (Anterior excursion greater than 3 mm in anterior drawer test under XR indicates ruptured ATFL; talar tilt greater than $10°$ is indicative of complete rupture of ATFL and CFL)
■ Peroneal tenography can also be used to look for CFL injury. Magnetic resonance imaging (MRI) is not routinely indicated, but can reveal concomitant osteochondral injuries not always easily visible on XR

4.2.1.2   Role of Arthroscopy

■ Indications:
- Osteochondral injury of talar dome
- Loose bodies
- Painful ossicles within the ankle ligaments
- Hypertrophied inferior border of the ATFL

4.2.1.3   Treatment

■ Conservative:
- Most cases treated conservatively
- Even grade-3 lateral ankle ligament injuries can be treated by conservative treatment with a combination of immobilisation and early protected mobilisation

- Operative:
  - Considered in highly competitive athletes, those with initial talus tilt greater than 15°, significant bony avulsion, significant injury to both medial and lateral ligaments, failed conservative treatment
  - In most cases, anatomical repair, such as by the Brostrom technique, can still be considered since the ligaments are not attenuated in the acute setting

4.2.2   Ligamentous Injuries and Chronic Ankle Instability

Types
- Functional – sometimes subjective with no laxity
- Mechanical – with objective laxity
  (Points often missed – assess carefully for proprioception, peroneal weakness, subtalar joint)

4.2.2.1 Differential Diagnosis of Chronic Ankle Pain
- Unusual if more than 6 weeks for chronic ankle sprain
- Subtalar joint origin
- Impingement and instability
- Superficial peroneal nerve neuroma
- Osteochondritis dessicans (OCD)
- Bony fracture – e.g. lateral process talus (snow boarder's ankle), anterior process calcaneus, etc.

4.2.2.2 Clinical Assessment
- Anterior drawer – more than 4 mm anterior subluxation talus on mortise in some 20° plantar flexion
- Varus stress testing
  More than 6 mm different (hold hind-foot, include subtalar)
  Mostly medial structures intact
  Careful exam, in many cases, reveals rotation instability in plantar flexion (since upon plantar flexion, less locked in mortise)
- Testing syndesmosis
  External rotation (ER) causes pain, XR assessment (e.g. medial clear space)
- Subtle cases
  - No laxity, functional instability
  - Subtalar joint surface has loss of parallelism

Differential diagnosis of negative stress test:
- Really negative stress test
- Not proper technique
- Subtalar unstable
  (Other investigations – e.g. MRI can see ligaments)

4.2.2.3 Conservative Treatment
- Strengthen peroneals
- Proprioception rehabilitation
- Brace/tapping/use of orthotics
- If successful, continue; later training is sports specific

4.2.2.4 Indication for Surgery
- Failed conservative treatment
- Not all cases need to have positive test to perform surgery

4.2.2.5 Selection of Arthroscopic versus Open Surgery
- ATFL intracapsular, arthroscopic intervention is possible
- CFL extracapsular, cannot use scope to intervene
- Sometimes ligaments are too attenuated and only scar remains; may need open surgery, especially in chronic cases
- (P.S. CFL contributes most to subtalar instability, if any)

4.2.2.6 Good Indications for Arthroscopic Interventions
- Lateral gutter impingement
- Anterior impingement
- Cartilage injury, e.g. flaps
- Loose bodies and OCD
- Chronic synovitis

4.2.2.7 Types of Open Surgery
- Anatomical – brostrum repair – direct ligament repair of ATFL/CFL
  - Advantages – anatomical; spares peroneal; good track record
  - [Post-operative: 2 weeks non-weight bearing (NWB); 2 weeks weight bearing (WB) cast; 8 weeks brace]
- Peroneal used/tenodesis procedure (e.g. Watson Jones)
  - Advantages – good if ligament replaced by scar; in cases with degenerative joint disease (DJD), gives more sense of stability
  - Disadvantage – sacrifice peroneal, not anatomical

■ Role of calcaneal osteotomy
  - Varus hind-foot
  - Cavus
  - Redo of lateral ankle reconstruction

4.2.3   Turf Toe

4.2.3.1   Pathomechanics

■ Commonly in football players; hyperdorsiflexion injury to first metatarsal-phalangeal joint (MTPJ) with planted foot
■ (MT head with changing radius of curvature = sliding becomes compression in dorsiflexion – explains the frequent concomitant injury to dorsal cartilage besides the plantar structures)

4.2.3.2   Structures that May Be Injured

Pathology
■ Dorsal side: sometimes compression injury to cartilage
■ Plantar side:
  - Proximal avulsion of plantar plate, sometimes displaced into the joint
  - Buttonhole of MT head through intersesamoid (ruptured) ligament
  - Buttonhole of MT head through medial sesamoid fracture

4.2.3.3   Management

■ Conservative, if mild (by taping to limit joint motion and compression; orthoses limit joint motion, e.g. Morton's extension, shoe-wear modification)
■ Operative, if significant injury to joint capsule and the sesamoid complex
■ Prevention
  - Avoid athlete foot wares that are too flexible
  - Return to grass playing field rather than using hard artificial turf

4.2.4   Sesamoid Dysfunction

4.2.4.1   Introduction

■ As usual, concomitant injury to turf toe
■ Types of injuries:
  - Separation of bipartite sesamoid
  - Sesamoid fracture

- Sesamoid dislocation – association with traumatic disruption of plantar plate
- Sometimes proximal migration of sesamoid with no MTPJ dislocation
- 'Sprain' – mild/moderate/severe sprain cannot return to sport; complete tear of capsuloligamentous complex; associated bony/sesamoid injury
- 'Dislocation' can be due to (i) volar plate avulsion, (ii) intersesamoid ligament injury or (iii) transverse fracture of medial sesamoid

4.2.4.2 Sesamoid Dysfunction Treatment
- Conservative – RICE, taping, orthotics, shoe wear
- Surgery – sometimes necessary even if close reduction is successful, since soft tissue (ST) injury (e.g. ruptured intersesamoid ligament) may need repair
  Common indications for operation (OT):
- Significant capsule avulsion
- Proximal sesamoid migration
- Displaced sesamoid fracture or displaced bipartite sesamoid
  Needs open reduction (OR) and repair of STs
- Complications (Cxs) of sesamoid injuries: persistent pain/DJD

4.2.5   Sand Toe
- Rarer than turf toe
- Plantar-flexion injuries in beach sports
- Reverse pathology – dorsal ST injury, plantar cartilage injury

4.3   Foot and Ankle OCD

4.3.1   Classification: Berndt and Harty (a Radiological Classification)
- Small area of compression
- Partial detached OCD
- Complete detached OCD, not displaced
- Complete detached OCD, displaced

4.3.2   Useful Hints
■ Osteochondral fracture can be anterior or posterior to dome – may even require PF/DF of the ankle to be visible on mortise view
■ If XR negative, consider repeat in 2 to 4 weeks

4.3.3   Other Investigations
■ Bone scan: negative scan rules out the diagnosis
■ Computed tomography (CT)/MRI: may, in fact, give more accurate staging

4.3.4   MRI Classification
■ Articular damage only
■ Cartilage injury and fracture beneath; (a) oedema or (b) no oedema
■ Detached and undisplaced
■ Detached and displaced
■ Subchondral cyst

4.3.5   Aetiology
■ Trauma
■ Idiopathic osteonecrosis

4.3.6   Location and Mechanism
■ Anterolateral: talus impaction when dorsiflexed ankle is forced into inversion; shape of fragment shallow and thinner
■ Posteromedial: talus impaction when plantar-flexed ankle is forced into inversion and ER; deeper and cup shaped (sometimes pain on palpation posterior to medial malleolus)

4.3.7   Treatment
■ Conservative – often involves NWB casting (though no definite evidence that NWB cast gives better result than WB cast and no definite evidence that patients need to be immobilised if they are kept in NWB cast)
■ Operative – frequently needed
   – Stage 1: *k*-wire drilling
   – Stage 2: drilling and/or BG
   – Stage 3 (separated, not displaced): refixation and bone graft (BG)
   – Stage 4 (loose body): r/o loose body and drilling of the crater

4.3.8 Useful Hints

Note: posteromedial lesions are difficult to access. For larger fragments, open reduction and internal fixation (ORIF) may be required with osteotomy of the medial malleolus for exposures (with direct visual and accurate repair). Note also that lesions are usually detectable earlier than with MRI and can be treated with retrograde drilling. In one study published in Arthroscopy, results of *k*-wire were not worse than cancellous BG)

4.4 Tendon Injuries Around the Foot and Ankle

4.4.1 Tibialis Posterior Tendon Dysfunction

4.4.1.1 Aetiology
- Most common cause of acquired adult flat foot
- Possible causes:
  - Pronated foot and lax ligaments increase stress on tibialis posterior tendon (PTT)
  - Inflammatory disorders such as ankylosing spondylitis
  - Intratendinous shear (between tendon fibres, owing to their multiple slips of insertion)
  - Attritional degeneration/rupture
  - Trauma
  - Iatrogenic after steroids

4.4.1.2 Presentation and Assessment
- History: pain, sometimes weakness, noted change in foot shape
- Examination:
  - Too many toe signs (from fore-foot abduction)
  - Local tenderness
  - Pain and/or weakness on resisted plantar flexion and inversion
  - Single leg heel raise test

4.4.1.3 Pathomechanics of Flat Foot Production
- Unopposed pull of peroneals
- Stretched medial ligaments
- Altered pull of tendo-Achilles (TA) lateral to midline

Result is fore-foot abduction, mid-foot pronation and hind-foot valgus

Cxs if untreated: impingement laterally at subtalar level and osteoarthritis (OA) of the subtalar joint

4.4.1.4 XR Assessment
▓ Anteroposterior (AP): may see fore-foot abduction or TNJ subluxation
▓ Lateral: may see mid-foot sagging
▓ Tenography: does not correlate well with operative findings
▓ MRI: only if the diagnosis is in question; not in every patient
▓ Ultrasound: may see size of tendon and changes in echogenicity inside the tendon; cheaper than MRI

4.4.1.5 Clinical Stages
▓ Stage 1: tendinitis, no deformity
▓ Stage 2: tendon degeneration with elongation, flexible deformity
▓ Stage 3: fixed deformity, hind-foot degeneration

4.4.1.6 Management According to Stages
▓ Stage 1: mostly conservative [rest, non-steroidal anti-inflammatory drugs (NSAIDs), TA stretching, PTT strengthening, arch support, even custom ankle foot orthosis or short leg cast]; operate if fails to respond by debridement, augment or repair and/or correct predisposing bony anomalies
▓ Stage 2: conservative means similar; most require tendon augmentation with flexor digitorum longus (FDL)/flexor hallucis longis (FHL), limited fusion (e.g. subtalar or double), and/or calcaneal medial displacement osteotomy/Evans calcaneal lengthening
▓ Stage 3: conservative as above with or without custom-made shoe; OT usually involves a triple fusion

4.4.2   Peroneal Tendon Injuries

4.4.2.1 Pertinent Anatomy
▓ The peroneal groove is, in fact, the fibula groove and there is a rim of cartilage at the lateral border. The depth of the groove is variable
▓ The superior peroneal retinaculum is the primary lateral restraint against peroneal instability; it is parallel to the CFL, hence, those inversion injuries affecting the CFL may injure the retinaculum

▓ The groove is traversed by the peroneal longus and brevis tendons. The brevis tendon lies directly posterior to the lateral malleolus, while the longus is lateral and posterior to the brevis. Both become tendinous prior to reaching the ankle area

4.4.2.2 Types and Sites of Injuries
▓ Common location of injury:
  – Peroneus brevis: mostly at level of fibular groove
  – Peroneus longus: more often at the cuboid tunnel
▓ Types of possible injuries:
  – Tendinosis/tenosynovitis
  – Rupture/split
  – Dislocation/subluxation

4.4.2.3 Common Mechanism
▓ Forced dorsiflexion while the ankle is in pushing off posture
▓ Ruptures/splints of the peroneal tendons likely to be underdiagnosed

4.4.2.4 Clinical Assessment
▓ History of inversion ankle sprain
▓ Resultant ankle pain and tenderness on the lateral side
▓ May be pain on clinical stretching or resisted eversion with or without weakness
▓ Tendons may be subluxable, as a click/pop on eversion against resistance
▓ One cause of recurrent ankle sprains with a negative anterior drawer test

4.4.2.5 Investigations
▓ XR: may see the fleck sign of avulsion from the posterior fibula; assess for talar osteochondral fragment
▓ MRI: good to delineate tendons; reveals intra-tendinous pathology
▓ Ultrasound: may reveal cases with possible subluxation that are not certain after examination or tendon rupture
▓ Tenography: seldom used

4.4.2.6 Conservative Treatment

- NSAID, rest, cast immobilisation, lateral heel wedge, peroneal strengthening exercises
- Cast for 4–6 weeks if presents with subluxation/dislocation; less useful if chronic on presentation

4.4.2.7 Role of Surgery

- Debridement and tenosynovectomy for tenosynovitis
- Side-to-side suture for splints
- If one tendon ruptured, may tenodese to remaining tendon; if both are ruptured, may need FHL/FDL transfer
- Subluxators: first check hind-foot alignment and assess the integrity of the lateral ankle ligament, especially the CFL; repair the superior retinaculum; may need to deepen the groove (bone block procedures have also been used)

  (Peroneus longus injuries near the cuboid tunnel may need CT for pre-operative assessment)

4.4.3   Acute Rupture of Achilles Tendon

4.4.3.1 Features of the Achilles Tendon

- A zone of relative poor vascularity is located 4–5 cm from the site of bony insertion
- The fibres of the tendon undergo a twist before insertion, causing the zone to be even under more stress
- Most normal physiological loads will produce a strain of less than 4%. At strains between 4% and 8%, the collagen fibres start to slide past one another and the inter-molecular cross-links fail. At strains greater than 8%, macroscopic ruptures occur

4.4.3.2 Location of Rupture

- The typical patient is a middle-aged weekend athlete. The most usual sites in these individuals is at 3–5 cm from the site of insertion
- Young and active athletes may rupture at the musculotendinous junction

4.4.3.3 Mechanisms of Injury
- Pushing off with the WB fore-foot while extending the knee (e.g. sprinting and jumping sports)
- Sudden unexpected dorsiflexion of the ankle
- Violent dorsiflexion of a plantar-flexed foot
  It can be seen that eccentric loading is an important mode of tendon failure, especially if the loading is obliquely oriented

4.4.3.4 Possible Predisposing Factors
- Previous steroid injection may weaken the tendon. It is suggested to avoid sports for 2 weeks after a recent steroid injection to the Achilles tendon
- Superimposition on a setting of repeated microtears, as in wearing inappropriate sports shoes that force the hind-foot into pronation as the heel strikes the ground, creating a whipping action of the Achilles tendon that can cause intratendinous microtears
- Other factors have been discussed, e.g. a region of relative hypovascularity and collagen degeneration. In addition, Sculco had proposed that possible malfunction or suppression of the proprioceptive elements of the skeletal muscle may play a role in some athletes

4.4.3.5 Clinical Features
- Sudden pain/give, usually during sports, as if the tendon was being kicked
- Weakness in plantar flexion
- Examination usually reveals a gap and a positive Simmond's test
- If the diagnosis is not sure, may consider ultrasound ± MRI

4.4.3.6 Goal of Treatment
- Not only to heal the tendon; but to avoid lengthening

4.4.3.7 Treatment Options
- Conservative: 6–8 weeks casting
- Open repair
- Percutaneous repair: only provides 50% of the initial repair strength of open repair and the chance of sural nerve damage is not low; only advantages include cosmesis and keeping the usually intact paratenon untouched

4.4.3.8 The Case for Operative Repair

- There is a lower re-rupture rate. In a recent paper analysing the literature from 1959 to 1997, Lo found that the overall rate of re-rupture was 3% with open repair versus 12% with conservative treatment
- Notice the aim of treatment to avoid lengthening the tendon cannot be easily achieved by conservative means. Healing with the tendon lengthened may cause functional disability later on, especially in an athletic individual

4.4.3.9 Operative Options

- Direct repair: suffices in most cases, except those found to have too high tension, or in delayed cases; no evidence to argue for routine augmentation in the setting of a fresh rupture
- Other choices: Lindholm augmentation, Lynn's plantaris augmentation, etc.

4.4.4 Achilles Tendinitis/Tendinosis and Management of Chronic Ruptures

4.4.4.1 Terminology

- Tendinosis: intratendinous degeneration. Seems to relate to overuse injury. High signal on T2 of MRI. Treatment with physiotherapy and bracing
- Paratendinitis: inflammatory cells in the paratenon. Presents with pain, swelling, etc.
- Paratendinitis with tendinosis
  (Note: presence of posterior heel mass is different from a nodule at the lower TA that is sometimes palpable with tendinosis. Common causes: Haglund's deformity and posterior spur. Another differential diagnosis is a bursa, but softer in consistency)

4.4.4.2 Chronic TA Ruptures

4.4.4.2.1 Clinical Features

- Palpable gap due to contraction and fibrosis of the triceps surae, e.g. in neglected cases
- Palpable tender mass in the tendon

4.4.4.2.2 Operative Indications
- Loss of effective plantar flexion
- Chronic pain

4.4.4.2.3 Operative Choices
- Using autologous tissue for repair: plantaris, turndown of proximal Achilles tendon tissue
- Augmentation: usually FHL
- Via transfer of muscles: plantaris, peroneus brevis, FDL, FHL
- Synthetic materials: polymer carbon fibres, dacron graft and mesh (Keep in short leg cast in 20° plantar flexion for 4 weeks post-operatively and use a heel-lift afterwards)

4.5 Hallux Valgus and Lesser Toes Deformity

4.5.1 Hallux Valgus (Fig. 4.1)

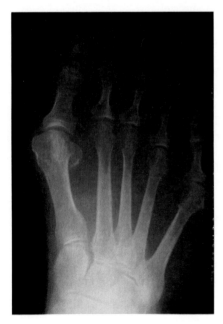

Fig. 4.1. Hallux valgus of the right foot

4.5.1.1 Introduction

- Hallux valgus (HV) is **not** a single disorder. It represents a complex deformity of the first ray that is frequently accompanied by deformity and symptoms of the lesser toes
- Elements of HV that may occur:
  - First MT varus deformity
  - Big toe in valgus
  - Bunion
  - OA of the first MTPJ, occasionally
  - Hammer toe, usually the second toe
  - Corns, calluses and transfer metatarsalgia

4.5.1.2 Predisposing Factors for the Production of HV

- Genu valgum with pronation of feet
- Pes planus
- Increased obliquity of the first MT-cuneiform joint
- Long first ray
- Excess valgus tilt of the articular surface of the first MT head [and proximal phalanx (P/P) articular surface]
- External factors: most important is shoe wear
  (Note: among the different factors, lateral deviation of the big toe is found to be most significant, although metatarsus primus varus may be an important factor in adolescents)

4.5.1.3 Pathomechanics of HV

- Increased HV angle at first MTPJ (especially greater than 35°) → pronation of first ray → abductor hallucis moves in plantar direction, i.e. medial capsular ligament as the only medial restraint → HV increases from unopposed adductor hallucis → MT head drifts medially from the sesamoid. The lateral sesamoid is displaced into the first MT space
- Valgus of big toe usually creates hammer of the second toe

4.5.1.4 Clinical Assessment

- Assessing the presence of symptoms (usually pain) and the exact location of pain is important, since not every patient with HV needs surgery
- Physical assessment is very important

- Overall limb alignment and the exact sites of tenderness
- Assess not only the fore-foot, but the mid-foot and hind-foot alignment and ROM
- Assess abnormal pressure areas, calluses, ulcers, pattern of shoe wear and WB and NWB posture
- Fore-foot: degree of valgus of big toe, any HV interphalangeus, degree of pronation of the first ray and status of the bunion. Any deformity of the lesser toes, such as hammer toe, claw toe, and the relative lengths
- Others: vascular status, neurological status

4.5.1.5 Radiological Assessment
▦ Weight-bearing AP and lateral ± sesamoid view
▦ Assess the following angles:
- HV angle normally less than $15°$
- Inter-MT angle normally less than $9°$
- DMAA (distal MT articular angle): angle of line bisecting MT shaft with line through base of distal articular cartilage cap (normal is between $10°$ and $15°$)
- Hallux phalangeus angle: angle between long axes of big toe P/P and distal phalanx bisecting their diaphysis (normally less than $8°$)
- Also assess the degree of congruency of the first MTPJ and any degenerative changes; any overall splaying of the foot should be noted

4.5.1.6 Options of Management
▦ Conservative: rarely successful
▦ Operative: many procedures reported; careful selection needed

4.5.1.6.1 Common Operative Options
▦ Chevron distal first MT osteotomy
▦ Proximal first MT osteotomy
▦ First MTPJ fusion
▦ Keller's excision arthroplasty
▦ Others

4.5.1.6.2 Chevron Osteotomy

- Indications:
  - Mild or moderate HV
  - Inter-MT angle less than 15°
  - HV angle less than 35°
  - Passive correctable
  - Minimal first ray pronation
    Advantage: quicker healing
    Disadvantages: AVN and cannot correct severe deformity
    Pearl: avoid performing concomitant lateral release since increases AVN chance

4.5.1.6.3 Proximal First MT Osteotomy

- Indications: always performed with lateral release and medial reefing
  - Inter-MT angle greater than 13°
  - Can tackle incongruent joints
  - Lots of potential for correction; but avoid varus
- Contraindications:
  - Small inter-MT angle (use lesser procedure)
  - OA of first MTPJ
  - Spastic cases (e.g. diplegic cerebral palsy where fusion is needed)
  - Increased DMAA
- Types
  - Crescentic: used by most surgeons
  - Others: e.g. closed/open wedge, etc.
- Complications:
  - Non-union
  - Mal-union (e.g. dorsiflexion)
  - Under-correction
  - Over-correction
  - Shortening
  - Transfer metatarsalgia

4.5.1.6.4 Keller's Operation
- A resection hemi-arthroplasty of the first MTPJ with removal of medial eminence
- Indications:
  - The typical candidate is a low-demand elderly with greater than 40–50° HV angle but inter-MT angle of less than 13°; incongruency of joint with degenerative changes and pronated first ray
- Complications:
  - Cock-up deformity, wound problems, hallux varus, etc.
- Salvage: first MTPJ fusion

4.5.1.6.5 Other Procedures
- Lapidus procedure
- Akin procedure
- Procedure for correcting abnormal DMAA
  (Note: first MTPJ fusion is a salvage procedure for HV surgery and first MTPJ OA)

4.5.2   Lesser Toe Deformity

4.5.2.1 Types of Lesser Toe Deformities
- Hammer toe: contracture (flexible or fixed) at proximal interphalangeal joint (PIPJ)
- Claw toe: contracture (flexible/fixed) at PIPJ with contracture (flexible/fixed) at MTPJ
- Mallet toe: contracture (flexible/fixed) at dorsal interphalangeal joint (DIPJ)

4.5.2.2 General Comments
- Most are acquired from improper footwear, but are sometimes acquired from muscle imbalance between the intrinsic muscles (lumbricals/interossei) and extrinsic muscles (FDL/FDB, EDL/EDB)
- Clinical and radiological assessments include other fore-foot deformities, especially HV (common cause of hammer), and the overall alignment of the fore-foot, mid-foot and hind-foot. Overall lower limb alignment is checked, as well as the neurovascular status and pressure points

4.5.2.2.1 Hammer Toe

▦ Most commonly due to either HV or fore-foot pressure from tight high-heeled shoes. More often in ladies. Can be flexible/rigid. Flexible ones mostly from FDL over-pull

▦ Conservative treatment: shoe with high toe-box, cushions and custom orthosis

▦ Operative treatment:
  – Flexible: transfer distal end of FDL to base of P/P; *k*-wire to realign the toe
  – Rigid: Du Vries arthroplasty (resect distal condyles at flare of P/P) if there is still high tension after resection, and/or flexor release. If MTPJ with residual hyper-extension, consider MTPJ capsulotomy, release collateral and lengthen/release the extensor tendon

4.5.2.2.2 Special Case

▦ Elderly with severe HV and rigid cross-over hammer toe can consider second toe amputation if it is deemed that it will fail to tolerate major reconstruction

4.5.2.2.3 Mallet Toe

▦ Mostly from shoe pressure, especially in a relatively long toe in ladies. Common to have callus formation at DIPJ dorsum

▦ Conservative: high toe-box shoe and/or orthosis

▦ Operative:
  – Flexible: FDL tenotomy
  – Rigid: resect distal condyle of M/P, FDL release, and/or plantar capsulotomy and *k*-wire fixation

4.5.2.2.4 Claw Toe

▦ Main Feature is hyper-extension of either flexible or fixed MTPJ (with associated PIPJ deformity); main symptom is metatarsalgia from pressure put on the MT head by the extended P/P

▦ Cause: seriously rule out any neuromuscular disorder (e.g. Charcot-Marie-Tooth). diabetes mellitus (DM), connective tissue disease

▦ Conservative: high toe-box shoe, custom orthosis for the frequently associated overall foot deformity (pes cavus with varus heel)

■ Operative treatment for claw toes:
- Flexible: again transfer of the long flexor. Residual MTPJ extension, if present, needs dorsal capsular release and tenotomy of the extensor
- Rigid: either or both MTPJ or PIPJ can be rigid. First perform Du Vries to correct the PIPJ, followed by MTPJ dorsal capsular release, collateral release and tenotomy of extensor including *k*-wire for stabilisation of the repair

4.5.3   Bunionettes
4.5.3.1 Types of Bunionettes
■ Enlargement of the fifth MT head
■ Lateral bowing of the fifth MT
■ Widened inter-MT angle between the fourth and fifth ray

4.5.3.2 Operative Options
■ Indications: for pain and deformity, and if conservative treatment fails
■ Type 1: use Chevron type osteotomy
■ Type 2: use mid-shaft oblique osteotomy
■ Type 3: use mid-shaft oblique osteotomy

4.6   Common Adult Foot Deformities and Management

4.6.1   Biomechanical Considerations
■ Only adult pes planus and pes cavus will be covered
■ The nature of these deformities were discussed in the section on paediatric orthopaedics and will not be repeated here
■ Following is a discussion of the underlying biomechanical changes and the rationale behind some of the more often used osteotomies

4.6.2   Adult Pes Planus (Fig. 4.2)
■ Aetiology:
- Tibialis posterior dysfunction
- TNJ capsular injuries
- Post-traumatic

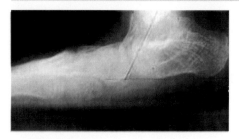

Fig. 4.2. Pes planus

■ Major surgical options (not mutually exclusive):
  - Tibialis posterior reconstruction
  - TNJ imbrication
  - Calcaneal medial displacement osteotomy
  - Evans lateral column lengthening
  - Subtalar arthrodesis
  - Triple arthrodesis

4.6.2.1 Biomechanics of Adult Pes Planus

■ The reader should understand the determinants of the normal medial longitudinal arch (Last's Anatomy)
■ In the normal foot during gait, there is a mechanical transition of a flexible foot during foot flat to a more rigid lever arm or platform at push-off
■ In moderate or severe flat feet, this does not occur. Instead, there is abnormal mid-foot dorsiflexion at the push-off (heel-off) phase occurring in the unlocked transverse tarsal joint. The second result of this change is that loss of the normally obligatory ankle dorsiflexion causes the triceps surae to contract, locking the hind-foot in valgus and making matters worse

4.6.2.2 Compensatory Changes

■ Given a valgus hind-foot, the foot attempts to become plantigrade at foot flat; the fore-foot has to be in some varus (relative to the hind-foot)

4.6.2.3 Clinical Application

- Having understood the biomechanics and compensatory changes led us to understand how to properly perform a triple in these subjects
- Simply correcting the hind-foot alignment from gross valgus to 5° valgus *without* due regard to the fore-foot can result in tilting of the talus after triple arthrodesis and rapid ankle degeneration from asymmetric surface loading of the ankle.
- Correction should be effected by everting the fore-foot through de-rotation of the transverse tarsal joint of Chopart prior to fixation. An occasional case of fore-foot correction may require plantar flexion of the first ray to re-establish the tripod of the foot. To this end, fusion of the first TMTJ may be required

4.6.3   Adult Pes Cavus (Figs. 4.3, 4.4)

- Many cases of pes cavus are associated with neuromuscular disorders, such as the Charchot-Marie-Tooth disease (Fig. 4.5). Common types include:
  - Calcaneocavus: a situation where the most prominent feature is an increase in calcaneal pitch. This is usually seen in disorders like poliomyelitis and spina bifida
  - Pes cavus with a plantar flexed first MT (though a handful of cases have more symmetric plantar flexion of all MT); this is the more common situation

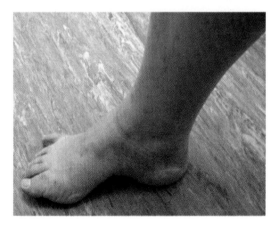

Fig. 4.3. Pes cavus foot – note the exaggerated medial arch

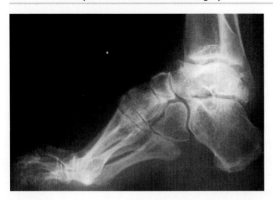

Fig. 4.4. X-ray of patient pes cavus

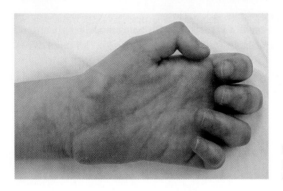

Fig. 4.5. Hand of a patient with Charcot-Marie-Foot

4.6.3.1 Compensatory Mechanisms

- With a significantly plantar flexed first MT, in order for the foot to become plantigrade, there will be obligatory hind-foot varus
- The result is that heel inversion in early foot flat causes lateral foot overload and other Cxs such as peroneal tendinitis, insufficiency of the lateral ankle ligaments and stress fracture of the fifth MT

4.6.3.2 Management

- Conservative: biomechanical orthosis to reduce the stress on the lateral foot
- Operative:
  - If plantar flexed first ray and flexible hind-foot as assessed by the Coleman Block test (Fig. 4.6): dorsiflexion osteotomy of first

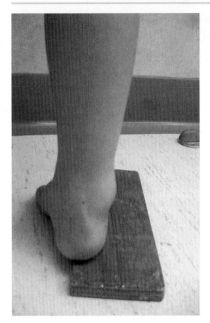

Fig. 4.6. The Coleman Block test

(± other) ray, muscle rebalancing by tendon transfers (e.g. pero-neus longus to brevis) and release of plantar fascia
- Above, and not totally correctable hind-foot: consider calcaneal os-teotomy
- Rigid pes cavus:
  May need a triple arthrodesis if the hind-foot is fixed in varus.
  Caution: when the varus hind-foot is corrected, the fore-foot is locked in varus; the talus must tilt for the foot to become planti-grade, resulting in ankle joint overload and OA

4.6.3.3 Appendix: Medial Displacement Calcaneal Osteotomy
▦ Indications:
- Severe tibialis posterior dysfunction
- Moderate to severe pes planovalgus
- Coronal plane hind-foot malalignment
▦ Contraindications:
- Normal hind-foot alignment

- – Advanced fixed pes planovalgus
- – Nearby OA of subtalar or TNJ
- – Fixed fore-foot abduction
- Advantages:
  - – Reduces valgus moment on medial mid/hind-foot STs
  - – Restoration of the arch
  - – No need for BG
  - – No effect on hind-foot motion
- Disadvantages:
  - – Common sural nerve injury
  - – Cast immobilisation and NWB needed

4.7   Degenerative Arthritis of the Foot and Ankle: Ankle Degenerative Arthritis

- Causes:
  - – OA
  - – Rheumatoid arthritis (RA)
  - – Old sepsis
  - – Post-traumatic
  - – Secondary to congenital foot deformity
  - – Secondary to neuromuscular diseases
  - – Secondary to previous foot or ankle surgery
  - – Secondary to advanced dysfunction of the tibialis posterior

4.7.1   Clinical Assessment
- Patient occupation, expectations and goal of treatment
- Pain level and precipitating factors
- Exact location of the pain and tenderness, as pain may arise from joints other than the tibio-talar articulation
- Gross lower limb alignment, any flexible/fixed deformities of the hind-foot, mid-foot and fore-foot
- XR assessment including WB views

4.7.2   Conservative Treatment
- NSAID
- Viscosupplementation

▦ Orthosis/brace
▦ Activity modification

4.7.3   Operative Options
▦ Arthrodesis (Fig. 4.7)
▦ Ankle arthroplasty (despite the different models available, not versatile enough to cater for severe deformity and revisions are difficult). Further discussion is beyond the scope of this book
▦ Distraction arthroplasty (based on the hypothesis that osteoarthritic cartilage, especially of the ankle, retains some reparative activity when there is concomitant release of mechanical stress and maintenance of intra-articular intermittent fluid pressure)
▦ Distal tibial osteotomy (only in the rarer case of distal tibia vara)

4.7.3.1 Position of the Ankle Arthrodesis
▦ Neutral dorsiflexion (a few degrees plantar flexion for wearers of high heels)
▦ 5° heel valgus
▦ No medial-lateral translation
▦ ER degree equal to the contralateral unaffected limb
(P.S. May accept mild shortening, slight posterior displacement of talus on the distal tibia (thereby increasing the moment arm of triceps surae) as proposed by some)

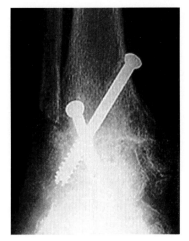

Fig. 4.7. Right ankle after ankle fusion

4.7.3.2 Methods of Ankle Arthrodesis

- Open arthrodesis: via, e.g. intra-articular BG, malleolar osteotomy, Blair's anterior tibial slide, compression arthrodesis of Charnley
- Less invasive methods:
  - Arthroscopic methods (not used if in the presence of ankle malalignment)
  - Mini-arthrotomy method (similar disadvantage)

4.7.3.3 Special Preference of Type of Ankle Arthrodesis in Relation to Underlying Aetiology

- AVN: Blair preferred
- Sepsis: external fixation; Charnley-type preferred
- Massive bone loss: needs special centre, as bone transport may be needed

4.7.3.4 Cxs of Ankle Fusion

- Non-union (common causes: AVN, smoking, sepsis, open fracture, alcoholism, DM/CRF)
- Mal-union
- Infection
- Stress transfer to more distal foot joints
- Stress fracture
- Nerve injury

4.7.3.5 Fusion of Other Foot Articulations and Their Indications

4.7.3.5.1 Triple Arthrodesis

- Indications:
  - Resistant congenital or neuromuscular foot conditions
  - Post-traumatic
  - Severe flat foot
  - Tarsal coalition with degenerative arthritis
- Contraindications:
  - Skeletal immaturity
  - Same pathology can be tackled by other lesser procedures, since long-term result after a triple is fair with much stress and hence possible arthrosis of adjacent joints
    (Those cases with associated significant ankle valgus tilt may need a concomitant calcaneal osteotomy)

Clinical Effect of Triple Arthrodesis
- Motion limitation for dorsiflexion and plantar flexion
- Motion limitation for inversion and eversion
- Much more stress, especially on the ankle joint after triple arthrodesis

Cxs of Triple Arthrodesis
- Ankle OA
- Ankle instability
- Mal-union
- Non-union

4.7.3.5.2 Subtalar Arthrodesis
- Indications:
  - Selected communited calcaneal fracture
  - Isolated subtalar OA
  - Selected cases of tarsal coalition (affecting middle facet)
  - Severe flexible flat foot
    Types: in situ versus bone block

4.7.3.5.3 Arthrodesis of Lisfranc Joint
- Indications:
  - Primary arthritis (most fuse only second, third and/or first rays, and leave fourth and fifth mobile)
  - RA
  - Post-traumatic
  - Some Charchot joints
  Complications:
- Non-union
- Mal-union – may cause secondary MT stress fracture, and metatarsalgia from the increase in stress
- Wound problems

4.7.3.5.4 First MTPJ Arthrodesis
- Indications:
  - Advanced HV with arthrosis
  - Salvage of hallux surgery
  - Hallux rigidus
  - Gout

- Inflammatory diseases
- Salvage of Helal
- Neuromuscular disorders, e.g. sometimes in diplegic cerebral palsy

Position of Arthrodesis
- 10–15° valgus
- 5–10° relative to ground in sagittal plane
- Neutral rotation (avoid pronation)

Complications
- Non-union: 10%
- Mal-union: too much dorsiflexion causes corn up deformity; too little causes difficulty with toe-off and hyper-extension/possible arthrosis of interphalangeal joint (IPJ)
- IPJ degeneration: predisposed by trans-articular pinning, not enough dorsiflexion and valgus

4.8   The Diabetic Foot

4.8.1   Introduction: Topics to Be Covered
- Neuroarthropathy and Charcot joint
- DM foot ulceration

4.8.2   DM Neuroarthropathy (Fig. 4.8)
- Definition: chronic destructive arthropathy of one or more articulations that develops as a result of DM neuropathy
- Unrelated to the severity and type of DM
- If not treated properly, may result in amputation

4.8.2.1 Aetiology
- 'Neurovascular' theory: autonomic dysfunction causes increased arteriovenous shunting and increased blood flow with resultant bone resorption
- 'Neurotraumatic' theory: joint with abnormal sensation can be subjected to repeated trauma, however minor, leading to joint destruction
- Abnormal glycosylation of proteins in DM may alter the mechanical properties of connective tissues such as collagen leading to breakdown

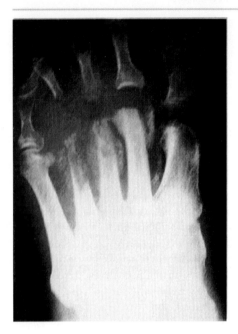

Fig. 4.8. Charchot type changes in a woman's foot

4.8.2.2 Stages of Development of Charchot (After Eichenholtz)
■ Stage 1: stage of development – featured by capsular distension with subluxation, bone and cartilage fragmentation, and much debris
■ Stage 2: stage of coalescence – featured by adherence and coalescence of bone fragments, absorption of debris and sclerotic bone ends
■ Stage 3: stage of reconstruction – featured by rounding and less sclerotic bone ends and attempts at reformation of the joint architecture

4.8.2.3 Sites of Involvement (After Brodsky)
■ Type I: NCJ and TMTJ affected
■ Type II: any or all of TNJ/CCJ/subtalar
■ Type IIIA: ankle (tibiotalar joint) affected
■ Type IIIB: fracture posterior tubercle of calcaneus with possible widened heel and pes planus

4.8.2.4 Diagnosis and Differential Diagnosis

- A combination of clinical and radiological parameters is needed for diagnosis and/or other investigations
- However, clinical findings can be difficult to differentially diagnose from infection, and sometimes a bone scan is needed to differentiate. Also, infection commonly leads to sudden loss of glycaemic control; infection without violation of the skin integrity is rare and unlikely
- It is also difficult to differentially diagnose a fracture associated with acute neuropathic collapse from an acute fracture in the patient with neuropathy

4.8.2.5 Principles of Management

- Prevention of recurrent ulcer and amputation is essential
- Patient education – he needs to actively participate in salvage of his own limb
- Protection from repeated injury is essential, mainly by casting, bracing and restricted WB. Total contact casting is contraindicated if there is peripheral vascular insufficiency. However, Charcot foot rarely occurs in any foot with a poor blood supply
- Selected cases sometimes need supplementary fixation to ensure maintenance of relative joint position and healing. Longer term immobilisation may be necessary to guide against late loss of fixation

4.8.2.6 Management Strategies with Different Brodsky Types

- Type 1: mid-foot affected. Most mid-foot neuropathic arthropathies can be treated conservatively by total contact casting and/or osteotomy only if there is severe deformity or instability
- Type 2: subtalar/transverse tarsal. Peritalar dislocation is mostly managed surgically. A properly performed triple will protect the foot from valgus collapse with or without TA lengthening
- Type 3: tibiotalar joint affected. Since this deformity is usually secondary to deformity/collapse of the mid-foot/subtalar joints, treatment is based on proper realignment of the foot. If a plantigrade foot can be attained, try to avoid fusion of the ankle

4.8.3   DM Foot Ulceration

▦ Factors in Aetiology
  - Abnormal pressure distribution (mechanical factors)
  - Neuropathy
  - Other factors: vasculopathy (especially small vessel disease), metabolic factors, etc.
    (An independent risk factor is history of DM foot ulcer)

4.8.3.1 Mechanical Factors

▦ Joint stiffness: the joint capsule stiffens from glycosylation of collagen. Loss of motion results in increased pressure/abnormal pressure distribution during gait

▦ Claw toes: possibly from motor denervation of the intrinsics. The result of clawing is that the MT fat pads are displaced distally, which uncovers the MT heads and concentrates pressure

▦ Tight TA has been under-estimated as a cause all along, but many ulcers heal after lengthening of a tight TA

▦ Cracking of skin and callosity: dry, cracked skin results from autonomic neuropathy. Also, the abundant calluses formed act as a 'foreign body' inside the shoe with unequal pressure distribution

▦ Changes in the body architecture/collapse and deformity from an associated neuroarthropathy may be contributory

4.8.3.2 Effect of Neuropathy

▦ Effect of Autonomic Dysfunction:
  - Plantar pressure during stance is usually high and exceeds capillary pressure. Even normal feet have difficulty perfusing all plantar tissues during stance and depend on perfusion at the short breaks of swing phase. Autonomic dysfunction causes abnormal auto-regulation and the vessels may not open fast enough in swing. Other effects mentioned are lack of sweating, dry and cracked skin and callosity formation

▦ Effect of sensory neuropathy: altered protective sensation predisposes to repeated injury and ulceration

▦ Effect of motor neuropathy: atrophy of foot mechanics leads to clawing and pressure increase under MT heads

4.8.3.3 Vascular Disturbances

▥ Ankle brachial index less than 0.45 is suggestive of significant disease
▥ Toe pressures of 50–60 mmHg are required for ulcer healing
▥ Transcutaneous oxygen greater than 30 mmHg is indicative of adequate blood flow
▥ Macrovascular disease is believed by some authorities not to have a major role in either pressure ulceration or neuroarthropathy
▥ Microvascular disease with basement membrane thickening, endothelial cell hypertrophy and increased capillary fragility are more important factors

4.8.3.4 Metabolic Factors

▥ Serum protein greater than 6.2 g/dl
▥ Serum albumin greater than 3.5 g/dl
▥ Lymphocyte count greater than 1500/mm^2
   In general, all are needed for proper healing

4.8.3.5 Wagner Classification

▥ Grade 0: callus only; no ulcer
▥ Grade 1: only superficial ulceration
▥ Grade 2: deep ulcer; exposed tendon/joint
▥ Grade 3: localised osteomyelitis
▥ Grade 4: gangrene of fore-foot
▥ Grade 5: gangrene of entire foot
   (In addition, take serial photographs and document exact size and depth of ulcer)

4.8.3.5.1 Role of Total Contact Casting

▥ Indications:
   – Grade 1–2 plantar ulcers
   – Width greater than depth of the ulcer
   – Adequate blood supply
▥ Contraindications:
   – Heel ulcers
   – Infected ulcer
   – Greater than or equal to grade 3 ulceration
   – Ulcer depth greater than width; fragile skin
   – Significant swelling and non-compliance

▥ Treatment rationale:
- – Decrease plantar pressure over the ulcer – decreases oedema and shear stresses
- – Protect ulcer

4.8.3.5.2 Other Surgical Options Sometimes Used
▥ Osteotomy of first MT; sometimes dorsiflexion osteotomy for first MT head ulcer
▥ Achilles lengthening
▥ Cheilectomy – resection of bony prominence
▥ Keller procedure for severe HV
▥ Procedures for lesser toe deformities

4.8.3.5.3 Pharmacological Manipulation
▥ Growth factor treatment: e.g. recombinant PDGF or cultured human fibroblasts
▥ Hyperbaric oxygen: need systemic application in a chamber
▥ Aldose reductase inhibitors: treat somatic neuropathy
▥ Drugs used to treat painful sensory neuropathy: gabapentine (stabilises neuronal membrane), tricyclics (central effect), etc.
▥ Future: c-peptide (improves autonomic dysfunction), inhibitors of glycosylation end-products

4.8.3.5.4 Prevention
▥ Patient education
▥ Prophylactic and meticulous care

4.9   Rheumatoid Foot

4.9.1   Comparison Between RA Feet and RA Hands
▪ Like the hand, feet anomalies are also common and frequently have initial presenting symptoms and signs
▪ Deformities of the toes and big toe are very common (just like the not uncommon finger deformities), if only because the fore-foot serves as a platform for push-off in walking/WB; notice that big toe deformity can be predisposed by foot pronation and valgus heel, whereas knee valgus can predispose to heel/ankle valgus posture (and sometimes possibly the other way round)

4.9.2   Natural History and Pathology

- Vainio review of 1000 cases: 80–90% with feet involved
- Spigel found that 65% had synovitis in the first 1–3 years; down to 18% at 10 years
- Ankle joint found by Spigel to be the least involved WB joint, but some synovitis does occur in 60% if followed long enough (around 10 years; down to 35% at 40 years)

4.9.3   General Comments

- While tarsal joints have a tendency to fuse spontaneously, the ankle joint does not and may be spared until later
- If the ankle joint is indeed diseased, the tarsal joints will already be as well, or will follow suit quickly
- The ankle, however, is usually quite significantly initially affected in JGA; also, degenerative OA will develop if the subtalar adopts a valgus (varus) posture with an increase in point pressure contact
- Significant valgus can cause talo-navicular dislocation/subluxation and WB on talar head and also will predispose to fracture of the malleoli, etc.

4.9.4   General Comments and Pearls

- Although most patients can still be treated conservatively, when it comes to surgery, most OTs are fore-foot surgeries, outnumbering that of hind- or mid-foot surgeries by 4–5 times
- Effect of proximal joints: patients with fixed flexion deformity of the hip and especially knees are predisposed to a disordered ankle with more DF than PF. However, in patients for whom knee extension is possible, equinus at the ankle sometimes develops (especially after a period of recumbency for medical reasons), which adds loading to the fore-foot

4.9.5   Pathomechanics of RA Foot Deformities (Figs. 4.9, 4.10)

- In the normal fore-foot, it provides a platform for push-off in walking and contributes to balance, especially when standing still
- The hallux plays a dominant role; the remaining toes make a significant contribution so that the fore-foot can be viewed as a single functional unit

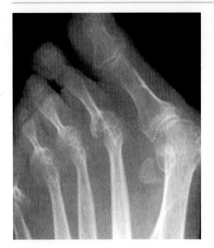

Fig. 4.9. Rheumatoid arthritis affecting the left foot

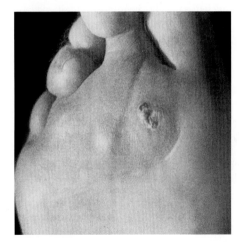

Fig. 4.10. Pressure sore at the metatarsal head in a Rheumatoid arthritic patient with forefoot disease

■ The fore-foot is splayed in RA, partly due to MTPJ synovitis that predisposes to HV. However, so does foot pronation 2° to heel valgus (sometimes itself 2° to knee valgus) and sometimes metatarsus primus valgus (IMA increased). Lax capsule and ligaments are also contributory

▨ The dorsiflexion force of walking (sometimes worsened by ankle equinus) with lax joint structure causes MT head herniates through plantar capsule, more distal position of plantar fat pad, callosities and dorsal joint subluxation and is worsened by imbalance of intrinsic and extrinsic muscles (hammer toe common, sometimes DIP also flexes, clawed toes; but swan-neck posture is rare)

4.9.6   General Treatment Principles

▨ Be sure there are no contraindications such as in acute flare of disease, vasculitis, poor general health (may need to step down steroid ± stop MTX 1 week before and 2 weeks after OT)
▨ Timing: avoid bilateral sequential (better to rely on the non-operated foot to ambulate) and concomitant upper limb and lower limb OT. If both fore- and hind-foot are deformed and painful, some experts advise to correct hind-foot first, since fore-foot deformities may recur in patients with significant pronation and valgus deformity of the hind-foot. Tackling ulcer, infected nail, etc. is minor, and it may be wise to first lower the sepsis rate. ST surgery should only be performed in early disease and may not last
▨ Total ankle is *only currently* for the subgroup with severe bilateral disease, where, if both ankles are fused in the presence of bilateral tarsal ankylosis and fused big toe, the knee is the most distal mobile joint – a severe handicap when attempting to arise from a chair or toilet seat. Here, a unilateral TKA is best indicated

4.9.7   Pathomechanics in the Causation of Fore-, Mid-
and Hind-Foot Disease

▨ Synovitis: distended capsule, lax ligament, bony destruction
▨ Enzyme bony destruction
▨ Muscle imbalance between intrinsics and extrinsics
▨ Stress of walking and of shoeing
▨ Duration and disease severity

4.9.8   Common Symptoms

▨ Walking on 'stones'
▨ Pain: fore-foot most common; if subtalar, sometimes near sinus tarsi; sometimes in TNJ distal to medial malleolus; ankle joint (seems to be in between both malleoli) – do not forget stress fracture whether or not referred

- Weakness: general or localised, e.g. with resisted eversion (peronei) or resisted plantar flexion in inversion/single heel raise (tibialis posterior), etc.
- Instability
- Ulceration and callosities
- ± Cosmesis

4.9.9 Other Points in the History

- Duration, activity, medical adequacy
- Other joints
- ADL and ambulation
- Symptoms of Cx, e.g. carpal tunnel syndrome (CTS) or tarsal tunnel syndrome (TTS)

4.9.10 Physical Assessment

- Fore-foot; description of deformity, i.e. whether it is passively correctable, callosity (plantar aspect of second/third MT head common, bunion, splay, HV, sometimes cog-up, toe overlap, hammer/claw toes common, if hammer callosity at tip and IPJ), ulcers, web space
- Mid-foot: loss of medial arch, mobility of TMTJ, subluxation, e.g. of TNJ
- Hind-foot: ST swelling along course of tendons (especially tibialis posterior/peronei), local tenderness/oedema, tenderness at sinus tarsi/TA insert/plantar fascia, TTS; check for heel valgus by measuring standing tibio-calcaneal angle
- Do not forget the knee/hip, upper limb, spine or other system
- General lower limb alignment
- Neurovascular status of both feet

4.9.11 Checking Motion and Gait

- Shoe wear and back of shoe, footprint, toe-box
- If prosthesis is available for patient, whether it can accommodate the deformity without undue pressure (P.S. prosthesis not meant to correct the deformity)
- Gait

4.9.12 Radiological Assessment

▦ Standing AP/oblique and WB lateral views are useful. Look for any deformities just mentioned, bony erosions, etc.

▦ Look for any ankle valgus in standing AP

▦ The occasional patient may have stress fracture as the cause of pain in the foot and ankle area

4.9.13 Conservative Treatment

▦ Optimise medical treatment of RA, which is a systemic disease

▦ Orthosis may be helpful, e.g. medial arch support for early pes planus or MT padding for clawed toes with painful callosities at the MT heads

4.9.14 Goal of Surgery

▦ Pain relief

▦ Prevention of deformity or correction of deformity (by treating its cause, if possible, and effect)

▦ Restore/preserve function

▦ Sometimes treatment for ulcers with or without cosmesis
Aim of surgery to change contour to wear usual shoes and correct deformity and pressure points/ulcers, not to reconstruct a normal foot
Try conservative first in terms of pain killers, RA control, arch support and foot orthosis

4.9.15 A Word About ST Surgery

▦ Tenosynovectomy and synovectomy: joint/tendon decompression, prevention of further cartilage/ligament/tendon damage, pain relief good – but not long-lasting; sometimes combined with other procedures and needs to be done early

▦ ST balancing: e.g. flexor-to-extensor transfer will correct isolated hammer toe if MCPJ is brought down to normal position after synovectomy; include extensor lengthening and collateral release to restore flexion of MCPJ

▦ Other examples include occasional tendon lengthening, e.g. sometimes of toe extensors

4.9.16 Management of Fore-Foot Disease

- Comparison between Keller's procedure and first MTPJ fusion:
  - Pain relief: fusion tends to produce more long-term pain relief than Keller
  - Deformity: rarely recurs after fusion; recurrence is possible with Keller and sometimes it produces cock-up deformity.
    Keller's excisional arthroplasty is simple and allows early walking, but weak push-off; fusion produces better stability and better balance, although it may be complicated by non-union or hardware problems

4.9.17 Lesser Toes

- MTPJ-excision arthroplasty mainly
  - Remove base of proximal one-half P/P; remove MT heads to gentle slope laterally
  - Extensor tenotomy/IM *k*-wire and interpose
  - Remove ellipse of plantar skin to reposition foot pad
  - Use a dorsal transverse/plantar incision (Clayton uses dorsal, Kates uses plantar)
- PIPJ (Mann):
  - Uses manual correction (or osteoclasis) together with first MTPJ fusion and lesser toes MTPJ-excision arthroplasty (sometimes may fuse the IPJ in hammer toes)

4.9.18 Other Fore-foot Procedures

- Silastic (interposition/Helal): not recommended since limited bone stock; results not better than excision arthroplasty; Cx of the silastic
- Helal's MT telescope (osteotomy): oblique osteotomy enables distal MT to slide proximally, relieves pressure; claims 70% good result, but cannot correct toe deformity
- Toe amputation: occasionally, for severe claw toes, disarticulate through MTPJ with trimming of MT heads (need toe block, MT support; not commonly done)

4.9.19 Results of Fore-foot Arthroplasty

- 80% Satisfactory result
- Results deteriorate with time and deformity may recur
- Fusion of first MTPJ might improve the good results with time in selected cases

4.9.20   Mid-Foot Disease in Rheumatoid Foot

▨ Hypermobility of first MT-cuneiform joint: if present, may sometimes need fusion
▨ TNJ (talonavicular joint) collapse and ankylosis: (1) may require simple fusion in the elderly low-demand patient and (2) consider double fusion (i.e. TNJ and CCJ) in younger active patients since might help prevent collapse of subtalar joint resulting from the natural course of the disease
(Note: maintain the longitudinal arch in TNJ fusion)

4.9.21   Hind-Foot Disease in Rheumatoid Foot

▨ For subtalar joint destruction, use isolated subtalar fusion
▨ For subtalar joint destruction and pronated fore-foot secondary to hind-foot valgus, use triple fusion
▨ Significant ankle joint involvement by disease is uncommon; ankle fusion may be indicated for varus/valgus deformity with or without pain
▨ An occasional patient with ankle valgus post triple fusion might require a supra-malleolar osteotomy or even pantalar fusion

4.10   Misellaneous Conditions

4.10.1   Morton's Neuroma

4.10.1.1 Clinical Features

▨ No neuroma, per se, really exists. An inter-digital neuroma-like swelling is likely to result from compression neuropathy caused by the common digital nerve passing beneath the transverse MT ligament
▨ Diagnosis is clinical (history and P/E) and does not use nerve conduction tests; it is difficult to confirm using MRI

4.10.1.2 Clinical Assessment

▨ History:
  – Occurs mostly in the third web area and second web space. Pain radiates from the plantar aspect of the foot towards the tip of the toes with numbness
  – It is made worse by tight shoes, but is better with shoe removed

■ Examination:
- Mulder's sign: one hand squeezes the foot in a medial-lateral direction; the other hand palpates the distal part of the plantar web space, pushing the thumb proximally to attempt to trap the nerve between the thumb and the MT heads. A positive test involves pain production, not just a click

4.10.1.3 Operative Treatment
■ Most surgeons use a dorsal approach
■ Identify the culprit lesion after spreading the MT heads and dividing the transverse MT ligament at the affected web space
■ Dissect the nerve out distally past its branches and transect it
■ Rate of recurrence is 15–20%

4.10.2 Tarsal Tunnel Syndrome

4.10.2.1 Clinical Features
■ Refers to compression of the tibial nerve in the tarsal tunnel
■ Tunnel formed by the flexor retinaculum
■ Contents: tibialis posterior, FDL, posterior neurovascular bundle and FHL
■ Three terminal branches of the tibial nerve in the tarsal tunnel: medial plantar nerve, lateral plantar nerve and calcaneal branch

4.10.2.2 Aetiology
■ RA synovitis
■ Ganglion
■ Accessory FDL muscle
■ Others: lipoma, neurilemomas

4.10.2.3 Clinical Features
■ Numbness in the sensory distribution of the involved nerves
■ Pain at the plantar aspect of the feet
■ Positive Tinel sign with or without wasting of intrinsics
■ Investigation: MRI and nerve conduction studies

4.10.2.4 Differential Diagnosis
■ Inflammatory joint disease
■ Plantar fasciitis

- Stress fracture
- Referred pain from the spine

4.10.2.5 Treatment
- If space-occupying lesion is present, decompress
- If RA, try conservative approach and decompress if no response

4.10.3 Os Trigonum

4.10.3.1 Nature of Os Trigonum
- Anatomical studies:
  - The os trigonum may be considered a developmental analogue of a secondary ossification centre similar to the posterior calcaneal apophysis (although there are histological differences)
  - Some consider it as an un-united portion of the lateral tubercle. (The os trigonum is an accessory bone found just posterior to the talus)

4.10.3.2 Differential Diagnosis
- Fracture tubercle of talus
- Enter into differential diagnosis of other post ankle pain:
  - Impingement pain of ballet dancers post compression syndrome – forced plantar flexion sometimes causes impingement of posterior talus between the calcaneus and distal tibia
  - Posteromedial tendinitis FHL or posterior tibial tendonitis

4.10.3.3 Other Features
- Oval, round or triangular and variable size
- 4–14% of normal feet
- May fuse with lateral tubercle or remain as separate ossicle

4.10.3.4 Mechanism of Pain Production
- The chondro-osseous border of the synchondrosis can be injured as:
  - Chronic stress fracture
  - Acute fracture (less common) – comparable to the injury patterns involving the accessory navicular

4.10.3.5 Clinical Features

▤ Posterior/posterolateral pain of the ankle, especially in sports or occupations that need forced plantar flexion of the ankle

4.10.3.6 Treatment

▤ Conservative
▤ Perhaps steroid injection with or without casting
▤ Operative:

Excision of bone block either due to os trigonum or osteophyte improves motion and lessens pain.

Consider lateral approach for isolated post impingement.

Intra-operatively, identify the sural nerve and FHL tunnel; identify the os after capsulotomy and check that there is no more impingement on PF before closing

General Bibliography

Helal B, Rowley D, Cracchiolo III A, Myerson M (eds) (1996) Surgery of disorders of the foot and ankle, 1996 edn. Martin Dunitz, London

Valmassy RL (ed) (1996) Clinical biomechanics of the lower extremities, 1996 edn. Mosby, Philadelphia

Selected Bibliography of Journal Articles

1. Vainio K (1991) The rheumatoid foot. A clinical study with pathological and roentgenological comments. CORR 265:4–8
2. Clayton ML (1998) Surgery of the forefoot in rheumatoid arthritis. CORR 349:6–8
3. Mann RA (1995) Disorders of the first metatarsophalangeal joint. J Am Acad Orthop Surg 3:34–43

Contents

5.1   Common Spinal Deformities

5.1.1   Scoliosis – An Introduction

5.1.1.1   General Comment on Scoliosis

▓ It is a three-dimensional (3D) deformity (Figs. 5.1, 5.2)

▓ To this, we may add a 4th dimension. This is because the scoliotic deformity changes with time

▓ The 3D deformity involves not only deformities in the coronal and sagittal planes, but is also featured by rotation of the vertebral bodies (commonly picked up by the appearance of the pedicles according to Moe's method of assessing vertebral rotation). Presence of vertebral rotation readily differentiates the structural from non-structural scoliosis

5.1.1.2   Basic Principle of Scoliosis

▓ According to Euler, the spine is regarded as a 'column'

▓ Concept of buckling of the column: a column loaded in compression experiences a deflection instability when a critical load is reached. Long and slender columns are especially prone to fail by buckling

▓ Formula: critical buckling load = constant/column length

5.1.1.3   Limitations of this model

▓ The spine is not a true column

▓ Non-homogeneous

▓ Buckles already present: with kyphotic and lordotic areas

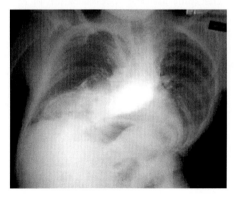

Fig. 5.1. Marked thoracic scoliosis with limited pulmonary reserve

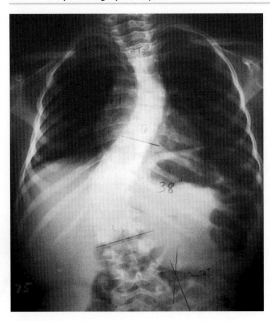

Fig. 5.2. Patient with thoracolumbar scoliosis

5.1.1.4 Possible Mechanism of Column Decompensation

▦ Most scoliosis occurs during the period of rapid growth. It is surmised that differential spinal growth can be a predisposing factor for this scoliosis, i.e. uncoupling of anterior and posterior growth
▦ What causes the rotation is uncertain. Theories include:
  – With differential growth, the spine assumes a combination of lordosis, rotation and lateral deviation
  – It is possible that, initially, a small curve develops – perhaps due to a defect of the neuromuscular control system – and during growth the curve may be exacerbated by biomechanical factors

5.1.2   Sagittal Malalignment of the Spine

5.1.2.1   Normal Sagittal Alignment

- Normal thoracic kyphosis measure from T1–T12 = 41–47° Apex T6–7, T7–8
- Normal lumbar lordosis measure from L1–S1 = 56–72° Apex L3–4 disc, two-thirds of lumbar lordosis occur at L4/5 and L5/S1 disc spaces. Try to preserve these two discs that confer most of the lordosis
- Normal sacral inclination = 50°

5.1.2.2   Lumbo-Sacral Sagittal Alignment

- There is a close association between sacral slope and lumbar lordosis
- Hip flexion decreases in total and segmental lordosis
- If segmental and total lumbar lordosis decrease – sacro-pelvis rotates around acetabulum – there is more vertical sacrum and hip extension on standing (or vice versa)
- Sacrum thought of (by some) as the 6th lumbar vertebra; translate along the arc defined by the pelvic radius centred at the hip

5.1.2.3   Changes with Ageing

- Degenerative spines have less segmental lordosis – L3–S1 more vertical sacral slope – and stand with more hip extension

5.1.2.4   Causes of Sagittal Imbalance

- Scoliosis
- Spondylolisthesis
- Localised kyphus – especially tumour, trauma, infection
- Iatrogenic causes

5.1.3   Spondylolisthesis – An Introduction

5.1.3.1   Normal 'Tug-of-War' Between Destabilising Versus Stabilising Forces of the Lower Lumbar Spine

- Stabilising Forces:
  - Anterior sacral buttress
  - Bony support (facets)
  - Posterior osteoligamentous structures (lamina, vertebral arch, etc.)
- De-stabilisation forces or destabilisation occurs if:
  - Slip angle increases for various reasons

- Deficiency of the bony posterior stabilising structures, e.g. spina bifida occulta
- Anomalies of other bony structures such as rounding off of the anterior sacrum, trapezoidal L5 etc.
- Involved in activities that put the posterior elements especially the pars under high cyclic stress or hyperextension stresses. Examples include gymnasts, soldiers carrying heavy loads on their backs, etc.

5.1.3.2 Keys to Understanding this Topic

▨ Three main components to be assessed:
  - Deformity – degree of lumbo-sacral kyphosis and forward translation
  - Degree of instability – say as seen on flexion and extension (F/E) films
  - Assessment of neurology – clinical and magnetic resonance imaging (MRI; good modality to assess any compression of the neural elements and also foraminal stenosis if any)
▨ In spondylolisthesis, there is more lordosis and no kyphosis, more at L1/2 and L4/5, but less at L5/S1. Owing to anterior translation of L5, the centre of gravity (C.G) moves forwards along the plumb line

5.1.4   Other Examples of Diseases Causing Sagittal Malalignment

▨ Ankylosing spondylitis with severe kyphosis, but LS spine cannot compensate; thus, lumbar osteotomy may be required
▨ Case of tuberculosis (TB) with severe acute kyphosis – anticipate lung/rib/central nervous system (CNS)/osteoarthritis (OA)/C.G/knee and hip problems

5.1.4.1 Spondylolisthesis (Fig. 5.3)

5.1.4.1.1 Classification

▨ Dysplastic
▨ Isthmic – lytic, pars elongation, acute fracture
▨ Degenerative
▨ Traumatic
▨ Pathological

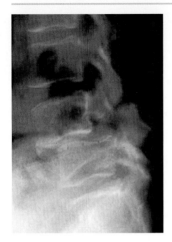

Fig. 5.3. A middle-aged woman with L4/5 spondylolisthesis

5.1.4.1.2 Important Points
- L5/S1 most common level for spondylolytic spondylolisthesis
- L4/5 most common level for degenerative spondylolisthesis
- Differential diagnosis (DDx) of the above two conditions important – that is why we always do oblique X-rays to search for pars defect even in spines with degeneration
- Most are developmental or acquired; really congenital in nature only in some of the dysplastic types

5.1.4.1.3 Natural History
- Degenerative type progresses 30% in 10-year follow-up study; most slips 30% or less
- Spondylolytic types are more likely to progress in female sex, high-grade slips, those with special anatomic features, e.g. hypoplastic L5 transverse process, spina bifida occulta, etc.
- In one long follow-up study in children it was observed that those with one-sided pars defect seldom progress. The disease in children is rather different from that in adults

5.1.4.1.4 Spondylolytic Spondylolisthesis
- Fatigue (stress) fracture of the pars interarticularis – due to repetitive trauma in a susceptible individual

5.1.4.1.5 Epidemiology
- Affects 6% of population
- Onset age 6–10 years
- Never noted at birth
- Greatest risk of progression 10–15 years
- High familial tendency
- High incidence in Alaska, and in those with spina bifida
- Common in athletes involved in sports; common in female gymnasts and soldiers carrying heavy weights

5.1.4.1.6 Pain Sources in Spondylolytic Spondylolisthesis
- Two theories
  - Pars defect may be the source of pain
  - Pain may be from stretching of neural elements in pars defect

5.1.4.1.7 Clinical Features
- Can be asymptomatic
- Pain on spinal extension
- Low back pain (LBP) with or without radiation to buttock and thighs
- May feel palpable step-off
- Higher grade slips, hamstring spasm common, flat buttocks

5.1.4.1.8 X-Ray Assessment for Spondylolytic Type
- Lateral view can reveal Dx in 80% of cases
- Sometimes may not see the defect with only a lateral or only an oblique view because angle of pars defect varies greatly

5.1.4.1.9 Other Investigations
- Bone scan (more sensitive than X-ray and the defect can be seen earlier)
  Single photon emission computed tomography (SPECT) scan, which is even more sensitive than bone scan, may be considered if high index of suspicion despite negative bone scan
- Computed tomography (CT) scan: may be useful in staging and predicting healing of lesions
  (Early lesions with hair-line defect, progressive lesions have wider defect, and late stage are featured by sclerosis)

5.1.4.1.10 Summary of Different Management in Different Ages

In Children

- Possibility of successful pars repair for very symptomatic spondylolysis since there is a normal disc
- Possibility of higher chance of further slip from ligamentous laxity, especially in girls and despite fusion in-situ [posterolateral (PL) intertransverse is the gold standard]
- Possibility of (seemingly solid) 'fusion mass' to slip further (especially if decompression procedures done) in children

Adolescent Spondylolysis

- Many think that pars defect (lytic) type does not occur at birth, and is hence developmental
- Direct repair can be considered in symptomatic cases with normal disc, especially if no slip
- Juvenile sportsmen/women are predisposed to develop this condition

Other Features of Adolescent Spondylolysis/Spondylolisthesis

- Disc mostly normal
- Even for high grades, may still get away with posterior in-situ fusion

Adults and Above

- The spondylolytic variety of isthmic-type spondylolisthesis is less likely to be associated with neurological deficit, since the posterior arch separates from both pars defects.; hence with significant neurology and/or acute/fast progressive neurology, we can rule out disc as the cause (especially in cauda equina, for example)
- Degenerative as the adult male/female ages; laxity is less and, here, despite an intact posterior arch (unlike isthmic), slip progression is mostly not too severe
- Dysplastic: real potential danger of neural injury, since there is a combined effect of intact post arch and a tendency for L-S kyphosis – e.g. rounding off of the anterior sacrum with loss of the anterior buttress

Low-Grade Middle-Aged Spondylolisthesis

- Pain – carefully diagnose where the pain is from, especially in worker's compensation cases, e.g. nerve blocks, and discogram is sometimes needed
- Neurology – the risk of cauda equina and severe neurology is much less than with the dysplastic type, since there is no intact neural arch in such cases
- Both pain and neurology – symptom/grade can worsen as disc subsequently degenerates. Beware, pain coming from nearby disc is also possible

Middle-Age High-Grade Spondylolisthesis

- In-situ fusion with or without decompression; versus instrumented fusion
- Fusion is more advisable to put in front [anterior spinal fusion (ASF)/posterior lumbar inter-vertebral fusion (PLIF)] especially for high-grades to increase fusion success, since the chance of fusion is higher with graft in compression

Spondyloptosis

- Clinical features: vertical buttock, typical gait sometimes deep loin crease present, marked hamstring spasm
- Choice of operation needs individual assessment. For severe cases, may consider Gaine's procedure; an alternative will be the use of fibula grafting

5.1.4.1.11   Prognosis in Severe Slip

- Age (worse in the young)
- Sex (more often in females)
- Slip degree >30°
- Slip angle >45°
- Trapezoidal L5 and dome shaped sacrum
- Spina bifida (possible weakened posterior tension band)

5.1.4.1.12   Rn Pearls – High-Grade Spondylolisthesis

- Special In/views
  - Long film standing anteroposterior (AP)/lateral, especially lateral to assess overall sagittal balance

- Measure slip angle, degree of slip, sacral inclination, etc. are musts
- Look for significant changes (translation and rotation) with F/E views
- Assess 'high-risk' factors that predispose to poor result

▓ Investigations to access extent/ease of reduction:
  - F/E view as mentioned
  - Hyperextension over bolster had been reported

5.1.4.1.13   Other Treatment Pearls: High-Grade Slips

▓ Many cases may need bone graft (BG) anteriorly – whether it be ASF or PLIF, → since higher chance of success with BG in compression instead of tension

▓ Those subgroups that have high chance of pseudoarthrosis despite posterior fusion: very high-grade slips, spina bifida (deficiency posteriorly), hypoplastic transverse process (hence likely flimsy iliolumbar ligament), dysplastic anatomy (trapezoidal L5, rounding off of anterior sacrum, etc.)

▓ Nerve monitor important if partial complete reduction is contemplated as well as multiple wake up test. Some experts nowadays tend to use direct stimulation, especially of L5 root, which is most commonly affected

▓ Intraoperative reduction/partial reduction – experts tend to reduce sacral-pelvic unit to the L5 rather than vice versa

▓ Many a times have to fuse from L4 to sacrum for high-grade slips

▓ If instrumentation needed to the sacrum, many add on iliac wing screws for added distal fixation

▓ Mere positioning can help reduction, as well as the use of instrumentation

5.1.4.1.14   How to Reduce Chance of L5 Root Injury With or Without Post-Operative Cauda Equina

▓ Nerve monitor/root stimulation and wake-up test

▓ Adequate decompression not only centrally, but sometimes need to dissect to see both L5 roots so that tension can be tested on table

▓ Those with tense roots clinically or evidence on table may choose to avoid total reduction – previous studies showed that the last 15% of reduction is most dangerous to neural structures

▓ Patients be primed of possible neurology post-operatively

▨ An occasional case develop cauda equina post-operatively from bulging disc – be sure to assess every aspect before proceeding to surgery

5.1.4.1.15   Treatment Pearls: Spondyloptosis
▨ Some authorities think fibula graft spanning sacrum to L4 may sometimes do the trick
▨ Otherwise the Gaines procedure is the way to go – involves vertebrectomy of L5 and anterior and posterior surgeries

5.1.4.1.16   Degenerative Spondylolisthesis
▨ Pathomechanics: (1) hormonal – creates ligament laxity, more common in women; (2) as L4/5 disc degenerates, increases micromotion of the said motion segment – facet joint degeneration, capsular laxity and facet orientation more sagittal relative to L5/S1 → forward slip occurs. Slip usually mild
▨ L5/S1 even less common than L3/4 – because of stabilisation effect of the iliolumbar ligament; facet here shows coronal orientation rather than sagittal, especially in cases with sacralisation of L5
▨ 5% of cases with both L4/5 and L 3/4 slips at the same time

Treatment Pearls: Degenerative
▨ 20-Year meta-analysis reported in Spine 1994: clinical outcome with added instrumentation not different, although fusion rate seemed higher; complication rate, however, is higher with instrumentation
▨ That fusion improves clinical outcome and prevents slip after the destabilising posterior decompression surgery is well reported by multiple studies with little controversy – but many stress the importance of a properly prepared bed and proper graft harvest
▨ Proper use of pedicle screws may help to restore lumbar lordosis (Fig. 5.4) and the more fusion levels needed with the rod/hook systems. Also, the fixation is stronger at pedicles in osteoporotic spines – there is lack of lamina to hold hooks anyway with the decompression

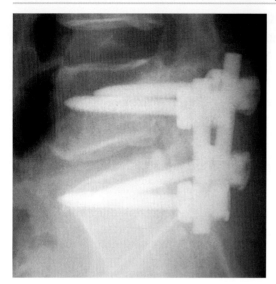

Fig. 5.4. Pedicle screw fixation in a middle-aged man

5.1.4.1.17 Appendix

BG Rationale

- Anterior grafting – favoured in Asian literature. Based on sound reason since graft is in compression. The snag includes more complex anatomy and special complications, e.g. retrograde ejaculation
- Posteriorly placed grafts: rationale is for lesser degree of slip. Graft may still be in 'compression' (and at least not tension) for slightly higher slips, may extend one level to L4, for example, for the PL fusion; however, in still higher ones and/or features of lumbo-sacral kyphosis, graft will be in tension increase chance of failure – severe cases may need A+P (PLIF also with disadvantages)
- Attempts to correct somewhat the L-S kyphosis include instrumentation and/or, in the extreme case, vertebral excision in the Gaines procedure: but there is trade off for a higher chance of neural damage

5.1.5   Adolescent Idiopathic Scoliosis

5.1.5.1   Differential Diagnosis
- Idiopathic – most common
- Congenital
- Neuromuscular, e.g. polio, spinal bifida, cerebral palsy, etc.
- Associated with syndromes, e.g. Ehlers Danlos, etc.
- Extraspinal: pelvic obliquity, sciatica, tumours (e.g. osteoid osteoma), leg length discrepancy, etc.

5.1.5.2   Possible Contributory Factors in 'Idiopathic' AIS
- Vertebral growth abnormalities: differentially faster anterior growth → hypokyphosis → buckling of spine
- Possible melatonin deficiency (as a result of conclusion from pinealectomised chicken)
- Genetic factors: 80–90% concordance in monozygotic twins; 40–50% concordance in dizygotic twins
- Possible role of decreased bone mineral density

5.1.5.3   Untreated Scoliosis
- Cardiopulmonary compromise if severe thoracic curves
- Back pain (AIS typically not painful, but back pain can occur when AIS patients go into adulthood)
- Truncal imbalance and altered bodily mechanics
- Cosmetic blemish

5.1.5.4   Prevalence
- 1–3% of curves are greater than 10°; male to female ratio is 1 to 1
- 0.1–0.3% of curves are greater than 30°; more common in females
- Likelihood of curve progression:
  - Age (some use bone age instead)
  - Menarche
  - Risser sign
  - Curve magnitude and type (thoracic more than lumbar)
  - Gender (more in females)
    (Factors 1 to 3 assess the amount of growth remaining)

5.1.5.5 Natural History of Curve Progression In Adulthood (after Weinstein)

- Rare if less than 30°
- Likely if:
  - Thoracic curve is greater than 50°
  - Lumbar curve greater than 30–40°
- LBP only slightly higher than controls

5.1.5.6 School Screening and Referral

- Adams forward bending test
- Refer if angle of trunk rotation (ATR) is greater than 7°

5.1.5.7 History Taking

- Family history (Hx)
- Degree of maturation
- Neurological symptoms
- Age at menarche
- Pain

5.1.5.8 Clinical Examination

- Severity and truncal balance → check level of shoulders and pelvis. Coronal imbalance by plumb line assessment; sagittal profile assessment important. Degree of truncal imbalance recorded (not just listing)
- Flexibility and range of motion. Flexibility testing can be by side bending and by suspension in the small child
- Clues as to the aetiology, e.g. (1) neurocutaneous stigmata – if present may indicate spinal dysraphism, (2) subtle neurological signs, e.g. asymmetric abdominal reflexes and (3) possible leg-length discrepancy or pelvic obliquity
- Maturity – secondary sex characters

5.1.5.9 Radiological Assessment

- Posteroanterior (PA) standing long film needed
- Lateral X-ray to assess sagittal profile sometimes indicated
- Degree of flexibility:
  - Side bending films
  - By calculation of the fulcrum bending index

5.1.5.10 King's Classification
- Type I – double curve, lumbar major
- Type II – double curve, thoracic major
- Type III – single thoracic
- Type IV – long C curve with L4 in curve
- Type V – double thoracic

5.1.5.11 Aims of Treatment
- To obtain a stable balanced spine, centred over the pelvis in the coronal/sagittal planes
- Stop curve progression
- Minimise patient morbidity and fuse as few segments as possible

5.1.5.12 Indications for Bracing
- Early Dx
- Mild curve (<30°)
- Skeletally immature, Risser 3 or less
  (Refer to landmark paper: 1995 SRS Brace Study [5])

5.1.5.13 Brace Wearing
- Dose-dependent effect at more than 20 h (preferably 23 h)
- Examples: Boston underarm (apex below T7); Milwaukee (apex above T7)
- When to consider weaning: when skeletal maturity is reached
  - Menarche over 2 years
  - Height assessment
  - Risser sign assessment
  - Hand (bone age)

5.1.5.14 Indications for Surgery
- Late Dx of significant curves
- Severe curves (>45°)
- Truncal imbalance
- Failed brace treatment, can be non-compliance or progression despite bracing

5.1.5.15 Surgical Treatment
- Approaches
- Anterior versus posterior versus combined
- Implant to use
- Steel versus titanium
- Screws, hooks, wires
- Levels of fusion
- Technique to achieve a fusion

5.1.5.16 Posterior Surgery
- Easier exposure, can treat almost all types
- Familiar
- Less morbidity, e.g. decreased pulmonary complications
- More choices of instrumentation options
- Longer fusion possible
- No de-rotation possible
- Full correction difficult

5.1.5.17 Anterior Surgery
- Shorter fusion
- De-rotation possible
- Shortening of spinal column
- Fuller correction possible
- Exposure difficult
- Technically more demanding
- Revision less straight forward than posterior approach
- Difficulty with sacral fixation

5.1.5.18 The Case for Combined Anterior and Posterior Surgery
- Rigid curves
- Crankshaft phenomenon
  - Young patients
  - Progression of deformity after posterior fusion
- Reduce length of fusion in double curves

5.1.5.19 Which Implant to Choose
- Harrington
- Luque and Harrington-Luque

- Third generation (3-D correction)
- Fourth generation
  - Top-loading
  - Titanium

5.1.5.19.1   Harrington Instrumentation

- Work on concepts of Harrington stable zone and stable vertebra (discussed elsewhere)
- Correction not bad but does not cater for re-establishment of sagittal profile; frequent cause of flat back syndrome
- Higher neurological complication rate with distraction
- Needs brace/cast even after operation
- Hooks not uncommonly cut out

5.1.5.19.2   Luque Instrumentation

- Truly segmental instrumentation with sublaminar wires
- No need for post-operative cast or braces
- Controlled lateral translation
- No axial load resistance

5.1.5.19.3   Cotrel-Dubosset

- A 3D approach to scoliosis
- Introduction of the hook/claw system – two hooks at the same or adjacent levels that allow either compression or distraction
- Sometimes may overcorrect and decompensate
- Said to be able to perform 'de-rotation' but true de-rotation does not occur, only simply lateral translational force

5.1.5.19.4   Current Trends

- Analyse curve segments independently
- Open closed disc spaces
- Careful analysis of sagittal profile
- Compression can induce lordosis
- Distraction can induce kyphosis
- Abnormal sagittal plane segments be included into fusion; and never stop at a kyphotic segment
- In lordotic thoracic curve, put in the concave distraction rod first
- In hyperkyphotic thoracic curve, put convex compression rod first

5.1.5.20 How to Achieve a Fusion?
- Proper bone grafting
- ±Immobilisation
- Not necessarily by instrumentation

5.1.5.21 Method of Grafting
- Bone harvesting at posterior iliac crest
- Recipient site preparation most important
- Facet fusion
- Decortication
- Transverse processes preparation
- Laminae preparation

5.1.6   Adult Scoliosis

5.1.6.1 Two Main types
- De novo (most >40, from disc degeneration, rotatory subluxation, etc.)
- Had scoliosis before skeletal scoliosis

5.1.6.2 Difference from AIS
- Stiffness common
- Disc degeneration
- More complications – more blood loss, more operative time, more sepsis, more rehabilitation time

5.1.6.3 Clinical Presentations
- Deformity
- Radicular pain
- Spinal stenosis
- Truncal imbalance

5.1.6.4 Pre-Operative Assessment
- Coronal – scoliosis, lateral listhesis
- Sagittal – kyphosis, any listhesis
- Degree of osteoporosis

5.1.6.5 Mechanical Problem Post-Operatively
▓ Kyphosis above rod/or instrumentation
▓ Flat back – to avoid flat back, segmental pedicle screw fixate restores lordosis, combined A+P (anterior support)
▓ Neurological compromise below rod – to prevent late stenosis below rod, fuse to sacrum
▓ Failure of sacral fixation

5.1.6.6 Treatment Options
▓ Conservative
▓ Surgical:
  – Decompress alone
  – Fusion and instrumentation
  – Decompression, and fusion plus instrumentation

5.1.6.6.1 Decompress Alone
▓ Indication – stable spine, < 40°, no rotatory subluxation, normal lordosis
▓ Complication – risk of increase in deformity

5.1.6.6.2 Fusion and Instrumentation
▓ No radicular or stenosis signs
▓ Curve progressive/marked/rotatory subluxation and lateral listhesis, etc.

5.1.6.6.3 Decompression Plus PSF and Instrumentation
▓ Can go posterior especially if reasonable disc status; no anterior osteophytes
  – Decompress the associated spinal stenosis
  – Instrumentation especially needed if wide post decompression needed
  – Occasional case may need A+P surgery

5.1.6.7 Indication for Intervention
▓ Progressive deformity
▓ Lung function worsening
▓ Significant deformity
▓ Pain persistent

5.1.6.8 Fusion Levels

▨ Similar argument to AIS
  – Include rotatory subluxation, spinal stenosis areas, etc.? Use of discograms
  – Sagittal: preserve lumbar lordosis, avoid end of fusion at the apex of kyphosis – upper and lower levels preferably in lordotic segment. Some say therefore the superior level not only includes the entire curve, but 2–3 segments above kyphosis
  – Indication for fusion to sacrum

5.1.6.9 Indication for 'Fusion to Sacrum'

In general, avoid 'fusion to sacrum'. Exceptions:

▨ Pelvic obliquity needs correction
▨ L5/S1 degeneration
▨ Provocative test L5/S1 +
Why avoid fusion to sacrum if possible:
▨ More pseudoarthrosis
▨ Flat back
▨ Loosening of sacral fixation
▨ Altered gait mechanics
Advantages
▨ Prevent later L5/S1 problem
▨ Better sagittal balance
Bridwell suggested that fusion short of sacrum is sometimes not so predictable – there is a possible higher complication rate should revision be required. The final answer not yet known

5.1.6.10 Selection of Approach

▨ Thoracolumbar (TL)/lumbar curves – if:
  – <70° with no kyphosis, anterior; posterior if need possible extended decompression
  – >70° cases, – can consider A+P
▨ T Curves – if:
  – <70° simple posterior, and fuse
  – >70° – A+P combined

5.1.7 Degenerative Scoliosis

5.1.7.1 Definition
▓ Adult scoliosis, no previous curve
▓ Mostly lumbar
▓ Spondylosis

5.1.7.2 Incidence
▓ On the increase at least in the USA (Shufflebarger)

5.1.7.3 Aetiology
▓ Multisegment asymmetrical disc degeneration
▓ Causing the coronal and sagittal plane decompensation and even sub-luxation – lateral spondylolisthesis

5.1.7.4 Pathomechanics
▓ Disc degeneration (asymmetrical multiple)
  – Causes both (1) decrease load share of the anterior column and (2) loss of efficiency of the posterior tension band
  – Results: increase shear forces and segmental instability
  – Vicious cycle (posterior structures overload and degenerate)
  – Asymmetrical disc degeneration; hence, cause translation and rotation deformity, and also can cause canal compromise

5.1.7.5 Pathomechanics: the Cause of Lateral Listhesis
▓ Normal function of the intact disc
  Both segmental mobility and segmental stability
▓ Normal disc resists compression (distractive device), decreases torsion and bending forces
▓ Intact disc motion – translatory + rotatory
▓ Here, asymmetrical disc affection not only causes coronal, but segmental kyphosis and decreases facet joint contact, – predispose to unilateral facet dislodgement/lateral listhesis

5.1.7.6 Classification (Bridwell): Four Types
▓ Depending on four parameters:
  – Coronal profile
  – Sagittal profile

- Spinal stenosis
- Subluxation – type 4 with 25% subluxation
  Additional associated factors to be considered: physiological age, co-morbidities, and family Hx
  (Other classification neglect sagittal, e.g. Isaza)

5.1.7.7 Natural Hx and Prognosis
- No good longitudinal studies
- No one knows
  One expert claimed that these are prognostic factors:
  - Cobb's >30°
  - Lateral listhesis
  - Moderate rotation
  - Decrease lordosis

5.1.7.8 Fixation Technique
- Overall: combinations of hook and screw; some use hooks in thoracic segment and screws in lumbar segment
- Fixation technique to the sacrum: structural interbody graft, LS fixation, iliosacral-lumbar fixation (Perhaps Galverston less used here) – adjunct orthotics

5.1.7.9 Complications
- Standard: neural, blood loss, medical, deep vein thrombosis (DVT), etc.
- Complications: those fusions to sacrum, especially pseudoarthrosis, instrument failure, pelvis stress fracture (Spine 1996); sagittal and coronal imbalance

5.1.7.10 Principles of Treatment
- Restore anterior column
- Restore lordosis
- Restore posterior tension band mechanism
- Decompress neural canal
- Restore coronal and sagittal alignment

5.1.7.11   Symbols and Signs

- Neural (paraplegia not reported?)
- Pain – many diagnoses
- Deformity and cosmesis

5.1.7.12   Investigation

- X-ray: usually see two lumbar curves, lost lordosis, lateral listhesis (especially L3/4 more common), thoracic spine can be normal for age of patient
- CT: see spinal stenosis, confirm facet arthrosis, etc.
- MRI: see spinal stenosis, black discs at multiple levels seen, nerve roots and foramen
- Others: possible discography and 3D CT

5.1.7.13   Conservative Rn

- Activity modification
- Non-steroidal anti-inflammatory drugs (NSAIDs)
- Corset
- Epidural

5.1.7.14   Surgical Intervention

5.1.7.14.1 Surgical Option 1:
Role of Minimal Surgery in the Flail Patient

- Occasional patient may need relief of stenosis – many caution that this approach can quickly invite recurrence and destabilises the spine further

5.1.7.14.2 Surgical Option 2: P → A → P surgery

- Rationale:
  - Wide posterior release (soft tissue includes Ligamentum flavum, and facet takedown), decompression and harvested BG (sometimes posterior osteotomy instead?)
  - Anterior inter-vertebral BGs (cages)
  - Go back to posterior again → posterior instrumentation → tension band restoration
    (The initial posterior step ensures ease and adequacy of re-establishment of lordosis during the anterior surgery)
    (Note: Realignment also helps to relieve lateral canal stenosis)

5.1.7.15 Fusion Levels
▓ Posterior usually from T11 – sacrum in Shufflebarger series
▓ Anterior usually from L2 – sacrum
(Most had lumbar lordosis restored to $40°$)

5.1.7.16 When to Stop at L5
and When to Include Sacrum and Upper Extent
▓ Stop at L5 (seldom) if: normal MRI at lumbo-sacral junction (LSJ), with negative discography here
▓ When stopping at lower T-spine is possible; $< 45°$
(Fusion extended if thoracic kyphosis is more than $45–50°$ and there is sagittal plane decompensation)

5.1.7.17 Conclusion
▓ The surgery described addressed the following:
  – Segmental instability
  – Spinal canal compression and soft tissue stiffness
  – Deformity
  – Curve balance
  – Sagittal profile

5.2   The Paediatric Spine

5.2.1   Congenital Scoliosis

5.2.1.1   General Principles
▓ Curves tend to be stiffer and less correction is possible relative to adolescent type
▓ No 'number rules' as in AIS
▓ Any thoracic-curve (congenital or otherwise) greater than $60°$ has a vast negative effect on the growing lung alveloli if age is less than 5 years – made worse if concomitant or pure lordosis (with airway compression) or kyphosis

5.2.1.2   Classification
▓ Failure of formation. Types:
  – Hemi-vertebra – fully segmented/semi-segmented/non-segmented
  – Incarcerated
  – Wedge vertebra (partial)

▨ Failure of segmentation. Types:
  – Unilateral unsegmented bar
  – Unilateral bar with contralateral hemi-vertebra
  – Bilateral segmentation failure = block vertebra
    Location: if lateral – scoliosis/bar; if posterior – lordosis; if anterior – kyphosis; if circumferential – loss of growth (block vertebra)
▨ Mixed

5.2.1.3 Natural Hx and How to Predict Prognosis

▨ Natural Hx depends on the type of deformity in each particular case
▨ Prognosis depends on:
  – Degree of deformity
  – Age of onset and effect on cardiopulmonary function (especially in those under 5 years of age for severe curve)
  – Remaining growth potential
  – Type of deformity

5.2.1.4 Natural Hx Versus Location and Type of Deformity

▨ Type: block vertebra is the best, unilateral unsegmented bar and contralateral hemi-vertebra is the worst; others that are prone to significant curves include: unilateral longitudinal bar, two consecutive hemivertebrae facing same side – especially if segmented
▨ Location: TL worse, upper thoracic best (according to proceedings of SRS)

5.2.1.5 Assessment of Unbalanced and Asymmetric Growth

▨ Dx work-up: X-ray and CT/3D CT (and MRI in all cases) to assess accurately the type of vertebral anomalies we are dealing with – e.g. whether hemi-vertebra is segmented, exact length of bar; it is not uncommon for both lesions by failed formation and failed segmentation to occur together. MRI will detect associated anomaly, e.g. diastematomyelia, tethered cord
▨ Observed deterioration important. There are no number rules as in AIS where if a 6-year-old child has 20° and then a year later 30°, you can be sure of a natural Hx of around 10° per year
▨ Unpredictability stem from affected growth plate's growth potential is difficult to predict (thus, even segmented hemi-vertebra do not always

progress since the retained growth plates may have poor growth potential)

▦ Some always have bad prognosis, e.g. unilateral unsegmented bar

5.2.1.6 The Worry of Growth Stunting with Surgery

▦ Many experts feel that the fear that too early a fusion will cause major growth stunting with short torso and long legs is unfounded, since allowing the curve to progress quickly may result in an even shorter torso in later life

▦ Two common ways to predict the effect of growth with vertebral fusion. (Methods used by Winter and by Dimeglio will not be discussed here)

5.2.1.7 Hx Taking

▦ Family Hx

▦ Possible aetiology: teratogens, diabetes mellitus, spontaneous abortion, neural tube defects

▦ Others: curve progression, old serial X-rays, past treatment, how noticed, etc.

5.2.1.8 Physical Assessment

▦ Spine: coronal and sagittal alignment; symmetry, compensation, even buttock contour (caudal regression syndrome)

▦ Upper limb (UL)/lower limb (LL): hand, forearm, radial hemi-melia; calf atrophy, cavovarus, leg-length discrepancy

5.2.1.9 Neurological Examination

▦ Standard exam

▦ Neurology especially more frequent with hemi-vertebra and contralateral bar

▦ High association of occult intraspinal anomalies

5.2.1.10 Common Associated Anomalies

▦ VATERL with or without hydrocelalus (H): V, vertebra; A, anal atresia; T, tracheo-oesophageal fistula; E, oesophageal atresia; R, renal; L, limb anomaly

▦ Especially need to rule out and treat renal anomalies since present in 20–30% of cases → by intravenous urogram (IVU) or by urodynamic studies (the latter said to be good especially for tethered cord)

- Others:
  - Head: cleft lip/palate
  - Neck: Klippel Feil, Sprengel
  - Chest: cardiac/rib
  - Abdomen: hernia
  - Skin – tags, lipoma, tuft of hair, naevi

5.2.1.11   Diagnostic Work-Up: Every Case Needs X-Ray, Renal Ultrasound and MRI

5.2.1.11.1   X-Ray Examination
- Standard erect PA, bending and lateral
  (but supine film for very young, also said to have better definition of vertebral anomalies from shorter focal length to the cassette)
- Traction films → to assess flexibility and alignment in curves over 60° (more useful again in the very young)
  Note: increasing role of 3D CT especially in the very young

5.2.1.11.2   Importance of MRI Assessment
- 30% Overall risk of occult lesions, e.g. diastematomyelia, tethered cord
- May also need pre-operative neurosurgical consult

5.2.1.11.3   Pre-Operative Lung Function if Indicated
- Cases with significant thoracic curve
- Thoracotomy planned

5.2.1.11.4   Intraoperative Monitor
- Wake-up testing: remains the gold standard for neurological testing
- Somatosensory evoked potentials (SSEPs) + motor evoked potentials (MEPs) are mandatory, especially if instrumentation is needed

5.2.1.12 Treatment: Prevention of Deformity with Timely Operation
- John Hall was noted to make this wise statement:
  " .... no spine with congenital scoliosis should need correction since it ought to be recognised early, and fusion performed before the curve progresses to the extent that correction is needed"

5.2.1.12.1   Aim of Non-Operative Treatment
- Monitor for progression
- Improve spinal balance in selected cases – decompression head tilt
- Modalities available: observation, orthosis

5.2.1.12.2   Which Curves Can One Observe?
- No role in congenital kyphosis and, in those lesions, very likely to progress like unilateral unsegmented bar
- Compare initial, previous, and current visits
- Follow for progression

5.2.1.12.3   Which One Can Brace (by Milwaukee)?
- Never use in congenital kyphosis, lordosis, and short stiff scoliosis, (and less useful for high curves; Winter says more useful in flexible TL curves to buy some time)
- Indications:
  - Long flexible curve
  - Compensatory curve
  - Post-operative bracing

  (P.S. Curves be $<50°$, 50% flexibility with side bending, traction. By compensatory curve, we mean above/below congenital curve; head tilt, lumbo-sacral curve)

5.2.1.13   General Surgical Options and Comments on Crank-Shaft
- Crank-shaft: well documented by Dubousset (JPO) – posterior fusion alone may arrest curve progression but creates a 'surgical tether' that, in the young child of less than 10 years (Risser 0, open TRC), can lead to significant, further rotatory and translational deformity and increased curvature
- This danger, however, depends on: anterior growth potential of these abnormal vertebrae
- Winter says crank-shaft incidence is much lower in congenital type than in idiopathics

  (P.S. In general, fusion needs to include all the vertebrae in the structural curve)

5.2.1.14 General Surgical Options

▦ Posterior fusion with or without instrumentation (gold standard, or at least time honoured)
▦ Convex A+P epiphysiodesis
▦ A+P surgery
▦ Excision of hemi-vertebra in selected cases

5.2.1.15 Surgical Timing Need to Individualise

▦ Intervene early in those types known to progress severely, e.g. unilateral unsegmented bar and contralateral hemi-vertebra
▦ Intervene early also in significant T-curve in those younger than age 5 years, since their alveoli are not well formed
▦ Other cases: intervene at onset of puberty if possible to prevent curve progression

5.2.1.16 Indications for A/P Convex Epiphysiodesis

▦ No kyphosis
▦ $< 50°$ (i.e. not so severe curve that still with growth potential)
▦ Younger than 5 years of age
First published by MacLennon. The concept involves: Convex anterior and posterior growth arrest and hemi-arthrodesis. Can be used in selected cases for both infantile and congenital cases

5.2.1.17 How to Perform Convex Epiphysiodesis

▦ Direct lateral position so that both the front and the back can be done at same time
▦ Although there are reports of transpedicular anterior surgery, the best results have been with a full anterior exposure. In the thorax, VATS can be done
▦ Post-operatively, need casting not brace for 6 months
▦ Follow-up until end of growth
▦ Loss of correction needs arthrodesis

5.2.1.18 Indication for Posterior Only Approach

▦ Usually regarded as gold standard
▦ Indications:
  - Curve progress under observation
  - Curve so large at presentation that operation is needed
  - Type of deformity known to have a poor prognosis

5.2.1.19 Use of Instrumentation

- In general, used to stabilise instead of overcorrect, since these are usually stiff curves of the child with congenital scoliosis
- Nowadays, newer instrumentation is available even for young child, but do not overdo it
- Disadvantage: increase in neural risks – SSEP is recommended

5.2.1.20 When Do We Need A+P Surgery?

- With greater mobility of the spine for further correction
- Elimination of anterior growth potential
- For severe curves, those with high chance of crank-shaft

5.2.1.21 Indications for Excision of Hemi-Vertebra (Resembles a Wedge Osteotomy)

- Fully segmented hemi-vertebra, quick progression
- Rigid angulated scoliosis
- Fixed decompensation
- Alignment not achieved with fusion alone
- Excision is a wedge osteotomy

  Advantages: (1) removes cause and (2) curve is corrected with only a short fusion

  Disadvantage: mainly neural complications

  (A hemi-vertebra is shown in Fig. 5.5. in a patient who also has spina bifida)

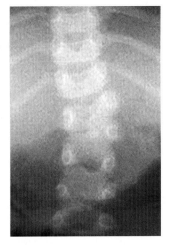

Fig. 5.5. Hemi-vertebra is noted in this X-ray of a patient with spina bifida

5.2.1.21.1   What Levels Possible to Do Excision of Hemi-Vertebra

- LS (+ lumbar) hemi-vertebra well described
- Thoracic levels have also been described but are technically more demanding, e.g. by Bradford and Kaneda
- Indication in the case of LS hemi-vertebra: oblique take-off, fixed decompensation, and trunk shift

5.2.1.21.2   Hemi-Vertebra Excision

- Pre-operative MRI: clarifies (1) local anatomy and (2) neural anomalies
- Technique: A/P resection mostly either in stages or sequential. Fuse whole curve, post-instrumentation

5.2.1.22   Complications of Treatment

- Paraplegia/neural deficit
- Blood losses
- Crank-shaft
- Pseudarthrosis
- Implant complications
- Sepsis

5.2.2   Congenital Kyphosis and Lordosis

5.2.2.1   Congenital Lordosis

- Caused usually by failed posterior segmentation in the face of active anterior growth
- Very bad prognosis, especially in the thoracic spine, since causes progressive respiratory failure and death (compression of the lung and bronchi)

5.2.2.2   Congenital Kyphosis

- Very high chance of paraplegia if left untreated for the group due to failure of formation (McMaster) being greater than defects of segmentation (less paraplegia and less severe) – half of the cases from failure of formation
- Less common than congenital scoliosis
- Apex commonly at: T10 → L3
- Lung function compromise can occur if severe
- Many treat these curves by fusion in situ since there are stiff and neural risks

5.2.2.2.1 Definition
▨ Deformity of one or more segments of the spine caused by developmental vertebral anomalies that impair anterior (or anterolateral) longitudinal growth in the sagittal plane

5.2.2.2.2 Aetiology
▨ Dysfunction of notochord tissue between day 20 and day 30 of mesenchymal phase of the embryo

5.2.2.2.3 Classification
▨ Failure of formation
  – Partial/complete affection one or more vertebra
  – Sharp angular → kyphosis/kyphoscoliosis
  – Rapid course: neural risk includes paraparesis
▨ Failure of segmentation
  – Slower course, less neural risk
  – Anterior bar one or more segments
  – More rounded kyphosis or kyphoscoliosis
▨ Mixed (rare, rapid course, high neural risk)

5.2.2.2.4 Natural Hx
▨ Although congenital kyphosis is less common than congenital scoliosis there is more paraplegia risk
▨ Type 3 has high progression and paraplegia risk
▨ Next is type 1 (failure of formation). Effect depends on percentage of missing anterior column and growth discrepancy; thoraco-lumbar most common
▨ Type 2 is less severe; affects length of defect and growth discrepancy. After more than 10 years, ossification of bar may cause spontaneous anterior epiphysiodesis

5.2.2.2.5 Differential Diagnosis
▨ Scheuermann, especially for failed segmentation type
▨ Others (e.g. neurofibromatosis, Marfan's, postural, post-operative infection, etc.)

5.2.2.2.6   Patient Evaluation

- Neural status
- Type of kyphus – flexibility, severity, balance
- Associated anomaly – renal again important (30%); others include cardiac, skin, cavovarus feet, MRI evidence of diasematomyelia/tether cord, etc.
- Investigation: X-ray and MRI
  (X-ray: erect AP + lateral)
  Intra-operative neural monitoring is a must

5.2.2.2.7   Conservative Treatment: Little Role

5.2.2.2.8   Bracing: Not Usually Effective

5.2.2.2.9   Surgery: Treatment Options

- Posterior in-situ fusion creates posterior epiphysiodesis. This procedure is best suited for those younger than 5 years old and for curves less than 50°
- A+P surgery: for higher curves greater than 50° and for any age group. Anterior spine here needs structural support, e.g. strut fibula and vascularised rib
- Excision of hemi-vertebra – sometimes excellent correction of large magnitude curve

5.2.2.2.10   How About 'Skeletal Traction'

- Most will not use it
- If used, MRI is needed to rule out tethered cord

5.2.2.2.11   What to Do with Someone who Presents with Neural Deficit

- Less severe deficit: indirect decompression that involves anterior release and strut graft; try partial reduction of the deformity and PSF/instrumentation
- Major neural deficit:
  - Vertebrectomy of abnormal level and partial resection of level above and below. However, results are unpredictable and always need to protect with PSF/instrumentation

5.3   The Degenerative Spine

5.3.1   Cervical Myelopathy

5.3.1.1   Definition
Refers to spinal cord dysfunction located at the cervical level arising from mechanical compression and vascular compromise

5.3.1.2   Mechanism of Injury to Cord
- Direct mechanical compression, e.g. hard disc, soft disc prolapse, ligamentum flavum, ossification of posterior longitudinal ligament (OPLL), etc.
- Dynamic compression and stretching, e.g. pincer action of osteophyte spurs produced on F/E
- Possible vascular factors

5.3.1.3   Symptoms
- Neck pain and/or weakness, numbness, wasting, and clumsy hands, difficulty in walking and unsteadiness, tendency to fall
- Sphincter disturbance rather uncommon

5.3.1.4   Signs
- Upper motor neurone – brisk jerks, Babinski [depending on level(s) of compression, can have combination of both upper motor neurone/lower motor neurone signs in the UL]
- Inverted supinator reflex
- Lhermitte signs
- Hoffman sign – one of the myelopathy hand sign
- Scapulohumeral reflex (Shimuzu 1993) – if positive, indicative of high lesion level around C3/4
- Myelopathic hand signs (10-s test, finger-escape test) – if positive, indicative of cervical myelopathy

5.3.1.5   Occasional Atypical Presentation
- If multiple level disease
- Needs to know the discrepancy between the bony level and the corresponding level of the neural tissue that can be affected, i.e. discrepancy between neurological and bone segment

■ Perhaps may be partly due to the complex pathogenesis: mechanical and vascular aetiologies

5.3.1.6 Causes of Cervical Myelopathy
■ Cervical spondylotic myelopathy (degeneration, especially in patients with developmentally narrow canal)
■ Prolapsed inter-vertebral disc (usually mainly affects 1 or 2 level)
■ OPLL (more common in the Japanese population)
■ Upper cervical instability (causing dynamic compression)

5.3.1.7 Natural Hx
■ About one in two cases will deteriorate
■ Most had episodic worsening (step-like fashion)
■ Some showed slow and steady progression
■ A few had a rapid onset and usually poorer prognosis
■ One-half of cases improve with conservative treatment

5.3.1.8 Clinical Assessment
■ Serial monitoring of patients and calculation of the JOA (Japanese Orthopaedic Association) score. Most need MRI (Figs. 5.5–5.7) to assess for any myelomalacia changes of the cord and together with CT assess the area of the canal and calculation of the compression ratio
■ Careful documentation by motor and sensory charting. Document any sphincter dysfunction
■ Trial of conservative treatment is useful in a majority of patients since 50% will improve

5.3.1.9 Indication for Operation
■ Progressive neurological deterioration
■ Failure of conservative treatment (6 months)
■ Before irreversible damage, especially in young patients with OPLL
■ MRI – check compression ratio (sagittal diameter/transverse diameter <0.4; cord area <40 mm^2; increased T2 signal)

5.3.1.10 Management
■ Have knowledge of natural Hx and discuss with patient the pros and cons of treatment options
■ With a JOA score <13, start to consider need for operation

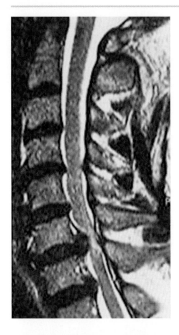

Fig. 5.6. Magnetic resonance imaging appearance of a woman with cervical myelopathy

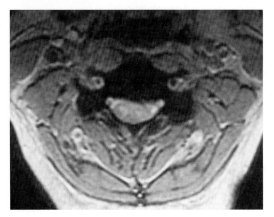

Fig. 5.7. Axial magnetic resonance imaging of the same woman with cervical myelopathy

■ Assess prognosis
Good prognostic signs: young age, less than 1 year of symptoms, unilateral motor deficit and the presence of Lhermitte sign

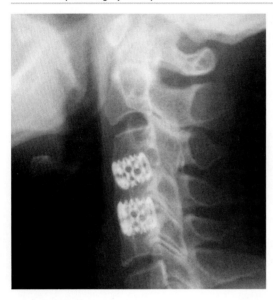

Fig. 5.8. Middle-aged man with 2-level anterior spinal fusion

5.3.1.11 Factors Influencing Choice of Anterior Versus Posterior Approaches

▪ Overall alignment of the cervical spine – avoid posterior approach in an already kyphotic cervical spine

▪ Number of levels to be tackled – if >3, it is more difficult to be tackled from in front, and also the fusion rate of BG spanning multiple cervical segments will be lower. Can consider ASF if 1–2 levels of decompression needed (Fig. 5.8)

▪ Especially in congenitally narrowed spinal canal, with space available for the cord (SAC) < 13 mm, it is advisable to go for the posterior approach

▪ Some conditions need special consideration on individual case-by-case basis; e.g. OPLL

5.3.1.12 Examples of Operative Intervention for Different Conditions

▪ One level significant cervical disc disease – can consider anterior approach and fusion

▪ Multi-level cervical spondylotic myelopathy – consider laminoplasty (single hinge or double hinge). An alternative will be multiple level laminectomy and fusion and instrumentation by lateral mass plating

■ OPLL – different approaches according to the type of OPLL, cervical alignment etc., will be discussed

5.3.2   Ossification of Posterior Longitudinal Ligament

5.3.2.1 Japanese Epidermiological Study

■ OPLL (Fig. 5.9) not a new disease: incidence (radiological) is 2% in Japan
■ Incidence in Asians 1%, much less in the white population, Caucasians 0.1%

5.3.2.2 Location

■ Cervical – most common (especially C456– the three most mobile segments)
■ T/L possible – 10% of all cases, but potentially may cause ambulatory/gait problems and more likely to be incapacitating. Thoracic most common at T5, and lumbar most common at L1 and L2
■ Equal in males and females; mean age at presentation 45–50 years

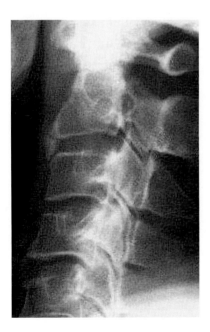

Fig. 5.9. A middle-aged man with ossification of posterior longitudinal ligament

5.3.2.3 Types of OPLL

▧ Segmental – most common 40%
▧ Continuous – less common 30%
▧ Mixed – about same as above 30%
▧ Others (e.g. localised/circumferential) – 7%
▧ Feature: although segmental type is most common; the narrowing created is less than those due to continuous and mixed types

5.3.2.4 Aetiology

▧ Uncertain. Some possibilities:
  – Generalised ossifying tendency, e.g. association with AS (2%), Ossified Yellow Ligament (OYL; 7%) and diffuse idiopathic skeletal hyperostosis (DISH; >20%). An example of DISH seen in Fig. 5.10
  – Diabetes mellitis/altered glucose metabolism (some say related to Asians due to huge rice consumption)
  – Possible abnormal calcium metabolism
  – Genetics – relatives have higher chance than general population (risk about 30%). Association with HLA BW 40, SA 5

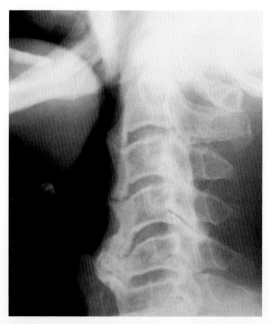

Fig. 5.10. An elderly man with diffuse idiopathic skeletal hyperostosis

5.3.2.5 Pathomechanics

- Many are asymptomatic
- Thus, many are incidental radiological findings
- Since most grow slowly, with thickening of the PLL, they are sometimes associated with ossified ALL, OYL, and even ossified dura; thus, extra care is needed in our pre-operative assessment
- Experiments and clinical experience show that the cord can tolerate compression of up to 70% reduction in diameter, if the compression is slow enough
- Some show symptoms at a much lesser restriction in diameter – here, there may be an element of instability of the spine or other factors, and triggered by accident, e.g. whiplash/hyper-extension type injuries. Hence, all OPLL patients need avoid hyper-extension
- An added mechanism to produce cord injury is irritation of cord by OPLL uneven surface with spinal movements beside compression

5.3.2.6 Histology

- Admixture of lamella and woven bone with undulating surface; underneath lies calcified cartilage columns (with tidemark) and underneath is some hypervascular tissue

5.3.2.7 Symptoms and Natural Hx

- Asymptomatic incidental X-ray finding – most common
- 25% Eventually have gait/ambulation problems; 10% cannot walk
- UL paresis/numbness, 40%
- LL paresis/numbness 15–25%
- Tetraparesis after minor trauma 20%
- Patient with frequent deterioration of symptom after hyper-extension injury of the neck

5.3.2.8 Sign

- Of thoraco-lumbar spinal stenosis (those OPLL localised in thoracic or lumbar region)
- Of cervical myelopathy
- Gait disturbances
- ADL difficulty
- UL/LL motor or sensory losses

5.3.2.9 Dx and Investigations
- Not too difficult to confirm with lateral C-spine X-ray
- High thoracic area ones may need tomogram or CT to diagnose
- Look for associated spondylosis
- Look for other associated features of ligament ossifying tendency, e.g. OYL, DISH

5.3.2.10 CT and MRI
- Good for assessing the canal diameter
- CT myelogram frequently needed before the anterior floatation method
- Associated pathologies may be seen, e.g. nerve root entrapment by facets
- MRI: cord signals changes, status of the disc and ligamentum, etc.

5.3.2.11 Treatment
- Always try conservative first
- Avoid hyperextension
- Rest with neck partly flexed, never extended
- Immobilisation
- With or without traction

5.3.2.12 Indications for Operation
- Failed conservative treatment
- Severe compression, moderate symptoms and signs, progression
- Anterior approach (floatation method): theoretically better, only for three or fewer vertebral level cases
- Posterior laminoplasties: no limitation of the level, most do at least C3–C7 levels

5.3.2.13 Problem of Re-Growth
- Can re-grow after operation, e.g. after laminectomy – documented
- Said to have less re-growth after the anterior floatation method, claims make it mature faster
- Even with no operation, progressive growth common

5.3.3   Ossified Yellow Ligament
- Most in thoracic and/or lumbar areas
- Beware ossified dura and dural tear during operation
- Three types: (1) separated, (2) fused and (3) isolated
- Investigation needs lateral X-ray and CT
- Treatment depends on whole picture

5.3.4   Lumbar Spinal Stenosis

5.3.4.1   Definition
- Involves narrowing of the central spinal canal (and usually also the lateral recess) with neural impingement that produces symptoms of neurogenic claudication or radiculopathy

5.3.4.2   Classification
- Congenital: usually in fact developmental, e.g. achondroplasia, idiopathic
- Acquired:
  - Degenerative stenosis (of the central canal, of lateral recess, or of the foramen)
  - Degenerative spondylolisthesis
  - Iatrogenic, e.g. post-laminectomy, post-fusion
  - Post-traumatic
  - Metabolic, e.g. Paget's disease

5.3.4.3   Pathophysiology
- Compression in extension
- Ischaemia and compression of cerebrospinal fluid (CSF) flow
- Cannot cope with nutritional demand
- Cannot remove product of metabolism
- Atrioventricular (AV) shunt on either side of compression
- Ectopic nerve impulse

5.3.4.4   Neurogenic Claudication
- Posterior (or anterior) thigh, and calf discomfort
- Pain, numbness, tiredness, heaviness
- Aggravated by standing or walking
- Relieved by many minutes of resting in flexed lumbar spine position

5.3.4.5   Dx of Spinal Canal Stenosis

- Clinical neurogenic claudication
- Clinical evidence of chronic nerve root compression
- Imaging confirms narrowing of spinal canal
- Absence of vascular impairment

5.3.4.6   Differential Diagnosis

- Vascular claudication
- Bilateral hip joint disease
- Spondylosis with leg pain
- Peripheral neuropathy

5.3.4.7   Key Feature of Lumbar Spinal Stenosis

- The clinical presentation can be best described by the phrase 'many symptoms but few signs'
- Sometimes the sign if present can be subtle, e.g. loss of an ankle jerk, and sometimes only brought on/made more obvious after walking for some distance when the claudication starts
- The following are the clinical comparison between neurogenic and vascular claudication (the major DDx)

5.3.4.8   Pain of Neurogenic Claudication

- LBP almost always
- Described as vague, and sense of heaviness
- Radicular or diffuse in distribution, to buttock, thigh and calf
- Precipitated by walking
- Pain relieved by flexion of spine, not relieved by standing alone

5.3.4.9   Other Features

- Walking uphill is better (spine flexed)
- Walking downhill is worse (spine extended)
- Time for pain relief with rest for many minutes
- Neurological symptoms commonly present
- SLR mildly positive or negative
- Mildly positive or negative neurological signs
- Pulses present
- No skin changes

5.3.4.10 Pain of Vascular Claudication
- Back pain rare
- Pain sharp, cramping
- At the exercise muscles
- Radiation not common
- Increase by walking
- Relieved by stopping muscular activities, even standing

5.3.4.11 Other Features
- Pain walking uphill worse
- Sometimes walking downhill better
- Quick relief on rest
- No neurological symptom
- No neurological sign
- SLR normal
- Absent pulse
- Skin atrophic changes quite common

5.3.4.12 Investigations
- Confirm Dx
- Define exact location of stenosis and pathology
- Plan what to do when operation is required

5.3.4.13 Conservative Treatment
- NSAIDs
- Flexion exercises and pain-relieving physiotherapy
  Epidural injections have been described

5.3.4.14 Operative Treatment Indications
- Progressive motor weakness
- Cauda equina syndrome (CES)
- Claudication not responsive to conservative treatment

5.3.4.15 Type of Operation
- Central laminectomy at stenotic levels
- Lateral recess not uncommonly also stenotic and requires decompression – can be caused by overgrown superior facet against posterior vertebral body/pedicle/bulging lateral annulus

▦ Fusion is considered if multiple level needs to be tackled and there is associated spondylolisthesis, severe back pain and cases with an element of dynamic instability

5.3.4.16 Those with Congenitally Narrow Canal

▦ Both the length and the width of decompression are important in performing decompression for these patients, and decompress all the stenotic level

▦ In dealing with patients with achondroplasia who develop lumbar stenosis at an earlier age than the usual patient, assess whether there is concomitant stenosis near the foramen magnum that may require decompression

5.3.4.17 Indication for Fusion in Lumbar Stenosis with Spondylolisthesis

▦ Narrow disc, age 70 years or more – fusion not usually required

▦ Wide disc, age 60 years or younger – decompress and fuse

5.3.5   Lateral Canal Stenosis

5.3.5.1   Relevant Anatomy

▦ Central canal of the lumbar spine – contains the cauda equina and thecal sac

▦ Lateral recess – abutted by the superior nerve root

▦ Intervertebral foramen – contains the dorsal root ganglion
(The spinal nerve is extra-foraminal)

5.3.5.2   The Three Zones of the Lateral Spinal Canal

▦ Entrance zone

▦ Mid-zone – under the pars interarticularis

▦ Exit zone – at the intervertebral foramen
(Lesions causing compression outside of the foramen are called extra-foraminal, or 'far out zone of Wiltze')

5.3.5.2.1 Entrance Zone

▦ Most cephalad part of lateral lumbar canal, synonymous with lateral recess

▦ Medial to or underneath superior articular process

▦ Anterior wall: PL surface of disc and vertebral body

- Posterior wall: superior articular facet
- Lumbar nerve root affected has the same number as the corresponding lumbar vertebral segment

5.3.5.2.2 Mid-zone
- Located under pars interarticularis and pedicle
- Anterior border: posterior aspect of vertebral body
- Posterior border: pars interarticularis
- Dorsal root ganglion and ventral motor nerve: covered by fibrous connective tissue extension of dura mater

5.3.5.2.3 Exit Zone
- Area surrounding intervertebral foramen, shaped like an inverted tear-drop, normal height 10–23 mm
- Bordered superiorly and inferiorly by pedicles of adjacent vertebrae
- Anterior border: posteroinferior and posterosuperior aspects of adjacent vertebral bodies and intervening disc
- Posterior border: lateral aspect of facet joint one level below the facet joint of the entrance zone of the same lumbar segmental nerve

5.3.5.3 Clinical Presentation
- Third or fourth decades of life
- Major complaint: radicular leg pain – exacerbated with lumbar extension
- Back pain: also exacerbated with lumbar extension
- Claudication is more frequent in central or advanced stenosis and rare in foraminal stenosis

5.3.5.4 Physical Examination
- Limited lumbar motion; particular extension
- Tension sign: normal
- Neurology
  - Motor:
    usually normal
  - Sensory:
    diminish in a radicular distribution
- Peripheral pulses
- Hip and knee joints

5.3.5.5 Differential Diagnosis

- Herniated disc
- Neoplasm
- Osteoarthritis of hip

5.3.5.6 Investigation

- Electromyography
    - Denervation in muscles innervated by lumbo-sacral nerve root
    - Differentiate from peripheral neuropathy

5.3.5.7 Pathophysiology of Nerve Root Compression

- Compression alone may not cause pain
- Compression of inflamed root causes pain
- Chemical mediators involved: substance P, phospholipase A2, neuro-peptides, etc.
- Other possible mechanisms: dynamic instability, ischaemia, venous stasis, nutritional deficit from abnormal CSF flow

5.3.5.8 Concept of Double Crush

- Two different nerve roots affected
- One nerve root compressed by two pathologies at two separate sites

5.3.5.9 Causes of Compression of the Nerve Root in the Three Zones

- Entrance zone = PL herniated disc, hypertrophic superior articular process, osteophyte from vertebral body, developmentally short pedicle, abnormal facet size/shape
- Mid-zone = pars interarticularis from spondylotic changes, soft tissue from a spondylolytic defect
- Exit zone = superior facet subluxation can compress the nerve against the pedicle/body/the bulging annulus. Foramen may also be narrowed by ligamentum, bulging annulus, osteophytes, etc.

5.3.5.10 Foraminal Disc Herniation

- Average age 60 years
- Severe radicular pain
- Neurological deficit always positive
- Most common at L4/5; rare at L5/S1
- L4 root

- Femoral stretch positive; SLR negative
- Sensation – medial shin
- Motor – weak quad and ankle dorsiflexor, spares EHL
- Reflex – decrease knee jerk

5.3.5.11 Causes of Extra-Foraminal Compression
- Far out disc prolapse
- 'Far out syndrome' caused by L5 transverse process and sacral ala in spondylolisthesis
- Iatrogenic by bone-graft, etc.

5.3.5.12 Conservative Treatment of Lateral Canal Stenosis
- Activity modification
  Mobilisation exercises
  NSAIDs
  Steroid injection

5.3.5.13 Operative Treatment
- Limit to the clinical symptomatic levels
- Laminotomy
- Undercutting hypertrophic superior facet
- Facetectomy
- Diskectomy

5.3.5.14 Indications of Fusion
- Instability when bilateral removal of facets over 50% each or a complete unilateral facet was removed
- Pre-operative instability; degenerative spondylolisthesis, degenerative scoliosis

5.3.5.15 Results of Surgery
- Satisfactory results; 79–93%
  e.g. Jonsson series reported in Spine
  e.g. Sanderson and Getty series reported in Spine
- Best results are achieved when a correlation is established between symptoms and radiographical findings, and the decompression appropriately addresses the cause of the symptoms

5.3.5.16   Treatment of Foraminal Disc Herniation

▨ Short trial of conservative treatment

▨ For older patient, decrease bed confinement

▨ For older patient, chance of nerve recovery

▨ Severe pain

▨ Operate if no improvement in 2–3 weeks

▨ Inter-transverse approach

▨ Avoid damage to inferior facet

5.3.5.17   Appendix: CES

5.3.5.17.1   Definition of CES

▨ CES = collection of symptoms and signs resulting from compression of nerve root bundles emerging from the end of the spinal cord below L1

▨ The classic feature involves severe LBP with bilateral sciatica associated with saddle anaesthesia, urinary retention, and bowel dysfunction

5.3.5.17.2   Introduction

▨ Relatively low incidence of only 1–2% of patients undergoing surgery for a herniated lumbar disc

▨ Important because delayed Dx of CES has negative consequence on the patient and surgeon

▨ Much increase in claims of negligence according to Medical Protection Society files in recent years, i.e. of medico-legal significance

5.3.5.17.3   Diagnosis

▨ Mainly clinical

▨ More investigations needed in more subtle cases

5.3.5.17.4   Clinical Types (Reported in Spine)

▨ Acute onset: acute LBP, sciatica, urinary disturbance, LL motor weakness, saddle anaesthesia

▨ Insidious onset: recurrent LBP episodes ranging from weeks to years – gradual onset sciatica, motor/sensory loss, with bowel and bladder dysfunction over a few days to weeks

5.3.5.17.5   Another Classification
(Reported in British Journal of Neurosurgery)

- Incomplete CES:
  Urinary difficulties such as altered sensation, loss of desire to void, poor stream, need to strain on micturation
- Complete CES (with retention):
  Painless urinary retention and overflow incontinence – bladder no longer under the executive control

5.3.5.17.6   Pathophysiology

- Mechanical pressure causes obstruction of the axoplasmic flow
- Element of ischaemia and venous congestion

5.3.5.17.7   The Neurological Lesion

- Cauda equina is composed of peripheral nerves; an injury causes a lower motor neurone type of flaccid paralysis
- Lesion usually patchy, difficult sometimes to diagnose since most common cause, such as L5/S1 prolapsed inter-vertebral disc, spares most of the lumbar roots!
- Since peripheral nerve injury, recovery possible unless complete

5.3.5.17.8   Complete Versus Incomplete CES

- An atonic bladder with overdistension, i.e. complete CES only occurs from muscular injury
- Preganglionic motor denervation only, i.e. incomplete CES result mainly in loss of reflex activity
  (N.B. partial loss of cauda equina function can cause little or no disability clinically)

5.3.5.17.9   Causes of CES

- Herniated IV disc (most common), Fig. 5.11
- Trauma
- Two to surgery, spinal manipulation, spinal or epidural
- Tumours, e.g. metastases
- Infection
- Others: vascular problems, spinal stenosis, late-stage ankylosing spondylitis

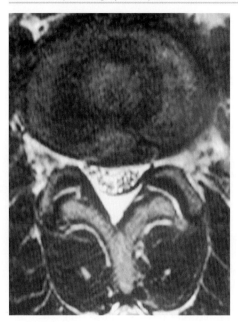

Fig. 5.11. Central disc prolapse in an elderly woman with cauda equina syndrome

5.3.5.17.10 Hx (Some Useful Questions to Ask)

▪ Saddle anaesthesia – 'does the toilet paper feel normal when you wipe yourself after going to the bathroom'
▪ Urinary symptoms - 'can you tell when your bladder is full?; any loss of control?; any difficulty passing urine?; or do you feel you want to go all the time?'
▪ Bowel symptoms – similar approach
▪ Screening sexual dysfunction – any loss of feelings of the genitals; any difficulty in ejaculation and erection should be asked
▪ Nature of pain – depends on underlying cause

5.3.5.17.11 Physical Examination

▪ Sensory: 'saddle' means the body areas that one would sit on a saddle – can be sacral, perineal and scrotal area
▪ Motor: LL motor loss may occur, even paraparesis, loss of ankle jerk is common
▪ Rectal exam: may be loss of tone and rectal sensation

- Bladder may be palpable, late cases can be painless retention (chart residual urine after Foley insertion)
- Findings can be quite asymmetrical

5.3.5.17.12 Summary of 'Red Flags' Signs
- Severe LBP with bilateral or unilateral sciatica
- Bladder and bowel dysfunction
- Anaesthesia or paraesthesia in perineal region or buttocks
- Significant LL weakness
- Gait disturbances
- Sexual dysfunction

5.3.5.17.13 Investigations
- Pre-operative X-ray
- MRI (urgent) should be ordered if suspect cauda equina compression
- Other investigations – e.g. urodynamic studies but should not delay emergent surgery

5.3.5.17.14 Other Possible Investigations
- Spinal angiography if suspect arteriovenous malformation
- Cystometry and/or fluoroscopy to assess detrusor muscle function
- Anorectal manometry and defaecography
- Some cases may use transurethral PG E1 application to rule out a vascular cause of erectile dysfunction
- Motor and sensory evoked potentials

5.3.5.17.15 Timing of Surgery
- Many retrospective studies – but most are small series giving widely different conclusions
  - Studies for urgent decompression have been reported previously by Shapiro and by Ahn
  - Studies with "no" correlation between timing of surgery and end result have previously been reported by Buchner and Kostuik and Delamarter
  - Studies for urgent decompression in incomplete CES only were recently reported by Gleave (Br J Neurosurgery 2002 [4])
  (No role of steroids)

5.3.5.17.16 Conclusion of Current Thinking on Operative Timing

- Proponents of early (< 48 h) and urgent (preferably within a few hours) seem to outnumber proponents that mention that 'exact timing not so important'
- Meta-analysis of more than 300 CES cases showed improved outcome can be performed by 48 h or less (but this meta-analysis did not realise that most of the papers cited in the literature did not distinguish complete from incomplete CES)
- Validity and usefulness to diagnose into incomplete and complete CES requires further study – if verified, then emergency surgery 'only' for incomplete CES is required
- Notice, in passing, that Kostuik and others has revealed outcome improvement in delayed decompression sometimes as late as a few years

5.3.5.17.17 Operative Intervention is the Rule

- Removal of large central disc can be more difficult than usual diskectomy
- May need extensive exposure
- Future resolution of 'best timing' studies is important, the reason being that when performed under less than optimal conditions, as in emergency operation, surgery may even add to rather than alleviate morbidity

5.3.5.17.18 CES Conclusion

- Beware of the red flags when dealing with patients with LBP
- CES patients do not always present with all the components of the syndrome as described in textbooks; in fact, can be very asymmetrical
- Most expert opinions in courts of law favour the use of urgent or early (< 48 h) decompression
- Despite prompt decompression, the prognosis of full recovery of sphincter and sexual functions are seldom more than 70%

5.4   Intervertebral Disc Prolapse

5.4.1   Function
- Support high compressive loads x few times body weight from muscle action
- Support high tensile loads by the annulus
- While maintain stability and flexibility of the spine

5.4.2   Functional Components
- Disc with nucleus pulposus – high water and proteoglycans especially in child
- Inner annulus; structure resembles fibrocartilage, more type-2 than -1 collagen
- Outer annulus, more type-1 than -2 collagen; resist tensile strain and disc bulge
- End plate – like hyaline cartilage, deforms on compression, and porosity to allow diffusion across to the relative avascular disc

5.4.3   Loading Conditions and Mechanisms to Resist Loading
- Normal disc can withstand very high compression stresses
- When an abnormal disc fails, it is believed that usually the failure starts at the end plate

5.4.4   Effects of Ageing
- ↓ Proteoglycans
- ↓ Chondroitin sulphate
- ↓ H_2O content
- ↑ Collagen content
  Result = ↑ Stiffness and ↓ shock-absorbing function

5.4.5   Differences Between Disc Degeneration and Simple Ageing
- Ageing alone will not decrease the disc space to any significant extent; ↓ disc space seen on X-ray seen with a degraded/degenerate disc
- Thus, some special triggers likely required to commence the process of disc degeneration. Likely triggers include possible end-plate rupture and/or an auto-immune process that resemble that of sympathetic opthalmia. Most recently, the role of genetic factors in controlling the relative proportion of collagen in the disc has been implicated

5.4.6   Natural Hx of Disc Degradation

■ The degenerate disc, unlike the normal but aged disc is prone to herniate
(the normal disc does not usually herniate easily even given a slit in the annulus)

■ Another possibility is that the degenerate disc may resorb its nuclear material, and there will be accompanying loss of disc space

5.4.7   Factors that Determine Whether Disc Herniation Will Occur

■ Degenerate disc not aged disc prone to herniate

■ May be triggered by trauma creating a tear of the annulus

■ Age since incidence rises from middle age

5.4.8   Differences Between Protrusion, Prolapse, Extrusion and Sequestration

■ Protrusion – still staying within the confines of the annulus

■ Prolapse and extrusion – extending beyond the confines of the annulus

■ Sequestered disc – the sequestered material is no longer in continuity with the parent disc material

5.4.9   Clinical Features and Dx of Disc Herniation

■ Back pain

■ Sciatica which may be accompanied by sciatic 'tension signs' on examination

■ Typically periodic nature of pain differentiates from other causes (e.g. unrelenting in pain from tumours) and night pain uncommon

■ Motor or sensory symptoms if nerve root compression occurred

■ Presence of numbness in the perianal region and of recent sphincter changes should arouse the suspicion of possible Cauda Equina Syndrome

■ Most cases confirmed by MRI (Fig. 5.12)

5.4.10   Dx of Discogenic Pain

■ Clinical Dx of 'discogenic pain' is in fact inaccurate

■ Investigations:
  - X-ray F/E view may show up subtle instability
  - Discogram helps differentiate whether the suspected disc level is in fact the pain generator
  - MRI

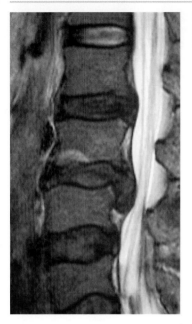

Fig. 5.12. Sagittal magnetic resonance imaging with disc prolapsing beyond the confines of the annulus

5.4.11 Discogram: Some Details (Fig. 5.13)
- Report details of needle placing at different levels
- Type and volume of dye
- Ease and difficulty of injection
- Patient assessment of pain level and character
- Pattern of dye distribute in AP and lateral, and sometimes axial CT
- 0.3 cc zinacef into each space at conclusion of the procedure

5.4.12 Useful Rules to Remember
- Disc herniation seldom:
  - Occurs in the very old (more commonly osteoporotic collapse fracture or tumours) or the very young (more commonly spondylolysis, benign tumours, sepsis)
  - Occurs at thoracic level, and if occurs, seldom higher than T8
  - Occurs at several levels at the same time, think of other Dx

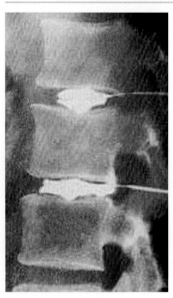

Fig. 5.13. Discogram with injection of dye at different levels to assess the level of the pain generator

5.4.13   What Does Literature Tell About Conservative Versus Operative Outcome

- Most cases can be managed conservatively
- Even for those cases where operation is needed for simple herniation (not counting the more sinister situation like cauda equina, etc.); the results after operation although is better at 1 year, the end result at 3–5 years are about the same
- Surgery can be accompanied by different types of complications, sometimes serious

5.4.14   Indications for Surgery

- Cauda equina syndrome – orthopaedic emergency
- Central sizeable disc herniation – danger of impending neurological loss, especially if neurological deficit already present
- Cord compression – in the rare thoracic disc herniation
- PL (or the less common far lateral) disc herniation, with failed conservative Rn, and especially associated also with neurological signs

▓ Intractable discogenic pain (need attention to Dx and pre-operative work-up as in general surgery for relief of sciatica more effective than back pain. The same holds for surgery for disc herniation besides discogenic pain)

5.4.15   Types of Operation for Disc Disease
▓ Fenestration and diskectomy
▓ Laminotomy and diskectomy
▓ Laminectomy – mostly for the large central herniation (as in causing cauda equina syndrome) may even need bilateral laminectomy
▓ Role of spinal fusion – (PL or even anterior) for discogenic pain cases. Seldom needed in the simple straight forward surgery for a disc herniation

5.4.16   Operative Complications
▓ Wrong level
▓ Persistent pain despite surgery (see the section on failed back surgery for management)
▓ Retained disc material
▓ Infection (superficial or deep)
▓ Injury to the dura and CSF leakage
▓ Complications peculiar to the surgery performed, e.g. if posterior instrumentation performed in an attempt to 'improve' fusion, then hardware complications, etc.

5.5   Spinal Tumours

5.5.1   Primary Spinal Tumours

5.5.1.1   Location of Spine Primaries
▓ Tumours with predilection for posterior elements (and/or spread to anterior): osteoblastoma, osteoid osteoma
▓ Tumours with predilection for sacrum: chordoma, giant cell tumour
▓ Tumours with predilection for anterior body: most of the rest
▓ Haemic tumours/Ewing: most are part of more generalised affection, and hence systemic Rn important
  [P.S. aneurysmal bone cyst (ABC) can be located at either anterior or posterior elements]

5.5.1.2 Terminology for Tumours Abutting the Central Nervous System

- Extraosseous paraspinal
- Extraosseous intraspinal extra-medullary, e.g. meningioma, neurofibroma
- Extraosseous, intraspinal intramedullary, e.g. astrocytoma, ependymoma

5.5.1.3 Osteoblastoma

- Pain not necessarily relieved by salicylates
- Can grow to quite large, some atypical variants
- Excision is mainstay

5.5.1.4 Osteoid Osteoma

- Painful scoliosis is typical presentation
- Pain relieved by salicylates
- Enucleation of Nidus is important

5.5.1.5 Chordoma

- Believed to arise from notocord rests
- Common at the two ends of the spine; skull base or sacrum – but other part of spine still possible
- Prognosis depends on level and size
- Surgery is mainstay
- Quite radioresistant – but radiotherapy (RT) useful in the usually unclear surgical margins

5.5.1.6 Giant Cell Tumour

- Giant cell tumour in spine quite aggressive in behaviour and one-half recurs (little correlate here between histological grade and behaviour)
- Can cause sacral root compromise and vertebral destruction
- Aim at en-bloc excision if possible
- RT risks malignant transformation

5.5.1.7 Myeloma (and Plasmacytoma)

- Prognosis better if solitary; 50% survive 5 years versus 10% if multiple
- Most common primary bone malignancy
- CT and skeletal survey may be useful

- RT for painful lesions
- Operation: only if large (>10 cm) and does not respond to RT

5.5.1.8 Lymphoma
- Can be osteoblastic as an ivory vertebra
- Can also be lytic as well
- RT and/or surgical decompression
- CT
- Sometimes cause much bone destruction and collapse

5.5.1.9 Osteosarcoma
- Neoadjuvant to tackle micrometastases with or without RT
- Many need neurodecompression
- En-bloc excision may be possible if diagnose early
- Rare (1–2% of all cases in spine)

5.5.1.10 Ewing's Sarcoma
- Most are from distant sites (real primary at spine very rare)
- Neural deficit/pain/sometimes as mass lesion
- CT and surgical decompression

5.5.1.11 Aneurysmal Bone Cyst
- Can involve either anterior or posterior columns
- <20 mostly
- Unlike giant cell tumour, occurs in younger and not aggressive – slow growth
- Excision versus possible curette/BG

5.5.1.12 Chondrosarcoma
- Primary or secondary to pre-existing lesion – exostosis (or enchondroma)
- Anterior column mostly (only 5% all cases)
- Aim at en-bloc resection
- RT for palliation

5.5.1.13 Osteochondroma (Exostosis)
- Most common benign tumour of bone
- Rare in spine

- Neural compromise very rare
- Treatment: observe and excise if symptomatic

5.5.1.14 Haemangioma
- Occasionally in spine and skull
- Lateral X-ray classic – snare drum vertebra (with prominent vertebral striations from rarefaction and honeycomb of cancellous structure of bone
- CT (axial) – possible 'polka dot lesion'
- Treatment: observe; recurrence likely even if curette and graft; RT not quite helpful and causes neuritis and morbidity

5.5.1.15 Eosinophilic Granuloma
- DDx Vertebra Plana or platysbasia (e.g. osteogenesis imperfecta, bone dysplasia)
- Common to affect spine – 10–20% cases
- Some say biopsy is not needed if < 10
- Most are self-limiting, symptomatic braces
- Vertebral height gets restored with time
- Bone scan r/o multifocal
- If progression – RT versus surgical curettage; possible CT for systemic disease
- DDx: TB, pyogenic osteomyelitis, neuroblastoma, Ewing, haemic malignancy, round cell tumours

5.5.2   Spinal Metastases
5.5.2.1   Epidemiology
- Metastases:primaries in spine = 40 : 1
- Blastic metastases = prostate, breast, kidney lymphoma, less commonly Ca Lung
- Lytic metastases = Ca Lung, etc.
- Do not forget that myeloma is the most common primary spinal tumour

5.5.2.2   Theories
- Seed and Soil – Paget
- Vascular theory – Ewing
- Batson vertebral vein system – Batson
- Angiogenesis theory – Fidler

5.5.2.3 Presenting Symptomatology
- Pain most common
- Neural deficit
- Possible deformity

5.5.2.4 Diagnosis (Fig. 5.14)
- If known multiple secondary metastases with known primary or the primary is very obvious, no need for biopsy
- Known source with suspected solitary metastatic lesion needs biopsy (since can be other pathology)
- Multiple metastases with no known primary – search for the occult primary

5.5.2.5 Types of Biopsy
- CT-guided needle (20-G needle in general for cells, compared with Trephine is 4G, versus trucut is 3 mm)

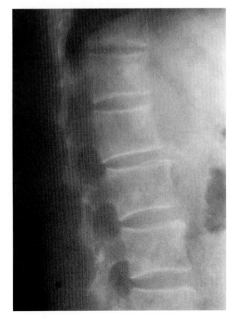

Fig. 5.14. Metastatic deposits to the lumbar spine

■ Open biopsy
  – Through the pedicle, other documented routes, e.g. extra-foraminal
  – Posterior lesions more accessible to open biopsy
    Pearl – need to plan biopsy before hand since may in fact be primary and need en-bloc resection

5.5.2.6 Investigation
■ Blood work
■ Search primary
■ X-ray spine and other relevant areas
■ CT and/or 3D sometimes required
■ MRI is good to assess possible neural compression, extent of marrow involvement, etc.

5.5.2.7 Response of Common Tumours
to RT/CT/Hormonal Manipulation
■ RT-sensitive tumours: lymphoma/myeloma more than breast/lung (e.g. small cell) more than renal/thyroid/GI tumours
■ CT-sensitive tumours: haemic malignancies/small cell lung/breast
■ Hormonal: prostate/breast/gynaecological tumours sometimes

5.5.2.8 Method of Delivery of RT
■ External beam – typical dose 4500 cGy
■ Targeted delivery
■ Useful if radiosensitive, especially in the spine since, in many cases, margin is involved or forced to do intralesional excision for tumours in the spine
■ Too high dose causes cord damage
■ Possible role of combination with vertebral plasty in the future

5.5.2.9 Surgical Indications
■ Neural decompression
■ For instability and/or deformity correction
■ Intractable pain

5.5.2.10 Main Surgical Options
■ Palliative decompression of neural structure; usually need instrumentation

- Intra-lesional excision of growth followed by RT/CT – especially if radiosensitive
- Aim is 'curative' – confirmed solitary metastases of known primary (stage-1 malignant Enneking) or stage-3 'benign' growth – e.g. giant cell tumour. Technically demanding; refer to works of Roy-Camille and Tomita – sometimes needs vertebrectomy

5.5.2.10.1   Option 1
- En-Bloc resection, vertebrectomy with curative intent
- Weigh risk:benefit ratio – since much blood loss and long operation
- Many do it front and back – e.g. Bologna/Italy group; Tomita uses his special saw to perform mainly from posterior approach, reported in Spine

5.5.2.10.2   Option 2
- Intra-lesional excision, followed by RT/CT if sensitive
- Even if margin involved (not uncommonly), RT can help
- Bologna group found possibly not much different from en-bloc but inhomogeneous study; may need larger scale study to tell

5.5.2.10.3   Option 3
- Decompress to relieve neural obstruction, e.g. laminectomy, frequently needs instrumentation

5.6   Inflammatory Diseases Affecting the Spine

5.6.1   The Spine and Rheumatoid Arthritis

5.6.1.1   Problem List and Scope
- Cranial settling
- Atlanto-axial instability/subluxation
- Subaxial subluxation
- (Periodental pannus)

  Scope: 30% of rheumatoid arthritis patients admitted with C-spine problems

5.6.1.2 Pathophysiology
▓ Discitis and synovitis leads to cartilage loss, bone erosion and lax ligament and to instability
▓ Upper cervical-spine more common because
 – C0/C1, C1/2 are essentially synovial joints
 – C1/2 facets oriented in axial plane, if ligament destroyed – no bony stability

5.6.1.3 Cranial Settling
▓ Vertical translocation of dens
▓ MRI: find the cervico-medullary angle
▓ Associations: chronicity of disease (6 years), poor survival, greater neurology (Atlas-Dens Interval 'ADI' paradoxical decrease)
▓ Signs: ↓ pain/touch trigeminal distribution; no corneal reflex, occiput pain, blackouts, brainstem sign, myelopathy sign (other lower CN palsy)
▓ Radiological: Ranawat's three stations, McGregor line and Wackenheim line

5.6.1.4 Atlanoaxial Impaction
▓ Cause: occurs with incompetent ligament since little bony stability
▓ Types: 70% anterior, 20% lateral, 10% posterior
▓ Prediction of neurology – correlate with posterior atlantodens interval (PADI) < 14 mm (SAC)
▓ Normal spine most motion C4/5, now C1/2

5.6.1.5 Natural Hx
▓ Atlanoaxial impaction (AAI) patients can die suddenly
▓ One in ten rate of undiagnosed medullary compression in one study
▓ X-ray progression can be more rapid than neural deficit progression by a factor of two- to threefold
▓ Most with severe neurology do poorly
▓ Poor prognosis if myelopathy is treated conservatively
▓ Paradoxical improved ADI with cranial settling

5.6.1.6 Periodontal Pannus
▓ Pannus now more widely believed as a reactive tissue resulting from instability rather than a direct consequence of inflammatory process

▓ Example – resolve after C1/2 fusion in 19 of 22 cases in one study
▓ Two-thirds of rheumatoid arthritis patients with AAI with >3 mm pannus

5.6.1.7 Subaxial Subluxation
▓ Case for operation
 – Canal diameter in X-ray < 14 mm
 – MRI F/E for the true space
 – If < 13 mm, then post-fusion

5.6.1.8 General Work-up
▓ Hx and physical examination (P/E)
▓ Early signs of cord compression: sudden increase neck pain, spasticity/hyper-reflexia; bowel and bladder, less ambulation
▓ Ranawat three classes:
 – Class 1: no neurology
 – Class 2: subjective weakness, hyperreflexia, dysaesthesia
 – Class 3: A ambulatory, B normal activity

5.6.1.9 Radiological Assessment
▓ Prediction of AAI: AADI >35%; PADI >97%
▓ Lines: McGregor, Chamberlain, Wackenheim
▓ Ranawat station – I/II/III
▓ F/E X-ray

5.6.1.10 MRI
▓ Best to assess craniocervical junction, soft tissue and ligaments
▓ Pannus
▓ Cervico-medullary angle: normal → 135–175°; abnormal: <135° → correlate with paralysis
▓ Sometimes MRI in F/E
▓ Overall indications of MRI:
 – Neurology and abnormal X-ray
 – Cranial settling
 – PADI < 14 mm
 – Subaxial canal < 14 mm

5.6.1.11 Other Investigations
▪ SSEP
▪ Note: sometimes good to confirm cervical myelopathy especially in cases of the very disabled; SSEP also can be abnormal in the subluxation group

5.6.1.12 General Treatment Goals
▪ Avoid irreversible neurology
▪ Prevent sudden death from unrecognised neural compression
▪ But no unnecessary surgery
   Perhaps treat gross instability

5.6.1.13 Prognosis for Neurological Recovery
▪ Severity of paralysis
▪ PADI <10 mm no recovery; >10 mm at least recover one class; all with >14 mm recover
▪ Subaxial subluxation (SAS) post-operative canal diameter >14 mm good prognosis
   Outcome in quadriparesis – age, degree of vertical translocation, early surgery
   Prognosis does not depend on sex, age, AADI, paralysis duration or percentage SAS

5.6.1.14 Indications for Surgery
▪ Intractable neck pain
▪ Myelopathy signs
▪ Progressive instability
▪ PADI <14 mm
▪ SC diameter <6 mm (normal 10 mm)
▪ Cranial migration distance – perhaps approximately 31 mm
   (Surgery may not be of benefit in cases of long-term bed-bound patients)

5.6.1.15 Controversial Group
▪ Patient with markedly abnormal X-ray in the absence of pain or progressive neurological deficit?
▪ Answer:
   – AAI: PADI <14 mm; check MRI (cord diameter <6 mm on flexing, or CM angle <135)

- AAI plus cranial settling: use MRI to assess (whether traction is
  (1) reducible – post fusion or (2) irreducible – C1 laminectomy or
  anterior decompression and C0/C1 fusion)
- Conservative for cranial settling if: isolated, stable, asymptomatic,
  without cord compression
- SAS: canal diameter on X-ray < 14 mm; MRI: F/E for true space –
  if < 13 mm post fusion

5.6.1.16 Other Special Circumstances
- Case for transoral resection of the dens:
  - Irreducible ventral extradural compression of the cervicomedullary
    junction
  - Irreducible cranial settling
  - Odontoid fracture with complex compression fracture fragments
    with large fibrous pannus
    [N.B. 80% of rheumatoid arthritis patients with cranial settling
    with reducible lesion that require only post fusion]
- Conservative treatment of subaxial spine
- Traction and halo vest for 4 months

5.6.1.17 The Operative Option
- Pre-operative traction – up to 3 weeks – leads to correction of deformity,
  reduction of translocation and might abolish need of anterior surgery
- Approach: anterior approach for anterior compression and anterior
  decompression usually also requires posterior fixation
- Bone quality: in osteoporotic bone, lamina may be strongest – sub-
  laminar wiring
- (Fixation with no fusion reported by Crockard)

5.6.1.18 Types of Surgery
- Gallie (and Brooks) fusion
- C1/2 transarticular screw; contraindications
  - Collapsed lateral atlantal mass
  - C1/2 comminuted fracture
  - Marked osteoporosis
  - Anomalous vertebral artery (20% cases according to Crockard)
- Co-C2 fusion (Fig. 5.15) in: cranial settling, fixed anterior subluxation,
  with or without resection of posterior ring of C1
- Technique of C0/C1: Swiss and Ranford's loop

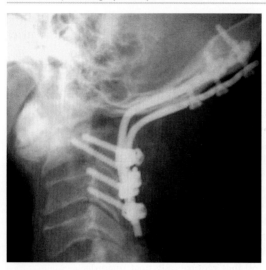

Fig. 5.15. Post-operative lateral X-ray of the cervical spine after C0-C2 fusion

5.6.2   Ankylosing Spondylitis

5.6.2.1   Nature
- Chronic inflammatory condition affecting the spine and SI-joint, with osseous proliferation (and ethesopathy) and associated with HLA B27

5.6.2.2   Pathomechanics
- Cause not known
- 95% HLA B27
- Most in males
- Can possibly run in families
- Potentially 1 in 1000 in Europe (less in the Black population in the US)

5.6.2.3   Diagnostic Criteria – Four of Five
- LBP >3/12
- Thoracic-spine: pain, stiffness, less chest expansion
- Lumbar-spine: less motion (limit extension first)
- Eye: iritis (past or present)
- X-ray evidence (earliest near TL region; early changes erosive followed by sclerosis at sites of attachment of annulus fibrosis), syndesmophytes (Figs. 5.16, 5.17)

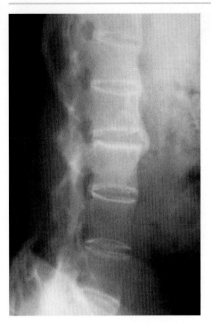

Fig. 5.16. The spine in a man with ankylosing spondylitis

5.6.2.4 Medical Treatment
▓ Drugs, including disease remitting agents, need to be optimised
▓ Physiotherapy and occupational therapy assessment

5.6.2.5 Surgery – Pre-Operative Planning
▓ Magnitude of deformity (correction needed)
▓ Chin-brow angle
▓ 30° more easy to achieve, 400 less reliable with single level (loss of correction more with open wedge)
▓ Correction by two 25° osteotomy of level >1 (at most 40°) and sometimes smoother lordosis with or without use of templates
▓ Measure hip mobility – usually do hip first (Fig. 5.18) if both hip and spine are significantly affected
  [P.S. AS patients are prone to develop pseudoarthrosis (Fig. 5.19) with trauma. The segment goes on to non-union due to the long moment arms of either side of the generally fused spine. Most try a course of conservative treatment and consider fusion if conservative treatment

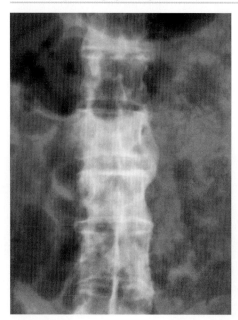

Fig. 5.17. Anteroposterior X-ray of the lumbar spine in a gentleman with ankylosing spondylitis

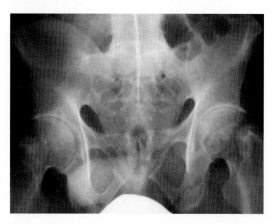

Fig. 5.18. Bilateral hip involvement in a patient with ankylosing spondylitis

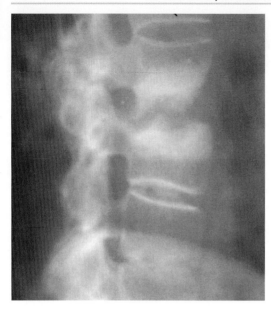

Fig. 5.19. Pseudoarthrosis in a patient with ankylosing spondylitis

fails. Recurrence is not uncommon, sometimes at another level that can escape solid spontaneous fusion]

5.6.2.6 Surgical – Consider Spinal Osteotomy if Creates Functional Deficits

5.6.2.6.1 Lumbar Osteotomy

▦ Smith-Peterson method: later modified by McMaster in '85
  – Many Cxs: aortic rupture, gastric dilation, mesenteric artery thrombosis
▦ Thomasen: modified it– by instrumenting the spine before destabilising it. Close the wedge:
  – Close wedge with decreased Cxs and deemed better
▦ Others: e.g. multiple pedicular closing wedges, fewer complications

5.6.2.6.2 Cervical Osteotomy

▦ Sitting position
▦ Decompress first (posterior laminectomy) and close defect after decompression

- Correction: 45–65°
- Cxs:
  - C8 root injury/sometimes cord
  - Non-union (less with modern technique)
  - Subluxation

5.7   Failed Back Syndrome

5.7.1   Aetiology
- Wrong Dx (patient, side, or wrong X-ray/MRI)
- Established neural injury or central pain syndrome – e.g. residual radiculopathy after disc herniates
- For operations done for decompression – inadequate decompression, e.g. missed lateral recess stenosis, lateral or far lateral disc, sequestrated disc, wrong level, recurrent disc
- For operations done for instability → inadequate fusion/pseudoarthrosis; sometimes iatrogenic (fracture pars, too much removal of lamina and facets)
- Cxs: declares early – e.g. infection; declares later – scar, arachnoid fibrosis, pathology of disc at one level next to fused level

5.7.2   Work-up
- Symptoms – new or old
- Category 1: improved for some period post-operatively; then, new symptom mostly implies new problem (e.g. other leg)
- Category 2: never any good period, e.g. inadequate/wrong Dx
- Category 3: if transient improved then (a) recurs early, e.g. sepsis/instability; (b) presents later – adjacent disc degeneration, new problem, etc.
- P/E: motor/sensory/SLR/gait – objective evidence of change
- X-ray: AP/Lat/oblique and always standing X-ray (look for disc space collapse, e.g. after sepsis). Oblique X-ray – picks up fracture Pars. Other things to look for: level of decompression, implant position, success of fusion, etc.
- CT: (a) position of implant, e.g. medial pedicle screw with nerve root impingement and (b)/ bony union – may need slightly oblique cuts and sometimes finer 1-mm cuts

5.7.3   X-Ray Assessment of PL and Anterior Fusion
▦ Accuracy for PL fusion 36–40% for X-ray/tomo/bending film/CT
▦ What if not sure?
- Finer cuts CT with reconstruction make oblique to the interface
- Definitive way to be sure about fusion of course is surgical exploration
▦ Anterior: assess continuity of trabeculae, F/E lack motion of graft. In longer term – evidence of remodel. (Some say fusion at anterior is less important – even pseudoarthrosis has not many symptoms if non-mobile)

5.7.4   Pitfalls and Pearls
▦ Avoid wrong Dx
▦ Do not forget SIJ can be cause of resistant LBP
▦ Choice of patient: psychiatric patient; worker's compensation, check for Waddell signs
▦ Established neural deficit – tell patient pre-operatively that deficit may persist despite decompression
▦ Inadequate decompression – especially lateral recess/medial facetectomy should be properly done
▦ Recurrent disc
▦ Segmental instability – may require fusion:
- To avoid fracture Pars, expose carefully and identify the Pars; leave at least 5 mm – decompress by undercutting (not overcutting) and medial facetectomy
- Realise pre-existing instability – clinical clues, e.g. significant mechanical symptoms; radiological clues, e.g. traction spurs, spondylolisthesis, motion on F/E – sometimes need fusion

5.7.5   About PL Fusion
▦ Instrumentation unlikely to improve fusion rate significantly if PL fusion was properly performed
▦ PL fusion alone: if single level, elderly (shorter operation, no cut out); mild mechanical pain
▦ Instrumentation considered if: >1 level; significant clinical symptoms; not enough BG

5.7.6   Overall Treatment Options in Failed Back

▥ Re-operate: for fusion/new disc – only 40% of re-operations had good results
▥ Pain management – epidural, nerve root block, epidural scope, radiofrequency, implantable pumps, gabapentin have all been tried
▥ Functional rehabilitation programme

5.7.7   Use of Epidural Scope

▥ Done by anaesthetist – pass a scope between coccyx to sacral canal to epidural space to problem area – infiltrate local anaesthesia/steroids and/or wriggle to break down adhesions

5.7.8   Use of Gadolinium-Enhanced MRI

▥ Radiologist DDx scar from disc by: recent scar diffuse enhancing; but disc fragment dark with rim enhancement
▥ Not reliable; found by recent studies especially in first 3±6 months – may still have mass effect like picture on MRI at site of original disc
▥ DDx = clinical + radiological + intra-operative finding
▥ Other MRI advantages: adequacy of decompression, new pathology, infection, sometimes more subtle pathology (e.g. pre-operative) like annular tear can be seen

General Bibliography

Vaccaro A, Albert T (eds) (2001) Master cases spine surgery, 2001 edn. Thieme, Stuttgart
Winter R, Lonstein J, Bradford D, Olilvie J (1995) Moe's textbook of scoliosis and other spinal deformities, 3rd edn. Saunders, Philadelphia

Selected Bibliography of Journal Articles

1. Luk DK, Cheung KM et al. (1998) Assessment of scoliosis correction in relation to flexibility using the fulcrum bending correction index. Spine 23:2303–2307
2. Fang D, Leong JC et al. (1988) Spinal pseudarthrosis in ankylosing spondylitis. Clinicopathologic correlation and the result of anterior spinal fusion. J Bone Joint Surg Br 70:443–447
3. Ducker TB (1992) Cervical stenosis: myelopathy hand. J Spinal Disorder 5:374–380

4. Gleave JR, Macfarlane R (2002) Cauda equina syndrome: what is the relationship between timing of surgery and outcome? Br J Neurosurg 16:325–328

5. Peterson LE, Nachemson AL (1995) Prediction of progression of the curve in girls who have adolescent idiopathic scoliosis of moderate severity. Logistic regression analysis based on data from the Brace Study of the Scoliosis Research Society. J Bone Joint Surg Am 77:823–827

6. McMaster MJ, Singh H (1999) Natural history of congenital kyphosis and kyphoscoliosis. A study of one hundred and twelve patients. J Bone Joint Surg Am 81:1367–1383

7. Dubousset J, Herring JA et al. (1989) The crankshaft phenomenon. JPO 9:541–550

6 Total Joint Surgery

Contents

6.1   Biomaterials

6.1.1   Definition of Biomaterials
■ "Biomaterials" refers to the synthetic and (treated) natural materials that are used to replace or augment tissue and organ function

6.1.2   General Requirements of Biomaterials
■ Adequate mechanical properties
■ Adequate wear resistance
■ Resists corrosion and degradation
■ Bio-compatible
■ High quality control
■ Cost not high
■ Maintains proper function and ability to predict mechanical function

6.1.3   Determinants of Proper Design
■ Understand working loads: mode of load, duration, frequency, magnitude
■ Mechanical properties: stress–strain; fatigue, isotropic versus anisotrophic; elastic versus viscoelastic; and the basic structure

6.1.4   Metals

6.1.4.1   History
■ 'Stainless steel' – with Co/Ni (18/8%) corrosion resistance not adequate until later on, molybdenum added to reduce pitting, and crevice corrosion
■ McKee introduced the first metal–metal joint with vitallium (Co–Cr–Mo)

6.1.4.2   General Structure of Metals
■ Made of crystals (i.e. metal atoms positioned in 3D periodic array)
■ Metal crystals joined by grain boundaries
■ Patterns of relationships of atoms:
    – Face-centred cubic (FCC)
    – Body-centred cubic (BCC)
    – Hexagonal close packed (HCP)

6.1.4.3 Types of 3D Layout in Metals
▦ FCC, e.g. 316L S Steel
▦ BCC, e.g. beta Ti
▦ HCP, e.g. CoCr, alpha Ti
  The above are the three most common ways, though there are 14 possible patterns

6.1.4.4 Drawbacks (*Defects*) of Metals
▦ Point – a lattice site not occupied by metal atom
▦ Line defect – dislocation. Improvements in metal design ought to prevent dislocations – a dislocation is the result of an extra half plane of atoms in a crystal – locally distorts the crystal structure (when a stress of sufficient magnitude is applied, these dislocations can move through the lattice – permanent change in shape of the crystal, and metal is plastically deformed)
▦ Area defects – at grain boundaries
▦ Volume defects – voids or cracks (even superficial scratches can lower the fatigue strength)

6.1.4.5 How to Improve the Defects
▦ Those processes that tend to prevent the motion of dislocation will act to strengthen the metal
▦ Grain boundary sliding is rarer – will not be discussed here

6.1.4.6 Methods to Strengthen the Metals
▦ Make an alloy: (solid solution strengthening) both interstitial or substitutional (if added atom is small, e.g. C/O/N/B) when we add one or more elements to the 'solvent' metal
  [Example of institutional – adding 0.1% carbon to iron = steel ($\times 10$ increased strength)]
▦ Cold working: the principle is to increase strength by increasing dislocation density, which entangles these dislocations into tight bundles – the resultant structure is much more difficult to move within the lattice
  Cold working is often performed on 316L stainless steel as strengthening – the metal can be cold worked by rolling, compression and other deformation mechanisms
  A process of annealing (heating) sometimes follows cold working and causes the alloy to return to pre-cold worked structure. The reason

for this process is to restore ductility and relieve internal stress, therefore decreasing grain size
▓ Hot working: deformation at high temperature, can sometimes reduce grain size, e.g.
  – Wrought – deformed into shape
  – Forged – high-temperature deformation to form a shape
▓ Grain size effect – alloy can be strengthened because if there are more grain boundaries per unit volume then it is more difficult to move dislocations
▓ Precipitation hardening – presence of a 2nd phase dispersed in the parent microstructure to inhibit the motion of dislocation, e.g. metal carbides forming in Co–Cr–Mo alloys to prevent dislocation motions

6.1.4.7 Protective Surface Layer of Alloys
▓ Passive oxide film is result of oxidation of outermost metal atoms on surface (very thin 2–10 nm)
▓ Stable in air and saline (formed by passivation treatment, e.g. by immersion in nitric acid bath)
▓ Barrier to release of metal ions, if absent metal will corrode rapidly
▓ If breached, metal is susceptible to hydration when bathed in metal ions in solution and the potential across the alloy–solution interface
▓ Examples:
  – Stainless steel ~ chromium oxide /Cr_2O_3 (FeO)
  – Co–Cr–Mo alloys, also chromium oxide mainly
  – Ti and titanium alloys → TiO_2 films (these are quite susceptible to hydration and changes in potential)

6.1.4.8 Other Possible Surface Modifications
▓ Ion implantation
▓ Chemical and physical vapour deposition
▓ Nitriding, diffusion hardening

6.1.4.9 Oxide Film in Relation to Wear
▓ Need to be thermal stable
▓ Need to be resistant to abrasion (mechanical strength)
▓ High adhesion to the substrate
  (Potential difference)

6.1.4.10   Stress–Strain Curve of Metals

▧ The linear portion of the stress–strain curve is less dependent on the presence of "dislocations" inside metals. The slope of the curve or stiffness depends on the relative ease or relative difficulty of stretching atoms from the equilibrium position in the lattice

▧ In the region of plastic deformation, as the stress increases, there is a point where dislocations begin to be created and move through the grains. Yield stress of the material is reached when the permanent deformation reaches 0.2%

▧ The amount of plastic strain prior to failure is a measure of ductility

▧ Fatigue life of a material is the number of cycles to cause failure at a fixed cyclic stress (in a classic cyclic stress versus number of cycles to failure)

▧ High cycle fatigue is when the number of cycles to cause failure $=10^4$ or more (in metals, during high cycle fatigue, most of the fatigue life is spent initiating a crack – factors to prevent crack initiation are important)

6.1.4.11   General Classes of Metallic Alloys

▧ Fe-based alloy, e.g. stainless steel

▧ Co-based alloy

▧ Ti alloy – especially Ti-6Al-4 V in total joint

6.1.4.11.1   Stainless Steel (Fe-Based Alloy)

▧ Fe-C based alloys

▧ 20% Cr, 12% Ni, 2.5% Mo, Mn and 0.08% C

▧ Some stainless steel is heat treatable, while some (like 316L) can only be cold worked

▧ 316L is the most commonly used stainless steel (L means low carbon)/called grade 2

▧ 316L stainless steel is found mostly in plates, screws, intramedullary (IM) nail, etc. for fracture fixations

▧ Why is low carbon good? – avoid formation of metal carbides that can adversely affect the corrosion resistance

6.1.4.11.2   Co-Based Alloy

▧ In addition to Co, also contains Cr/Mo/C and others (e.g. Ni, silicon, iron)

- HCP and/or FCC
- Used in total joint since it has high strength, hardness (resists surface deformation) and corrosion resistance (and/or hardened by precipitate of carbides, less wear and more surface hardness)

6.1.4.11.3 Ti-Based Alloys

- Advantages – high strength, low modulus, excellent corrosion resistance, biocompatible
- Drawback: notch sensitivity (sensitive to surface flaws) → can accelerate fatigue process and avoid sharp edges of geometry, e.g. porous-coating junctions, both of which raise the stress
- Type commonly used in total joint: Ti-6Al-4V (V is vanadium, not vitallium) → high strength and high fatigue resistance (due to the bimodal microstructure – with alpha and beta phases)
  [New: beta Ti (under investigation) – lesser E (elastic modulus)]
- HCP
- Four grades that vary in oxygen content (function as institutional strengthening element)
- Why is pure Ti not used in total joint? – not enough strength to carry the large stresses

6.1.4.12   Crevice (and Other) Corrosion

- Corrosion process – limited by the passive oxide film; – if the rate is low enough for the body to eliminate the generated corrosion debris, then this ionic and particle release may not be clinically significant
- There are situations, as in the modular junctions, where mechanically assisted crevice corrosion (fretting) has been reported; this corrosion is a conjoint effect of mechanical abrasion of the oxide film that covers the surface of the alloy in the taper and the restricted crevice environment
- Besides a local effect, this corrosion can cause systemic levels of Co and Cr
- Modular taper corrosion can sometimes cause fatigue failure of Co/Cr stems

6.1.4.13   Fatigue

- Fatigue in orthopaedic implants is now less common with improved materials and processing

▓ It can still occur since it is dominated usually by high-cycle fatigue, and crack initiation plays an important role in that process. Most cracks start at surface of the implant, hence the importance of the surface conditions (roughness, degree of cold work, etc.) and role of patient factors (e.g. weight and activity)

6.1.4.14 Wear
▓ Metal–metal couples – conjoint effect of corrosion and wear
▓ Systemic actions of wear particles not yet known but with possible mutagenic actions

6.1.5   Polyethylene

6.1.5.1   History
▓ Charnley's originally used polytetrafluoroethylene: though with low friction and inert; but it does not stand abrasion
▓ Quick wear: 1 cm in 3 years

6.1.5.2   Structure
▓ Ultra high molecular weight polyethylene (UHMWPE) is different from high-density polyethylene in terms of molecular weight (MW), density, impact strength and abrasive wear (better in all respects)
▓ Polymerisation of ethylene – synthesis conducted with catalyst, (made from Ti chloride and Al alkyl compound)
▓ Condition needed: 4- to 6-bar pressures and between $66°$ and $80°$
▓ Aim: increase MW, but minimise branching
(N.B. commercial polyethylene also may have calcium stearate, but does not always affect clinical performance as seen in Charnley's acetabular cups)
▓ 100% crystallinity cannot be achieved (because of large size of the polymer); crystallinity can be increased using high temperatures ($>250°C$) with no degradation and high pressure (2800 atm)
▓ The smallest structure in a crystalline region of a polymer is the unit cell; groups of unit cell form lamellae – sometimes folded, each with $150-CH_2$ groups

6.1.5.3 Fabrication – Three Methods

▦ Direct moulding: power into mould that compresses into the final shape; then heated under pressure (advantage – can make complex shapes and high glossy surface finish; disadvantage – slow and property varies with moulding conditions)

▦ Ram extrusion into cylindrical bars from 1 inch to 6 inches in diameter – implants are then machined from this cylindrical bar stock (widely used)

▦ Large sheet moulding: 8 inches thick and 8 feet long

6.1.5.4 Factors Determining Its Properties

▦ MW – just discussed

▦ Crystallinity – both crystalline (50–70%)and amorphous phases present; newer ones are more crystalline (note: modulus increases with crystallinity; more crystallinity may increase strength, improve oxidation resistance and increase resistance to fatigue crack propagation)

▦ Degree of X-links – sterilisation with no oxygen and newer technical use of electron beams. However, too many X-links make the material more brittle

6.1.5.5 Effects of Oxidation

▦ Recombination

▦ Chain scission – fragment of the original polymer chain is removed

▦ Cross-linking – two radicals from different polymer sections combine to form chemical bonds between two polymer chains (a cross-linked polymer may be harder and more abrasion resistant)

6.1.5.6 Current Sterilisation

▦ Vacuum

▦ Use ethylene oxide gas or gas plasma to sterilise the component (poorer penetration power)

6.1.5.7 Disadvantages of Polyethylene

▦ Fracture – rare, but it does occur

▦ Fatigue – after cyclic loading

▦ Creep
  – Note – subsurface white band can occur especially in those with a shelf life of more than 4 years

- Oxidative degradation may increase the modulus and brittleness of the polyethylene

6.1.6   Cement (Methyl Methacrylate)

6.1.6.1   History
▦ In olden days, as cranioplast, plexiglass, judet hip, etc.
▦ Previous examples were all transparent; now they can be seen on X-ray with barium sulphate

6.1.6.2   Basic Structure
▦ Methyl methacrylate (MMA) is one member of a group of polymers widely known as polyethylene, polyvinyl chloride, polystyrene – repeating carbon-based units of variable chain length
▦ Monomer with MW of only 100
▦ Longer chain length and greater viscosity; ultimate chain length of the polymer depends on the manufacturing process – initiators and activators

6.1.6.3   The Chemical Reaction
▦ Powder: pre-polymerised polymethyl methacrylate (PMMA) beads and initiator (dibenzoyl peroxide)
▦ Liquid: monomer and activator (N/N dimethyl-p-toludine)
[Main reaction is benzoyl peroxide radical reacting with monomer to begin the polymerisation process]
(Note: 47 °C bone necrosis, 56 °C protein denaturation; modern cement with 1-mm to 4-mm-thick mantle does not however appear to produce excess temperature enough to cause necrosis)

6.1.6.4   Physical Stages After Mixing
▦ Stage 1 – lumpy after mixing (monomer–polymer conglomerates)
▦ Stage 2 – liquid stage; can then be transferred to cement gun
▦ Stage 3 – dough; less viscous, further swelling and polymerisation (time where cement no longer sticks to gloves; prone to produce laminations at this stage); average time for doughy state formation is 5–8 min
▦ Hardened and exothermic (on average 2600 calories/20 g) – a combination of the bulk polymerisation of the monomer MMA and matrix

polymerisation of the MMA in the presence of pre-formed polymer particles.

(Normal cement also has hydroquinone to prevent spontaneous polymerisation)

6.1.6.5 Systemic Toxicity of the Monomer

■ Can cause hypotension due to cardiac depressant action, etc. (mechanism not yet certain; initially thought to be related to the monomer, newer theories include emboli during pressurisation in the cementation process)

■ Need close monitoring during total hip replacement (THR) cementation process in particular, especially in elderly patients with limited cardiopulmonary reserve

6.1.6.6 Shrinkage

■ About 6% shrinkage upon polymerisation

■ About 5% monomer evaporates during preparation especially if not done under vacuum

6.1.6.7 Factors Determining the Setting Time

■ Temperature – higher start temp, shorter set time (but ultimate exothermic reaction same); cool components before mixing delay set time

■ Humidity – data on simplex P – more humid faster set time

■ Vacuum – shorten the setting time a bit (reduced oxygen that normally can inhibit the reaction)

6.1.6.8 Choice of Viscosity

■ Modern trend is for retrograde filling and pressurising to allow flow to interstice; to this end, use of cements in a lower viscosity and less dough state recommended

■ Porosity – can be decreased by vacuum and centrifugation

■ Concept of "pseudoplasticity": higher pressure during administration causes better flow and penetration, which suggests rapid and sustained insertion of prosthesis (for better interdigitation)

■ Note: high viscosity cement is needed if manual handling is preferred by surgeons, e.g. Palacos; simplex P is an intermediate, example of low viscosity, e.g. Zimmer LVC, Sulfix 6)

6.1.6.9 Strength of Cement

■ In general cement is stronger in compression than tension
■ Better strength with:
- Porosity reduction (open bowl causes 10% porosity, reduce beats/stand – 5%; vacuum 1%)
- Higher initial MW
- Lack of defects
- Possible lack of barium
  (Vacuum method works by exposing as much of the surface area as possible to the vacuum to release the bubbles – minimise stirring which can entrap bubbles in the mixture.)
  (Addition of fibres blocks the flow of cement and is not recommended.)
  (Effect of antibiotics: prerequisite is the antibiotic used; reasonably heat stable; may cause some weakening since they act as a discontinuity in the cement, especially in large doses (5–10 g) – much lesser effect with a small dose (0.5–2 g). In addition, rapidity of elution is quicker for tobramycin than vancomycin)

6.1.6.10 Longevity of Cement

■ Fatigue life – increases with porosity reduction (lesser voids); pores are stress concentrators and crack initiators. Avoid blood inclusions and laminations
■ Proper timing/viscosity necessary to get the proper interdigitation
■ Quality of mantle – Harris/O'Neil classification and proper thickness (2–5 mm distal to tip, 2 mm around, 3–5 mm on acetabular side)
■ Generation of cementing method used
■ Placement/alignment of prosthesis (avoid varus implant alignment since it increases stress)
■ Design of prosthesis: avoid sharp corners
- (Some evidence that debonding of metal–cement interface with prior heating of femoral implant to 44 °C is less likely – causes the cement nearer the stem to polymerise earlier)

6.1.6.11 Creep

■ Under strain, over time, the material can undergo permanent change and deformation – creep

▦ Example – Exeter prosthesis subsidence since a smooth shape stimulated interest on the changes of PMMA over time under load – the presence of the polished tapered stem leads to maintenance of a tight bond between the cement and bone with a Taper lock effect
  – (Previous approach in the other direction to improve metal–cement interface with the use of PMMA 'precoat' and even irregular surface: found not to be successful)

6.1.6.12 The three Generations of Cementation Techniques
▦ 1st generation – hand mixed, cancellous bone left alone, vented, minor canal preparation, finger manual insertion in doughy stage, femoral stem shapes with high stress transmission (e.g. sharp corners)
▦ 2nd generation – distal restrictor, pulsatile lavage, dried canal, retrogradely injected with cement gun, stem rounded corners, removal of cancellous bone to near endosteal surface
▦ 3rd generation – vacuum/centrifuge of cement, retrogradely injected with cement gun and pressurised; distal and proximal centralisers for an even cement mantle and neutral stem position; cement precoating (removal of cancellous bone to near the endosteal surface, pulsatile lavage, packed with adrenaline-soaked gauze and dried the canal)

6.1.6.13 Rationale Behind the 2nd and 3rd Generations of Cementation
▦ 2nd generation – aim to improve the bone–cement interface
▦ 3rd generation – aim to improve the metal–cement interface

6.1.6.14 Cement Grading (Harris and O'Neill)
▦ Completely fill medullary cavity and white out
▦ Slight radiolucency
▦ Radiolucence of 50–99% of cement–bone interface or defective/incomplete mantle
▦ Stem tip not covered or radiolucencies of 100% of interface

6.1.7 Ceramic

6.1.7.1 Nature
- Several classes of materials known for their biocompatibility under a wide range of physical, mechanical, chemical and electrical characteristics
- Most of these materials with substantial quantities of oxygen and quantities of carbon, calcium, phosphorus, aluminium and zirconium
- The above elemental combinations result in reduced densities, and lowered E (elastic modulus)

6.1.7.2 Common Types
- Oxides of aluminium, zirconium and titanium (the alumina in use are primarily fine grain-sized alpha alumina)
- Carbon and related –C–Si, graphite, diamond
- $CaSO_4$ (plaster)/fill bone lesion, phosphates/as grafts and aluminates
- Glass and glass ceramics
- Sulphates aluminates and calcium phosphates

6.1.7.3 Biomechanical Features of Ceramics
- Strongest in compression
- Brittle
- Fracture prone
- Low wear because of: decrease in abrasion (e.g. alumina femoral head and ceramic–ceramic bearings), scratch resistance, increased hardness to indentation and decreased coefficient of friction

6.1.7.4 Ways to Improve Physical Properties
- Ceramic grain-size control
- Minimise porosities (since this can cause fracture and 3rd body wear)
- Meticulous manufacturing and processing
- Larger component sizes (less stress) – this may cause technical difficulties at surgery, however; thus beware of using smaller sized ceramic femoral head, for instance, as they break more easily
- In future, techniques to produce more uniform surface coatings

6.1.7.5 General Uses of Ceramics
- Total joint
- Grafts

- Insulation
- As bioactive coats (bone on-growth)

6.1.7.6 Advantages of Ceramics Used as Biological Coating
- More normal in physiological environments, e.g. C/Ca/P/O
- Elastic modulus more similar to nearby tissues (decrease the magnitude of interfacial microstrain differences)
- Very biocompatible
- In dentistry, off white/intraoral application
- An interfacial barrier to transfer of elements, heat or electrons from the substrates

  If direct contact and integration with bone is attained, there is improved force transfer

  [If used as coatings, the initial active response with bone is short term (less than 1 month), and most of the active biomaterial (other than the surface zone) is intended to remain as an implant over the long term (years). For example, porous and particulate material is used in bone grafts (BGs) intended for long-term augmentations, and implant coatings are intended for attachment to bone and soft tissue]

  [Some are degradable – as scaffold to deliver growth factors, for example]

6.1.7.7 Summary of Advantages of Ceramics
- Inert, stable
- Biocompatible
- Low friction
- High strength – especially fully dense ceramic biomaterials such as aluminium and zirconium oxides in total joints

6.1.7.8 Summary of Disadvantages of Ceramics
- Brittle (better to use larger bulk/component size) – they are brittle (non-ductile) because of their atomic bond responses to mechanical forces
- Prone to fracture, since they are mechanically weak when loaded cyclically under high magnitude tension and shear-stress conditions. (Hence often used in larger bulk structural forms, where mechanical stresses will be lower)
- Sensitive to hoop stress

6.1.7.9 Types of Bioceramic Bone Interactions
- Type 1: inert – no attachment except through surface topography
- Type 2: active – attachment with chemical interaction, e.g. $CaPO_4$-based hydroxylapatite classified as bioactive. Over time, the dissolution/deposition interaction result in micro-interlock and possibilities of regionalised biochemical bone-ongrowth attachments, which will enhance force transfer

6.1.7.10 Use in the Morse-Taper Junctions
- Surface modifications or ceramic inserts have been used at morse tapers and screw connections to minimise component corrosion, fretting corrosion and, hence, wear
- Type of ceramics used here are hard, dense and stable, as they are non-conductors of electricity

6.2   Modes of Wear in Total Joint

- Adhesion
- Abrasion
- Third Body
- Fatigue
- Corrosion

6.2.1   Adhesive Wear
- When the atomic forces between two articulating surfaces under load are greater than that between inherent material properties of either surface, continued motion of the surfaces require breaking the bond junctions. Each time a junction is broken, a wear particle is created. In practice, this process may create pits and voids mostly on the polyethylene

6.2.2   Abrasive Wear
- Occurs between surfaces of different hardness. In most cases, roughened areas or asperities on the harder surface plow onto the softer surface

6.2.3   Third Body Wear

■ Can be thought of as a form of abrasive wear when a free particle gets entrapped onto a pair of articulating couple, or sometimes the particle gets embedded onto the softer surface

6.2.4   Fatigue Wear

■ Occurs when subsurface/surface cyclic shear stress in a material exceeds the fatigue limit of that material

■ Cases with significant wear can result in delamination, not just microscopic or macroscopic pits. In the case of polyethylene, it is believed that oxidative degradation (if present) can be an added predisposing factor

6.2.5   Corrosion Wear

■ Can be thought of as a form of third body wear, the liberated corrosive debris acting as an abrasive free body. Since the motion of an articulating couple removes corrosive products, liberation of such products exposes a greater surface (less resistant to corrosion) to even further corrosion

6.2.6   Effect of the Wear Particles

■ With the millions of cycles we walk each year, the plentiful submicron particles generated can induce periprosthetic osteolysis (discussed in the next section), which is a significant causation of aseptic loosening of the total joint replacement

■ Arthroplasty surgeons have also discovered the concept of effective joint space. For example, wear particles can find their way between the bone–implant interface in the non-circumferentially porous-coated femoral component, and osteolysis can occur in spaces far beyond the joint itself, aided in part by the continuous pumping or fluctuating hydrostatic forces between the bone and the implant.

[Note: the major modes of wear in both THR (Fig. 6.1, showing eccentric wear of acetabular polyethylene) and total knee replacement (TKR) include adhesion and abrasion. However, in TKR, the fatigue mode of wear is important, and delamination can occur]

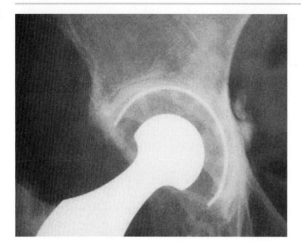

Fig. 6.1. Eccentric wear of the right acetabular component
of the total hip replacement

6.2.7   Ways to Lessen Wear

- Increased surface hardness of biomaterial used in the articulating couple, e.g. ceramic is noted for its hardness although it is brittle
- Decreased friction forces by research into the different methods of joint lubrication, e.g. those surfaces with more 'wettability' may fare better in this respect. This topic will be discussed later
- Develop better, more wear-resistant, polyethylene. The newly highly cross-linked polyethylene seems promising. However, the method of sterilisation of polyethylene is the absence of oxygen and is important as it decreases the chance of oxidative degradation
- Other factors: the surface finish and the sizing of the implants by the manufacturers; attention to details of the surface finishes of the morse-taper junctions; and the geometry of the implanted components are important, e.g. metal–metal articulating couples. Needless to say, surgical technique and a thorough understanding of the design of the prostheses as well as the nature of the biomaterial on the part of the arthroplasty surgeon are also very important

6.3   Lubrication of Joints

■ Human synovial joints are noted for low wear via the following mechanisms:
- Very low coefficient between hyaline cartilage rubbing on hyaline cartilage (see section on cartilage in basic science)
- Nature of the synovial fluid secreted (containing glycoprotein lubrican), which serves the function of lubrication. Also the fluid may change in viscosity depending on the different rate of joint motion and loading
- In the human hip joint, for instance, it is believed that different methods of joint lubrication mechanism are at work, including elastohydrodynamic lubrication and squeeze film lubrication

6.3.1   Types of Joint Lubrication

■ Boundary lubrication: involves adsorption of a single monolayer of lubricant on each surface; lessens wear by preventing direct surface contact
■ Fluid film lubrication: separation of bearing surface increased with thin film of fluid
- Hydrodynamic – occurs when rigid bearing surfaces are not parallel
- Squeeze film lubrication – this method may carry high loads for short period; the viscosity of the fluid in the gap produces pressure that tends to force lubricant out (as in articular cartilage)

6.3.2   Other Methods Used by Synovial Joints

■ Elastohydrodynamic lubrication: as in human joints, where the bearing surfaces are not absolutely rigid as in metals; pressure in the fluid film deforms the soft articular surface – this deformation causes increased surface area of the bearing surface. The advantage of this deformation is that it helps reduce the escape of fluid between the bearing surfaces, and the film will last longer
■ Weeping lubrication: occurs in human joints, since hyaline cartilage is fluid filled, porous and permeable and can exude fluid when the joint is under load (can also imbibe back when joint unloaded as in the swing phase of gait)

▨ Boosted lubrication: it is surmised that the solvent part of the joint lubricant fluid enters the cartilage during squeeze film lubrication, and it is possible that the hyaluronic protein complexes are left behind between the surfaces, resembling an ultrafiltration process

6.4   Periprosthetic Osteolysis

6.4.1   Nature of Periprosthetic Osteolysis
▨ Mainly macrophage and fibroblast response to wear particles especially polyethylene
▨ The cellular response stimulates osteoclasts, and bone resorption ensues

6.4.2   Importance and Clinical Relevance
▨ Important cause of long-term failure of implant
▨ Causes implant loosening (aseptic type)
▨ Loss of bone stock, making revisions difficult
▨ Predispose to fracture, i.e. periprosthetic fractures
▨ Prevalence: can reach 50% by 10 years

6.4.3   Clinical Features
▨ Mostly no or minimal symptoms (if symptomatic can be from associated synovitis)
▨ Pain produced, however, if there is complication such as fracture (be it macro fracture or micro fracture)

6.4.4   Common Radiological Patterns
▨ Balloon lysis in the periacetabular region of innominate bone, and endosteal scalloping in the femoral cortex
▨ Lytic/radiolucent areas, e.g. around the greater trochanter (GT)/lesser trochanter (LT) in THR implants, with bone losses; tend also to occur in TKR, although less common (Fig. 6.2). Notice that the average size of the wear particles in THR is much more likely to excite a histiocytic response than the larger average size of the particles in TKR

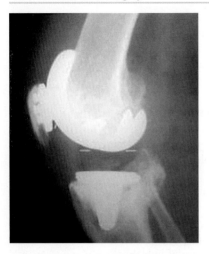

Fig. 6.2. Failed total knee replacement. Note the radiolucency surrounding the loosened tibial tray

6.4.5   Pathogenesis (Jacobs)

■ Not the cement disease as originally thought, but an adverse response to phagocytosable particulate wear debris and corrosion debris; possibly facilitated by local hydrodynamic effects (see Discussion on effective joint space)
■ Involved complex interactions of cellular mediators

6.4.6   Pathogenesis – Cells Involved

■ Osteoclasts
■ Macrophages
■ Fibroblasts
■ Osteoblasts

6.4.7   Pathogenesis – Mediators and Pathways

■ Tumour necrosis factor (alpha)
■ IL-1 and IL-6
■ PGE_2
■ Others – under investigation (cytokines, enzymes, prostenoids). Stimulation of the RANK/RANKL ligand pathway for osteoclast activity and/or more osteoclast precursors
■ Possible tyrosine kinase pathway as well

6.4.8 Classification for Acetabular Osteolysis and Its Treatment (Cementless Cases)/Maloney

- Type 1: liner exchangeable, cup stable; graft and exchange the liner
- Type 2: liner not exchangeable (not modular) and cup appears stable; revision of whole component mostly needed (at the expense of bone loss)
- Type 3: component unstable; revision

6.4.9 Timing of Surgery in General

- Tendency towards earlier intervention before too much loss of bone stock
- Have to prime patient before the index operation of such subsequent procedures

6.4.10 Future and Possible Prophylaxis

- Role of biphosphonates (recent animal experiment in canines showed preventive role; more recently, another rat animal model showed a possible added therapeutic role even after osteolysis was established)
- Role of drugs counteracting the mediators
- Changes in design
- More durable articulating interfaces, e.g. higher X-linked polyethylene (and compression moulding), etc.

6.4.11 Mechanism of Action of Bisphosphonates

- The drugs show some promise in animal studies to reduce osteolysis, but they do not reverse the action of the inflammatory mediators. They bind to hydroxyapatite (HA) and interfere with ruffled border formation of the osteoclast/acidification process. However, they do not act by interfering with the formation and maturation of osteoclasts
- Will not work in instability-induced porosis

6.5 Primary TKR

6.5.1 Pearls to a Successful TKR

- Patient selection
- Choice of implant

- ▨ Surgical technique:
  - – Correct bone cuts and restoration of a favourable mechanical environment and alignment
  - – Correct component placement
  - – Correct ligament balancing
- ▨ Attention to extensor mechanism restoration

6.5.1.1 Patient Selection
- ▨ Realistic expectations
- ▨ Consideration can be given to other treatment options in younger adults. Examples: high tibial osteotomy (HTO) in the young adult high-demanding labourer, unicompartmental knee replacement in isolated medial compartment disease for selected patients around 60 years old. The details of the different surgical options in the middle-aged patient with knee arthritis will be dealt with later

6.5.1.2 Choice of Implants
- ▨ There is a tendency towards the use of mobile-bearing knee replacements in younger middle-aged subjects (the pros and cons of this implant will be discussed in detail). No long-term results over 15 years are available, however.

  In general, it should be remembered that use of the least constraint possible, taking into consideration knee and the surgeon's ability, will result in the best long-term outcome
- ▨ More traditional fixed-bearing knee designs may suffice for the low-demand, elderly subjects, as these implants have a good long-term track record. However, how do you choose between posterior cruciate ligament (PCL) retention and substitution?
  - – Posterior stabilised implants. Advantages include: lower articular stress from increased conformity, facilitated deformity correction since PCL is excised (since if PCL tight, serves to remove a constraining force), reliable stability for most models and good range of motion (ROM) attained in the majority (especially the newer generation of posterior stabilised implants). Disadvantages include: femoral side bone loss from the cutting of the inter-condylar box, theoretical bone–cement interface stresses and increased patella complications recorded in the past, such as patella-clunk syndrome associated with the posterior stabilised (PS) IB II implant. However,

this problem is much less in the newer generation of posterior-sta-bilised total knee implants with a more posteriorly situated inter-condylar box

- PCL – retaining TKR. Advantages include: theoretically more likeli-hood of maintaining femoral roll-back (not borne out in laboratory experiments), less femoral side bone loss since no need for cutting the inter-condylar box, theoretically better proprioception and en-hanced quadriceps function, and a lesser stress at the bone–cement interface. Disadvantages include: theoretical ease of earlier loosen-ing from the femoral glide (see-saw action), especially in the older models with a flat-dish polyethylene associated with high stress to the plastic; and technical difficulty in re-establishing the correct tension of the PCL, which in fact is often attenuated anyway in the patients with osteoarthritis (OA) of the knee (especially if OA is advanced, and PCL retention not always feasible)

6.5.1.3 Surgical Technique

6.5.1.3.1 Making the Appropriate Bone Cuts

Alignment of the Normal Lower Extremity
  The mechanical axis of the normal lower limb passes from the centre of the femoral head through the knee to the dome of the talus
  The anatomical and mechanical axes of the femur varies by the angle made due to the offset of the hip. According to Moreland, the mean difference of the two axes is 5.9° or about 6°. There is usually no vari-ation between the anatomical and mechanical axes of the Tibia

The Classic Versus the Anatomic Methods of Alignment Restoration: Two Main Philosophies of Bone Cut in TKR
  Two schools of thought
  - Classic cut – perpendicular to the mechanical axis, both femoral and tibial cuts perpendicular to the mechanical axis (used by most surgeons)
  - Anatomic cut – popularised by Hungerford and allows for the fact that the natural medial joint line is 2–3° varus (since this is how the leg views the forces in a one-legged stance; not very popular since high chance of a varus cut, seldom used)

Why Are There Classic and Anatomic Methods?

- The classic representation of the lower limb is correct for a double leg stance
- Normal joint line is at an angle to the mechanical axis of 87° on the lateral side and 93° on the medial side
- The obvious next question is why does the knee joint line tilt 3° off the perpendicular, i.e. 93°?

The Answers

- We know the highest loads on the knee in walking are during a single leg stance
- As the body shifts from a double to single leg stance, the centre of gravity (C.G) shifts over the supporting foot and the weight-bearing (WB) line falls medial to the hip, through the medial compartment of the knee to the ankle. With this shift in single leg stance, the joint axis becomes perpendicular to the mechanical axis

How to Choose As a Surgeon?

- As a surgeon, you can aim for the joint line to be correct in the double leg stance, i.e. 90° to the mechanical axis, passing through the hip, knee and ankle (the classic alignment)
- You may aim for the joint line to be correct in the single leg stance (the anatomic alignment).
  Most surgeons use the classic alignment (and hence classic cuts in TKR). This is based mainly on the fact that the anatomic method increases the chance of a varus cut, and the individual variation is too great to consider it important

Elaboration of the Classic Method

- The classic method causes a valgus over-correction of the lateral tibial plateau, and is compensated by a relative under-resection of the lateral femoral condyle
- If the joint line is cut at 90° or the classic cut, more tibia will be resected laterally than medially. In extension, more femur will be resected medially than laterally. In flexion, the femoral cuts must be externally rotated 3° in order to avoid asymmetry of the flexion gap

Main Principles of Instrumentation
- Flexion and extension (F/E) gap
- Measured resection method

A Practical Note
- Many current instrumentation systems use a combination of the F/E gap and measured resection methods
- Those systems that combine the classic alignment method with the measured resection method characteristically externally rotate the femoral component from its anatomical reference by $3°$ (e.g. NexGen TKR)

Elaboration of the Measured Resection Method
- Here, the distal femoral resection and the posterior femoral resections equal the thickness of the components to be implanted, thus preserving the joint line near to original
- This method was shown in cadavers to reproduce perfectly the kinematics of the intact knee using a minimally constrained prosthesis that preserves the PCL. Any ligament imbalance is therefore caused by osteophytes, scar, contractures, etc.

Measured Resection Versus F/E Gap Method
- The measured resection method carries out all bony resection first and then balances ligament – it can be used with either the classic or anatomic methods
- With the F/E method, the tension of the soft tissue must not be changed by the bony resection (e.g. if the post-capsule is contracted, it becomes the principal determinant of the space between femur and tibia when the knee is extended. However, with knee flexed, the post-capsule is no longer under tension, the collateral laxity can now become evident and the knee is unstable)
- With the F/E gap method of ligament balancing, bone resection level and ligament balance are determined at the same time (here, the surgeon has to be careful that such problems as structural abnormalities, contractures, etc. do not lead to incorrect resection levels)

What to Do if F/E Gaps Are Not Well Balanced?
- General rule: balance symmetrical problems (i.e. problem occurs both in flexion and in extension) with adjustment on the tibial side (such as thickness of the polyethylene or level of the bone cut on the tibial side)
- Flexion gap satisfactory but tight in extension: resect more femur distally
- Extension gap satisfactory but flexion is loose: upsize the femoral component or even increase the polyethylene thickness to balance flexion, and resect an equal amount from the distal femur in extension

6.5.1.3.2 Correct Component Placement

Common mistakes in component placement include:
- Femoral component
  - Coronal plane varus/valgus malalignment relative to the mechanical axis
  - Sagittal plane malalignment with excess flexion or extension
  - Axial plane malalignment with excess internal rotation (IR) or external rotation (ER) relative to the epicongylar axis
- Tibial component:
  - Varus or valgus component alignment in the coronal plane
  - Tibial component internal or ER
  - Excess cutting of the posterior slope, and rarely anterior sloping alignment in the sagittal plane
  - Other problems:
    Anterior and posterior translation of the femoral component
    Proximal or distal translation of the joint line
    Medial or lateral translation with implant overhang
    Improper cut of the patella and improper placement of the patella button
    Refer to the section on TKR Alignment for the details of how to tackle these problems

6.5.1.3.3 Proper Ligament Balancing

- The following is a guideline to ligament balancing for the varus and valgus knees, based on expert teachings by Whiteside
- This does not mean this is the only method or sequence of soft-tissue release. It should be stressed that proper pre-operative planning and

intra-operatively proper bone cuts should be performed before correct ligament balancing can be performed

Soft-Tissue Release for the Varus Knee

- Before discussion, one must know what soft-tissue structures are tight medially in knee F/E
- Structures tight in full knee extension: posteromedial capsule, posterior portion of medial collateral ligament (MCL)
- Structure tight in knee flexion: anterior portion of the MCL

Example

- If, intra-operatively, the knee is tight medially in extension only, only need to release the posterior MCL and posteromedial capsule with curved osteotome
- If, intra-operatively, the knee is tight medially only in flexion, we only need to release the anterior portion of MCL

Soft-Tissue Release for the Valgus Knee

- Before discussing the topic, one must know which soft-tissue structure(s) is/are tight in knee extension and knee flexion. One should beware of the frequently encountered collapse of the lateral femoral condyle and make the proper bone cuts
- Knee extension: tightness is noted in iliotibial band, lateral collateral ligament (LCL), popliteus and posterolateral capsule
- Knee flexion: tightness occurs in the popliteus and LCL

Example

- Intraoperatively, if the knee is tight laterally only in extension, do not release structures that are tight in both flexion and extension. Thus, only release the iliotibial band and the posterolateral capsule, etc.

6.5.1.3.4 Restoration of the Extensor Mechanism

- Proper restoration of the extensor mechanism function depends on:
  - Proper restoration of the patella thickness and correct sizing of the femoral component
  - Proper trochlea design of the femoral component
  - Avoid malrotation of the femoral and tibial components

- Proper restoration of soft-tissue balancing and assessment of the need for lateral release

  Patella-clunk syndrome is commonly associated with posterior-stabilised designs. Its occurrence can be minimised by careful debridement of the peripatella retinaculum, avoidance of proximal placement of the patella button, and use more modern PS knee designs with a more posteriorly situated intercondylar box (Ip D, Int Orthop 2002 [2])

6.6   Alignment in TKR

6.6.1   What Constitutes Alignment
- Most people talk mainly about varus/valgus alignment in TKR
- This is over-simplified; the knee has three axes with many degrees of freedom
- Alignment involves not only varus/valgus, but any F/E of component, rotational alignment and also translational alignment along each axis

6.6.2   How About Patella?
- The 6 degrees of freedom apply to the patella as well, but since patella oriented in the coronal plane, the nomenclature is different

6.6.3   The Importance of Joint Line Restoration in TKR
- Proper restoration of joint line needed for proper collaterals functioning
- Effect of patella baja – needs to be prevented in TKR. Patella baja not only predisposes to patella-clunk, but also anterior knee pain and/or motion restriction

6.6.4   Four Main Reasons to Ensure Good Alignment
- Biomechanics – more symmetric bone loading
- Prevent premature failure of polyethylene (note catastrophic failure can occur when too much force on one compartment)
- Prevent premature loosening – bone prosthesis and bone–cement prosthesis interfaces
- Prevent undue strain on ligaments that can cause gross instability

6.6.5   What Alignment Can Be Assessed on X-Ray?

▨ X-ray can visualise: varus/valgus alignment if we do scanograms, F/E of the total joint components if we take a true lateral translation – may sometimes be seen (if gross)

▨ X-ray cannot adequately visualise – rotational and subtle translational malalignment
(To measure accurately, ensure neutral rotation of the knee and no flexion contracture)

6.6.6   On Coronal Varus/Valgus Alignment

▨ A straight line from the centre of hip to centre of knee and ankle centre is called neutral alignment. A positive value indicates a varus deformity, while negative indicates valgus deformity in degrees

▨ Most of the instruments use the femoral shaft for varus/valgus orientation – with a joint line to femoral shaft axis angle of about 9°. Most systems use the IM guide. The extramedullary (EM) guide is useful if canal is blocked. However, if femur is deformed, use the mechanical axis – in this case, using the femoral head as reference is needed, and the position of the femoral starting hole may need to be adjusted accordingly

▨ For the tibia, we may use the EM versus IM alignment guide, although there are studies claiming comparative results between the EM and IM guides for the tibial cut; IM guides may risk suboptimal tibial cut especially in bowed tibiae

6.6.6.1 Varus Knee

▨ Avoid varus cut at all costs since this can lead to early catastrophic failure of the TKR

▨ Most of the varus/valgus posture for the femoral component is determined by the femoral IM guide

6.6.6.2 Valgus Knee

▨ Do not leave the post-operative knee in significant valgus since this will put excessive strain on the MCL, causing its further attenuation

▨ Again, varus/valgus posture for femoral component is usually determined by the IM femoral guide

6.6.7   F/E of the Total Knee Components

■ Normal posterior tibial slope: 7–10°
■ Excess slope: lowered resection level encounters weaker bone
  Unstable in flexion

6.6.8   Effect of an Anterior Slope of Tibia

■ Anterior subsidence of the tibial component can produce recurvatum deformity – bad news for the PCL if retained
■ Quadriceps weakness and knee instability in general are expected
■ The IM femoral guide determines both the varus/valgus and the F/E of the femoral component
■ For deformed femurs, the EM guide may be useful (severely deformed femurs need concomitant osteotomy or staged osteotomy followed in a second stage by TKR)
  (Improper F/E of the femoral component affects the functioning of the patella joint/patella tracking/quadriceps mechanics; as well as ROM of the knee post-TKR)

6.6.9   Rotation Alignment of Tibial and Femoral Components

6.6.9.1   Tibial Component Rotation in Total Knee Arthroplasty

6.6.9.1.1 Ways to Ensure Proper Tibial Component Rotational Alignment

■ Best to align the intercondylar eminence of the tibial component with the tibial crest in the sagittal plane (Merkow)
■ Deliberate ER should be avoided (Hozack)
■ Recent Japanese study showed tibial torsion to vary from 12° internal to 30° of external torsion, some cases also associated with proximal tibia vara as well
■ Provide good exposure and excise tibial osteophytes (Insall)
■ Allow less reliance on less reliable bony indicators (e.g. feet deformities are not uncommon in the elderly OA knee patients)
■ Another way is using a pegless tibial trial, the knee taken through a full ROM several times – rationale is hopefully that the tibial trial will seek its correct rotational alignment, based on femoral component alignment and overall ligament balance (Hozack)

6.6.9.1.2 Summary of Guidelines for Tibial Component Rotation

- Aim at tibial tubercle medial 1/3
- Use tibial crest as a guide
- ROM method – put in the trial tibial and femoral components and bring the knee through a ROM to let the tibial component find the most suitable rotational position (assuming the femoral component is properly implanted)
- Do not use the foot as a guide, as foot deformity is common and may make our assessment inaccurate

6.6.9.1.3 Causes of Malrotated Tibial Component in TKR

- Inadequate exposure
- Reliance of unreliable/less reliable bony landmarks – e.g. foot is a poor land-mark for tibial rotation (Ranawat)
- Excessive internal or external tibial torsion
- Deliberate external rotation of the component by the surgeon

6.6.9.1.4 Effects of Externally Rotated Tibial Component

- Mismatch of the arc of knee motion as determined by the ligaments and that imposed by femorotibial congruency
- Increased wear
- Kinematics: causes the tibia to rotate internally on flexion and shift the patella medially
- Relative ER of the tibial component relative to the femoral component was found to be not uncommon in one recent study; may account for the relatively high incidence of posteromedial polythene wear reported in many retrieval studies

6.6.9.1.5 Effects of Internally Rotated Tibial Component

- Patella dislocation/subluxation
  Q angle increases; more wear/fracture/dissociation; subluxation not common, owing to the expanded lateral flange of femoral component (Nagamine)
- Kinematics: tibia externally rotate on flexion

6.6.9.2 Elements of Proper Design of the Femoral Component

- Reproduce proper trochlea topography to ease proper patella tracking
- Maintain retinacular balance and enhance stability

▨ Maximise contact area with the patella at different angles of knee flexion by a patella-friendly trochlea design

▨ Avoid excessive anterodistal build-up which may overstuff the patellofemoral joint (PFJ) and limit deep knee flexion

▨ In posterior-stabilised designs, avoid positioning the inter-condylar box too anteriorly as this may predispose to the development of patella-clunk syndrome

6.6.9.2.1 Guides to Correct Femoral Component Rotation

▨ Epicondylar axis – some say not easy to palpate since partly covered by fibres of the collaterals

▨ Whiteside's line – useful

▨ Posterior condyle – favoured by Hungerford, but not reliable in the valgus knee

(Most systems build in 3° of ER)

6.6.9.2.2 Effect of Femoral Component Malrotation

▨ Too much ER causes subluxation or even dislocation of the patella and maltracking

▨ Abnormal knee kinematics will result from excessive femoral-component IR

6.6.9.2.3 Femoral Component Rotation

▨ A femoral component that is too internally rotated tightens the medial flexion space and opens the lateral flexion space; an excess externally rotated femoral component causes the patella to track medially, and the gap in flexion is larger medially

6.6.9.3 Translation of the Tibial and Femoral Components

▨ Proximal–distal:

 – In the measured resection method, either the medial or lateral distal femoral condyle can be used, since this method seeks to re-establish the anatomical level of the distal cut – the exact resection level is system specific as different prostheses differ in thickness

 – In the F/E gap method, the ligament tensioning is used to determine the proximal–distal position of the femoral component. In general, a displacement of femoral component that is too proximal and anterior can cause mid-flexion instability, despite sometimes showing stability in full extension and flexion

6.7   TKR Designs

6.7.1   General Areas
▦ Aspects of design to reproduce more normal biomechanics
▦ Aspects of design for better fixation
▦ Aspects of design for lower wear
▦ Aspects on biomaterials (e.g. choice of material for the base plate) – see section on Biomaterials

6.7.2   Wear Reduction
▦ Conformity: much more of an issue for the TKR (than THR) – more conformity of the articulating surfaces implies more constraint and risk of torsional stresses of the implant–bone interfaces
▦ Polyethylene thickness: 8 mm minimum
▦ Different E (elastic modulus) of the articulating pair – in the case of TKR, between CoCr which has an E value of 200× that of polyethylene. Other methods:
   – Decreased adhesion – probably less dominant wear mode in TKR than abrasive and subsurface wear
   – Decreased abrasion – beware of backside wear under polyethylene and between polyethylene and metal base plate; higher quality polyethylene and better sterilisation
   – Decreased 3rd body wear – better surface finish, etc.
   – Fatigue wear – one of the dominant wear modes, the long-term problem of conformity constraint seems to be "solved" by the new mobile-bearing TKR – but only time can tell whether there is more or less osteolysis, and wear at the added mobile interface

6.7.3   The Fixation Interface

6.7.3.1   Cemented TKR with Good Track Record
▦ Cemented TKA has a good track record – e.g. total condylar, and Insall-Burstein (IB) total knee
▦ Survivorships >90% at 15–20 years

6.7.3.2   Uncemented TKR with Unsatisfactory Track Record

▦ Based on the poor results of PCA (porous-coated anatomic) for several reasons:
  - Bad plastic – heat pressed, severe osteolysis and wear
  - Metal-backed patella – many needed revision
  - Too flat-on-flat (e.g. the Ortholoc), contributed to the high amounts of wear

6.7.4   Present Status of Cemented TKR

▦ Still preferred by most
▦ Preferred especially since most are aged over 65 years with medical co-morbidities; should be durable enough for just one operation in their life time, especially for the high-risk elderly patients
▦ In older subjects, some had used all poly tibial component – no back-side wear

6.7.5   Present Status of Uncemented TKR

▦ It is important to note the resurgence of some interest in uncemented TKR after reported good results at 18 years of low contact stress (LCS) mobile-bearing – with slightly superior results in survivorship than in cemented TKR
▦ Proponents interpreted the above as indicating – a knee design that had a good articulating surface that did not cause accelerated wear, and osteolysis could perform as well as knees with cemented fixation
▦ Other reasonable results of uncemented include – Ortholoc (Whiteside, no metal backed patellae) and natural knee (Sulzer)
▦ According to Dorr, uncemented TKR can be considered for those younger than 60 years old

6.7.6   Present Status of Revision TKR

▦ Most surgeons use cemented metaphyseal fixation and uncemented stems
▦ Problem
  - Metaphyses usually weak and bone losses
  - Poor rotational support especially for the femoral side (cf. total hips) – premature femoral side loosening can occur
▦ Dorr mostly used the press-fit stem on the tibia; deemed rather more durable, although sometimes cement the stem in selected cases

6.7.7   Future

■ More use of mobile-bearing, especially for younger and more active patients

■ For younger patients, some experts are now starting to go for hybrid/uncemented fixation

■ Fixed-bearing uncemented TKR can sometimes be useful as seen in the results of natural knee

■ Need to await longer term results and wear, e.g. backside/osteolysis issues with these knees (also general tendency to use better plastics, and avoid metal-backed patellae)

6.7.8   Mobile-Bearing TKR

6.7.8.1 Types

■ IR–ER design allows the knee to locate to a preferred rotational orientation (backward motion of one condyle associated with forward of the other)

■ IR–ER about a medial axis better simulates anatomical knee motion, as the normal knee rotates through a longitudinal axis on the medial tibial plateau

■ Allow IR/ER and anteroposterior (AP) translation so the knee can locate at a preferred rotational and translational orientation – this design relies especially on ligamentous structure for stability and kinematics

■ 'Guided motion type' – IR/ER and AP translation is guided by intercondylar cams or guide surfaces in an attempt to produce the AP motion of the normal knee, i.e. roll-back with flexion and roll forward with extension. This includes the posterior stabilised mobile-bearing knee arthroplasty (MBKA) devices and designs that have an intercondylar, saddle-shaped cam

P.S. designs produce roll back only with flexion; saddle design attempts to produce roll back and roll forward with extension with flexion and extension, respectively. The guided rollback achieved with these designs in high flexion is preferable to that achieved with rotation-only designs, but it does require a partially conforming femoral/tibial articulation surface

6.7.8.2   Mobile-Bearing Knee Kinematics

- Roll-back occurs primarily as a function of PCL, optimising the quadriceps lever arm in flexion, thereby increasing the flexion. The increased quadriceps lever facilitates downhill walking and stairs descent
- One original aim of MBKA was to reproduce normal kinematics, but no current knee designs really reproduce the normal knee kinematics

6.7.8.3   Kinematic Abnormalities that Can Occur

- Example: paradoxic anterior translation (more with multidirectional); reverse axial rotation pattern (normal tibial IR with flexion reduced in both fixed-bearing and rotating-only, mobile-bearing total knee; PCL-substituting and -sacrificing only designs show tibial IR with knee deeply bent)
- Example: femoral condylar lift-off

6.7.8.4   Contraindications to Implantation of Mobile-Bearing Knees

- Malalignment – gross, but extent of lesser degree of malalignment that may be accepted is unsure
- Marked fixed flexion contracture – avoid use of PCL retaining multidirectional MBKA

6.7.8.5   Results So Far of Mobile-Bearing TKR

- Currently, results at intermediate to long-term follow-up are equal to the best results reported for fixed-bearing knees

6.7.8.6   Concept of the "Conformity-Axial Constraint Conflict" in Relation to the Surgeon's Choice of TKR

- Many modern fixed-bearing knees are more conforming than the earlier round-on-flat TKR. By increasing conformity to diminish wear, theoretically more axial torque is applied to the prosthesis–bone interface. The threshold of axial torque stress at which prosthesis loosening occurs is unknown; however, minimising this stress appears to be an advantage. Improvements in polyethylene wear properties and quantification of the acceptable degree of constraint may even allow fixed-bearing prostheses to outperform MBKA devices, according to Insall. Only time will tell

6.7.8.7 Theoretical Advantage of MBKA

- Less linear wear since more conformity
- The dreaded increase in axial torque with increased conformity decreased with ability to rotate; some designs allow AP translation, others even multidirectional, retaining the cruciates
- CoCr used as the tibial base-plate decreases wear from the rotating forces (compared with Ti implants), as it is stiffer
- Rotating platform. Said to be better tolerant to minor degrees of tibial base-plate malrotations, but is not a substitute for good surgical technique
- Theoretically, the self-aligning ability of MBKA might improve PF mechanics, but there is no concrete evidence

6.7.8.8 Advantages in Summary

- Self-aligning [especially in cases with anterior cruciate ligament (ACL) and PCL still intact]
- Less contact stress (more conformity – at least during the phases of gait cycle with high loading such as the stance phase)
- Less contact stress means less surface and subsurface wear
- Decreased peak stresses which are better distributed
- Slightly more forgiving with respect to minor degrees of rotational malalignment

6.7.8.9 Disadvantages of Mobile-Bearing Knees

- Possibility of more backside wear; some series report some osteolysis possibly from the smaller wear particles produced
- Bearing dislocation – attention to technique, design and especially not excessive flexion gap
- Kinematics also not normal
- Overall, possibly less tolerant to instability
- Sometimes soft-tissue impingement especially the polyaxial ones, and questionable smooth mobility of platforms/bearings
- The best result longer term, e.g. with LCS, matches but does not surpass the best results of fixed-bearing designs. In Callaghan's study, the ROM attained with LCS in fact is less than that with most good series of fixed-bearing designs
- Possibility of more backside wear, especially with designs with multi-directional motion and meniscal-bearing ones – i.e. despite linear

wear, decreased with increased conformity; volumetric wear may be higher

▦ Some studies, such as the series by Callaghan, found that: rotating platform and meniscal-bearing MBKA designs have a similar or lower flexion range than fixed-bearing; the least amount occurs with the cruciate-sacrificing rotating platform design, which often exhibits anterior femoral roll-back

▦ Meniscal-bearing TKR dislocation is common (2–7%) and that of rotating platform less so (0.2% in a large series of 600 knees). The former is said to be related to meniscal bearing that uses curved tracks without stops.

Many MBKAs now use platform stop mechanics of various kinds to decrease dislocation

▦ No evidence that MBKA with less back-side wear than fixed-bearing knees, if not more. In fact, there are some claims that multi-directional polyethylene platforms have wear rates nine times the wear rate of unidirectional platforms.

Another mechanism of possible excess wear from MBKA is from malalignment and poor ligament balancing that can produce cyclic polyethylene impingement on constraint stops in gait and more wear

6.7.9   Unicompartmental Knee Design (Figs. 6.3, 6.4)

6.7.9.1 Indications

▦ Mostly for elderly with mainly medial (sometimes lateral) compartment disease who have the following:
  - Both cruciates intact
  - No rheumatoid arthritis (RA)/diffuse inflammatory joint disease
  - No flexion contracture (>10–15°)
  - No significant laxity of the collaterals
  - Not too active especially if aged younger than 65 years
  - Not excessively obese

6.7.9.2 Why Do It?

▦ Advantage over TKR – better proprioception and/or better mobility

▦ Advantage over HTO – much shorter rehabilitation

▦ General reason – it is a basic principle of orthopaedics to save all normal tissue, knowing that any device used will be mostly inferior to the natural joint

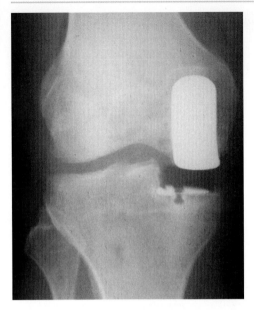

Fig. 6.3. Post-operative AP view of right unicompartmental total knee replacement

(Note: the most traditional indication for the unicompartmental design was for osteonecrosis of the femoral condyle)

6.7.9.3 Pre-Operative Assessment

▦ Clinical tests – e.g. rule out significant PFJ disease, RA, gross obesity, poor motivation, significant flexion contracture, etc., or factors that can produce bad result

▦ X-ray: (1) AP WB in extension – degree of deformity, overall alignment; (2) AP in 20° flexion (Rosenberg) – see more clearly the status of the cartilage; (3) lateral WB view in extension – see flexion contracture or recurvatum, level of patella; and (4) Merchant's view – help assess PFJ

▦ Template the knee: to see the extent of the defects on the femoral and tibial sides, and define the area of bone cuts – the position of the tibial implant should follow the joint line

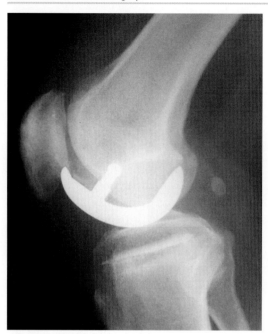

Fig. 6.4. Post-operative lateral view of right uni-compartmental total knee replacement

6.7.9.4 Three Major Types of Designs
▓ Resurfacing
▓ Resection type
▓ Mobile-bearing type (Goodfellow)

6.7.9.4.1 Resurfacing Type
▓ Advantages: minimal bone loss, slow rate of loosening
▓ Disadvantages: need experience, more wear – especially in implants using inlay with 6 mm or less polyethylene
▓ Hence, use more than 6 mm polyethylene and surface hardening

6.7.9.4.2 Resection Type
▓ Advantages: technique more familiar and guided by instruments; position can be accurate; shorter learning curve
▓ Disadvantages: greater bone loss; higher loosening rate (due to fixation in the softer cancellous bone)

6.7.9.4.3 Mobile-Bearing Type
- Advantages: theoretically less wear; less stress on implant
- Disadvantages: higher rate of dislocation; longer learning curve

6.7.9.5 Principles of Surgery
- Adequate exposure to view also the opposite compartment as a reference for resection level and cutting angles
- Most are medial replacements (implantation in the lateral compartment is done by a lateral or medial parapatella approach; usually no tibial tuberosity take down)
- Tibial cut beside the cruciate ligament insertion at the eminentia intercondylaris; femoral preparation should allow for fixation in the subchondral bone for optimal bone stock and load transfer. Restore proper joint line relative to the opposite compartment. Minimal polyethylene thickness should be 6 mm, but it is better to use 8 mm. For femoral side, use the smallest implant that covers the pre-existing defect; on tibial side, use the implant that provides full coverage of the resected area, not too proud as to affect the collateral

6.7.9.6 Complications
- Over-correction – painful tension in MCL in the case of varus deformity
- Under-correction – some experts will tolerate mild under-correction unless excessive – otherwise rapid deterioration of the non-replaced compartment is expected
- Prevention of early failure – e.g. make sure intra-operative implant stability can be achieved without cementing, especially in the flexed-knee position. If any lift-off or rotation of the tibial plateau can be seen, pressure on the implant has to be reduced and one must ensure proper ligament tension (collateral) and preserve the ACL

6.7.9.7 Early Results
- Most report good to excellent results especially in the first 10 years, especially in terms of mobility, proprioception, etc., for the different designs

6.7.9.8 Long-Term Results Depend on the Design (in Addition to Techniques)

- Resurfacing: the best, e.g. For Marmor implant, after 10 years more than 90% survival reported
- Resection type: worse, e.g. Miller-Galante 14% progressive radiolucent lines occur rather early at 2–5 years
- Mobile-bearing type: results not homogeneous, e.g. Goodfellow's Oxford design – more than 90% after 10 years, but some series fare worse, e.g. Swedish ones (deterioration at 6–7 years)

6.7.9.9 Revision

The key is to always revise to TKR. Revision to another unicompartmental TKR results in a low success rate unless solely polyethylene problem. (During revision, the holes should be filled with autograft)

6.8 Treatment of the Young- and Middle-Aged Knee OA Patients: Clinical Work-Up

- History: job, activity level, sports involvement, degree of pain, mechanical symptoms, body weight and likelihood to comply with prolonged rehabilitation
- Physical examination: instability, adductor thrust, one versus multiple compartment, overall limb alignment, disease in nearby joints, PFJ, Q angle and aetiology of OA, RA, etc.

6.8.1 Patient Categories

- Middle-aged OA knee patients with instability (ACL) especially if sports active
- Middle-aged OA knee patients with instability, with alignment problems or adductor thrust
- Young/middle age with large chondral lesion, symptoms getting worse
- Heavy-manual labourer/very active middle-aged OA patients with mainly one-compartment disease
- Sedentary obese middle-aged OA patients with or without alignment problems

6.8.2   Suggested Treatment for the Five Groups

▦ May consider ACL reconstruction and arthroscopy

▦ May consider ACL reconstruction and realignment (single operation or staged)

▦ See cartilage repair strategies, but these techniques may be futile if already generalised chondrosis

▦ HTO and/or sometimes distal femoral osteotomy to buy time

▦ May consider TKR/unicompartmental knee replacement

6.8.3   Summary of Main Treatment Options

▦ Arthroscopy debridement and/or ligament reconstruction

▦ Realigment osteotomy

▦ Unicompartmental knee replacement

▦ TKR

6.8.3.1   Section 1: Use of the Scope

▦ Arthroscopic debridement is suggested mainly for those with normal or near normal alignment and mild to moderate degeneration (unicompartment) disease – if a non-operative programme was not successful (especially those with acute onset of well-localised joint line pain, persistent effusion, catching and locking; sometimes advanced OA with mechanical symptoms may also need the scope)

▦ Example: excise loose chondral flaps, resect the unstable portion of degenerated meniscus, remove osteophytes – if causing painful impingement

▦ Mechanism proposed: wash out inflammatory mediators; the Cl^- ion in normal saline may interrupt pain impulses

6.8.3.2   Studies on ACL Reconstruction in Middle Age

▦ Each patient needs individual assessment – the middle-aged patient is not an ideal candidate (especially one with previous partial menisectomy and early post-traumatic arthrosis)

  – Patient understands the limited goals

  – Goal – pain relief, restore stability, improve activities of daily living (ADL; options, e.g. reconstruction/osteotomy/combined/meniscus transplant)

▦ Contraindication: unrealistic goals, advanced OA. In knees with full-thickness cartilage, with loss on opposing cartilage surface, secondary bone changes and instability

▦ Do have some literature to support ACL reconstruction (e.g. by Shelbourne) – improved objective and subjective stability, decreased pain and increased activity level (but no control group in either paper). Frank Noyes had similar results

6.8.3.3 Study on Combined Osteotomy and ACL Reconstruction
▦ Proceed to osteotomy first if indicated; proceed to ligamentous reconstruction if patient with give way episodes (Noyes)

6.8.3.4 Ways to Salvage the Young Post-Meniscectomy Patient
▦ Indication of Meniscus Transplantation:
  – Previous total/subtotal meniscectomy
  – Isolated unicompartmental joint line pain
  – Failed conservative
  – Closed physes
  – Normal/near normal alignment
  – Stable knee or stabilising operation planned

6.8.3.5 Current Status of Meniscus Transplant
▦ Experimental technique and salvage procedure for the younger patient with refractory pain
▦ Save the meniscus whenever possible; transplant is sometimes considered in those under 45 years old, with pain, normal alignment, and stable joint – they need to be advised not to return to high-demand contact sports
▦ 75% success rate, peripheral healing reliable, failures due to: 'shrinkage, posterior horn rupture and extrusion'. No studies are yet beyond 5 years – allograft meniscus heals to capsule; revascularisation by host cell occurs; no evidence of native meniscus function and hyaline cartilage protection

6.8.3.6 Section 2: HTO (and Distal Femoral Osteotomy)
▦ Contraindications of HTO:
  – Adductor thrust
  – RA/general inflammatory joint disease (and generalised arthrosis)
  – Incompetent collaterals and tibiofemoral subluxation
  – PFJ disease (and PF pain as the major complaint)

- Obese (1.3× ideal body weight)/active should not be a contraindication. Coventry stated: "Best in less active/less heavy people" – however, it is exactly the group of patients who are heavy and active' that need HTO since prosthesis in this group fails very early
- Unrealistic goals and those who cannot co-operate with rehabilitation – note that rehabilitation is longer than with unicompartmental TKR
- Others: diffuse knee pain, meniscectomy in the compartment intended for weight bearing
  (Relative: aged over 60 years, poor rotation arc less than 90°)

6.8.3.6.1 Advantages of HTO for Varus Knee and Medial Compartment Disease

▦ Transfer weight-bearing forces from the arthritic portion of knee to a healthier part of the joint. This re-distribution of mechanical forces increase the knee life-span in contrast to other modalities (though neither osteotomy nor arthroplasty provide a 'normal joint')
▦ Goal: (1) pain relief; (2) better function and (3) permitting heavy demands otherwise precluded by prosthetic replacement (key to success: proper alignment; proper technique; proper patient selection)
▦ Correction near maximum point of deformity; cut between knee joint and tibial tubercle confers advantage of broad cancellous area for union
▦ Buy time

6.8.3.6.2 Disadvantages of HTO
▦ Results decline after 7 years (Coventry)
▦ Need proper technique/selection/alignment

6.8.3.6.3 Coventry's Results of HTO
▦ Results decline after year 7
▦ Better if initially there is some over-correction
▦ Those who are obese and very active do worse

6.8.3.6.4 Pearls for Success After HTO
▦ Proper restoration of alignment – aim at 3–4° over-correction
▦ Proper patient selection
▦ Good surgical technique, avoid complications

6.8.3.6.5 Surgical Pearls

▦ The rule of thumb that 1 mm of wedge height equals $1°$ of angular correction results in under-correction for tibial widths more than 56 mm (after mathematical analysis done in Mayo Clinic)

6.8.3.6.6 Complication

▦ Neurovascular complications important; non-union rather uncommon since there is a large area of cancellous bone as the bone cut is above the tibial tubercle; adequate skeletal fixation is important (a special method of compression by staples was previously described), use of EF has been described in the past – but pin track sepsis is common; open-wedge type risks intra-articular fracture. Aiming at slight over-correction is the important teaching of Coventry, with utmost care to avoid disruption of the medial periosteum and cortex

6.8.3.6.7 The Medial Open Wedge Method

▦ Pros: do not violate the fibula or tibio-fibular joint; and dissect away from the peroneal nerve
▦ Cons: need BG since opening the wedge is not without morbidity, and risk graft displacement and loss of correction; intra-articular fracture is a common complication.
  (Some say that this method may be used in some young patients in whom joint line obliquity and malalignment require correction with concomitant ligamentous reconstruction of the knee)

6.8.3.6.8 Distal Femoral Osteotomy for Valgus Knees

Important note: "many valgus knees have inherent superolateral obliquity of the joint line". Hence, use classically distal femoral osteotomy for valgus deformities exceeding $12–15°$ or when the joint line obliquity would exceed $10°$ after correction

6.8.3.6.9 Reason for Avoiding HTO in Valgus Knees

The danger of a varus proximal tibial osteotomy is that the magnitude of joint line obliquity is increased by the wedge resection and is likely to cause clinical failure. (Note: excess joint line obliquity produces ineffective weight transfer as some weight is applied as shear forces against the intercondylar eminence when the femur subluxes on the tibia. This is further aggravated by MCL laxity after such osteotomy – produces the so-called 'teeter effect' of the femur toggling on the intercondylar eminence during gait)

6.8.3.6.10 Reasons Why Distal Femoral Osteotomy is a Non-Forgiving Operation

- Difficulty cutting the wedge effectively
- Need effective stabilisation of the closed osteotomy
- Need to predict accurately the wedge size necessary to ensure proper correction of the limb

6.8.3.6.11 Rare Situation for Considering HTO for Valgus Knees

- 12–15° is the upper limit for consideration; exceeding 12–15° of valgus correction or 10° of resultant joint line obliquity tends to result in lateral subluxation of the tibia and gives poor results (Coventry J Bone Joint Surg Am 1985 [2]; also Maquet CORR 1985 [3])
- MCL laxity can also result from removing a bone wedge from above MCL insertion

6.8.3.6.12 Pros and Cons and Results of Distal Femoral Osteotomy

- Pros – conversion to TKR result quite good; may need stem to span screw holes; union mostly good
- Cons – not a forgiving operation (done less nowadays), need bulky blade plate hardware, and sometimes impinges on the vastus medialis

6.8.3.7   Section 3: Unicompartmental Knee

- Advantages
  - Mimimal bone resection
  - Easy to revise
  - More physiological, since cruciates retained (might be able to dance, golf)
  - Rehabilitation much quicker than with osteotomy
  - Results in the 1st 10 years better than with HTO (Coventry – HTO results decline after 7 years)
  - Less blood loss
- Disadvantages:
  - Learning curve – some models (resurfacing type instead of resection type; no elaborate instrument or blocks that may be unfamiliar to TKR surgeon)

- Good results only obtained with proper patient selection, proper alignment, and proper and adequate surgical technique
- As with other arthroplasty techniques, an occasional case of infected joint or implant failure can cause problems

6.8.3.7.1 Ideal Candidate for Unicompartmental Knee

▥ Middle aged or older (usually < 60 years), especially females who are not too active in sports and unlikely to put too heavy a demand on the prosthesis, who have predominant OA in one medial/lateral compartment; who do not have any significant degree of flexion contracture, varus/valgus deformity, PFJ OA or pain or incompetent collateral ligaments
▥ Best considered as the first arthroplasty in the middle-aged OA knee patient

Mistakes made in the Past

- Over-correction – opposite compartment degeneration
- Under-correction – can lead to loosening and subsidence
- Medial–lateral component malposition – can cause iatrogenic subluxation
- Lax MCL – contraindicates lateral compartment replacement
- Poor patient selection

Design Mistakes and Improvements

- Narrow femoral component can subside in heavy patients; too narrow causes increased loading
- Lack of secure posterior condylar prosthetic fixation promotes femoral component loosening
- More femoral resection allows less tibial bone to be resected, yet enough space for adequate polyethylene thickness in extension. However, not enough femoral resection lowers the joint line and requires more tibial resection
- Tibial polyethylene thickness – 2 mm in metal-backed prosthesis is inadequate; 4 mm at most lasts 10 years; 6 mm or more is needed for long-term survival
- Too high constraints must be avoided (unless mobile bearing is used), because the wear pattern appears to be dictated by the retained ligaments and opposite compartment. Increased constraints lead to increased interface stress of the implant

Other Pearls

- Soft tissue: medial–lateral congruency is assessed in extension rather than flexion since, in flexion, the everted quadriceps artificially externally rotate the tibia on the femur
- Lack of secure posterior condylar fixation promotes loosening
- Revision: almost always to TKR, unless only polyethylene wear; femoral side defect is rarely encountered in revision, tibial bone defect in revision depends on the initial resection level. Results of revision are similar to primary TKR if initial resection is not excessive

6.8.3.7.2 Outcome of Unicompartmental Knee
- Result is good in 1st 10 years = TKR (if not better)
- Declines after the 2nd decade
- Hope for better results with better designs in future

6.8.3.7.3 Pearls for Success in General of Unicompartmentals
- Proper realignment
- Proper surgical technique
- Proper patient selection

  Choose designs to avoid the three common modes of failure. These would include: (1) less loosening (e.g. better component design, by use of mobile bearings, better fixation lugs), (2) less degeneration of opposite compartment (do not select RA patients, do not over-correct); and (3) polyethylene wear (e.g. by adequate thickness and high quality polyethylene)

6.9   Overall Complications of TKR

- Related to component malposition
- Related to improper bone cuts
- Failure to restore the extensor mechanism function and special PFJ complications
- Instability
- Infection
- Periprosthetic fractures
- Aeptic loosening
- Others, e.g. use of an improper implant, skin flap necrosis, hardware related and other mechanical complications

6.9.1   Complications Due to Component Malposition

▦ The malposition can create malalignment in the coronal, sagittal, and transverse planes
▦ The details of the effects have been discussed in the section on 'Alignment of Components'
▦ Rotational malalignment, unlike malalignment in the coronal or sagittal plane, may not be immediately obvious in post-operative X-ray and sometimes requires CT to diagnose. Rotational malalignment is a frequent cause of PF complications and may result in abnormal knee kinematics (discussed already)

6.9.2   Complications from Improper Bone Cuts

▦ Improper bone cut of the distal femur can result in abnormal Q angle
▦ Anterior notching of the distal femur can predispose to periprosthetic fractures
▦ Improper referencing from posterior condyles is a frequent mistake in valgus knees in which a defective lateral femoral condyle is common. This can result in improper rotational alignment of the femoral component
▦ The amount of posterior slope of the proximal tibial cut depends on the implant we use. The effects of excessive cut or even the reverse (i.e. anterior slope) have been discussed
▦ In most cases, the patella bone cut should be such that the original patella height be restored. Excessive bone cut creates too thin a patella for the patella button. Inadequate cut results in overstuffing the PFJ

6.9.3   Complications of the Extensor Mechanism

▦ Patella fracture
    – This complication can be minimised by avoiding overzealous bone cut of the patella, overzealous soft-tissue release with resultant avascularity or too tight PFJ post-operatively with increased PFJ stresses
▦ Patella-clunk syndrome
    – Seen mainly in PS TKR; causative factors include proximal placement of the patella button, inadequate debridement of the peripatella synovium and implants with more anteriorly located intercondylar box. These factors are discussed in the published works of the author

- Patella Maltracking
  - There are many causes of patella maltracking, including improper bone cuts, hence malrotated femoral or tibial components, improper soft-tissue balancing of the extensor mechanism or lateral release not done if indicated, overhanging tibial tray, and implant-related factors, such as those femoral components with excessive anterodistal buildup (e.g. IB II) or in the absence of a patella friendly trochlea surface
- Avulsion injury of the patella ligament and/or the tibial tubercle
- Patella alta or baja

6.9.4   Instability

- Most of the time due to improper soft-tissue balancing
- It should be noted that delayed onset varus/valgus instability, despite being deemed to have normal soft-tissue balance post-operatively, can be due to implant (usually polyethylene) wear
- Valgus instability can result from inadvertent injury to MCL. Intra-operative MCL cut may necessitate the use of varus/valgus constrained prostheses besides repair. Absence of the MCL in a revision setting needs hinges
- Others: bearing spin-out of meniscal-bearing type of mobile-bearing TKR, jumping of the cam-post mechanism of PS knees with hyperflexion or poor soft-tissue balance; and frank dislocation of the patient with inadvertently cut PCL given a PCL-retaining TKR

6.9.5   Other Complications

- Infection (septic loosening) has been adequately covered in Chap. 7
- Periprosthetic fractures will be discussed in the coming book on Traumatology by the same author and will not be discussed here
- By and large, the overall alignment is of paramount importance for the survivorship of TKR: 'notice that malalignment can ruin the best of knees; proper restoration of alignment and mechanical environment can make a bad knee regain satisfactory function'

6.10   Difficult Primary TKR

6.10.1   Problems with RA

■ General comments:
  - Systemic work-up important in RA – cervical spine, medical opti-
    misation, other systems
  - Locally for the lower limb: do the hip first if concomitant signifi-
    cant hip and knee disease
  - Uncommon for knee to be involved in early disease, but 90% even-
    tually. Two-thirds are bilateral
■ Problems with TKR in RA:
  - Osteoporotic bone-cemented TKR usually preferred
  - Ligamentous laxity
  - Valgus knee is common (more than general population) – difficult
    if fixed valgus is encountered: needs gradual release of the con-
    tracted tissues, progressing from a lateral retinacular release with
    division of the IT band, to LCL release at femoral origin. If MCL is
    attenuated, high constrain implants are needed (Fig. 6.5)
  - Flexion contracture – occasional, but can be severe – may need VY
    or quadriceps snip; post-release important not just bone cuts (not
    only elevate joint line, but risks delay worsening of collateral lax-
    ity); beware of neural damage. Rehabilitation important

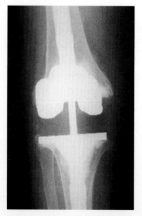

Fig. 6.5. Varus-valgus constrained type of total knee
replacement

- Type of implant – unless ligaments are very poor, too high a constraint transmits shear and rotation forces to the bone–cement interface. Scott recommends PCL-retaining some reports of PCL commonly still intact in 90%
- Other problems – cysts (sometimes large) commonly need grafts and stemmed prosthesis for protection
- More complications arise from infection, wound and, since patients tend to be younger when they need joint replacement, they are more likely to need revision and undergo component loosening and wear, etc.

6.10.1.1 TKR in RA – Long-Term Result
- Several series report 85%+ survivals at 10 years (Ranawart)
- Some argue that this is partly due to the lower functional demand of most of these patients
- Not much data at more than 10 years
- Laskin reported 50% high late failures with PCL retention (CORR 1997 [4]) – PCL was found to be absent at revision, although many other series do not report similar problems (e.g. Whiteside JA and nationwide Swedish studies)
- There have been some reports of common (>60%) incidence of a tibial component in radiolucent lines with PS implants (e.g. Laskin, J Bone Joint Surg 1990), although a few others claim a good result.
  (Currently, it is not settled beyond doubt whether to retain the PCL, and whether PS implants are good or not)

6.10.2 Fusion Take Down
- Complications – more infection, wound healing problems, poor ROM – frequently needs manipulation under anaesthesia (MUA). Incidence of loosening and revision is higher
- Pearls – beware, ligaments can be gone (may need increased constraints), very scarred, and tibial tubercle osteotomy may be needed. Post-operative continuous passive motion ensures the motion achieved intra-operatively is maintained, releasing adhesions under the quadriceps
- Outcome depends on: degree of pre-operative deformity, aetiology of ankylosis and patient's age (and likely also on status of ligaments)

(Note: do not overdo MUA – in these cases, quadriceps extensor mechanics are usually contracted, and vigorous MUA can cause tendon ruptures and/or fracture.)

6.10.3 Post-Patellectomy Knee

▪ Normal patella function – contributes to the extensor moment arm; reinforces the AP stability of the knee, smooth articulation for the extensor mechanics; thick hyaline cartilage also helps to bear compression loads; cosmetic; shields the knee from trauma

▪ Explanation for AP stability – the knee is viewed as a '4-Bar Linkage system' with the patella tendon parallel to the PCL and the quadriceps parallel to ACL; the PCL prevents anterior translation of the femur on the tibia during flexion, and the forces directed through the patella tendon parallel to the PCL reinforce this stabilising function of the PCL, hence lessening AP stability of the knee during flexion

▪ Explanation of the extensor moment arm – the patella gives the quadriceps mechanical advantage for knee extension, by displacing the quadriceps tendon anteriorly. Contributes to 10–30% of the quadriceps moment arm, depending on the degree of knee flexion; by increasing the perpendicular distance between the applied force and the centre of rotation of the knee joint, the patella decreases the amount of force required of the quadriceps to get enough torque to straighten the leg. Torque decreases by 15–50% after patellectomy

▪ Results in general for TKR in post-patellectomy patients is inferior, e.g. lesser ROM, decreased quadricep torque, extensor lag, less stairwalking ability and pain

▪ Implant choice – Sledge proposes retention of cruciate ligaments to maintain the intact portion of the 4-Bar linkage system; others favour the use of unicompartmental replacement if unicompartment disease – if bi-compartment, try to use a prosthesis that preserves both cruciates. Cameron agreed with this proposal but later reported a good result from using IB II. Laskin also thinks that 'PCL may be an unreliable source of stability in post-patellectomy patients', since loss of patella caused stretching of the post-capsule and PCL in the 4-Bar linkage system. Success with PS knees here is not surprising – the PS designs ensure that the centre of rotation moves toward the posterior aspect of the tibial plateau during flexion – rollback, which improves the quadriceps moment arm

6.10.4   TKR After Previous HTO

Problems:

- Patella baja common
- ROM is less post-operatively in some series (HSS reported 80% good result)
- Be prepared for:
  - Removal of hardware
  - May need an offset stem
  - Restore tibial posterior slope
  - Tibial stemmed implant to bypass screw holes
    (Also bypass screw holes with stem after removal of old supracondylar plate)

6.10.5   After Femoral Supracondylar Osteotomy

- Bypass the screw holes
- Otherwise good results

6.10.6   After Maquet Procedure

- May need to use extra long blades
- Beware of tibial rotations
- When using the EM guide, be aware of proper posterior slope restoration

6.10.7   Take Down of Previous Infected Knee

- Figure from Mayo shows at least 5–10% infection rate
- Higher still if previous osteomyelitis
- Pre-operative adequate work-up includes different scans
- Intra-operative frozen section is helpful

6.11   Total Hip Replacement

6.11.1   What are the Great Differences of THR from TKR

- Wear particle size smaller – closer to the 10-μm mark – osteolysis quite common (although itself may be asymptomatic, the process weakens the bone)
- Ball-socket articulation has more intrinsic stability than the knee that rolls and glides. Sometimes get away with milder degrees of soft-tis-

sue imbalance (although the power of the abductors and re-establishment of proper offset are important for success)

▦ Major wear mechanics rather different– in knees, more abrasive and de-lamination kind of wear as well as fatigue

▦ Pain occurring after THR is diagnosed more differentially and can be referred from many other structures such as the spine, sacroiliac joint, etc. In the setting of sepsis, early effusion developing after TKR is easier to detect than after THR since the knee is more superficial

▦ Unlike TKR, lesser worry even if there are many previous incisions, since better vascular supply

6.11.2   General Keys for Success

▦ Getting the right biomechanics – get the appropriate centre of rotation; the right offset, GT location, size of head, size of socket (larger area, less stress), and/or medialisation needed but not excessive

▦ Getting good fixation (cemented, uncemented, hybrids) will be discussed later

▦ Getting the best interfaces – so many choices are available of articulating couples and proper choice of biomaterials – see section on Biomaterials

▦ Minimise wear (and friction)

6.11.3   Ways for Wear Reduction

▦ Factor 1: conformity (much less of an issue here than say TKR, since highly conforming ball and socket)

▦ Factor 2: adequate polyethylene thickness (if polyethylene is used)

▦ Factor 3: relative E (elastic modulus) of the articulating couple

6.11.4   Other Methods to Decrease Wear

▦ Decrease adhesion – low friction and good lubrication

▦ Decrease abrasion – low friction principle and methods to decrease backside wear – e.g. screw holes and sharp edges

▦ Decrease 3rd body wear – surface finish and hardness

▦ Decrease fatigue wear – adequate thickness of polyethylene; this wear mode is much more important in TKR, since much sliding and gliding motions are involved

6.11.5 Basic Hip Biomechanics in Relation to the Understanding of THR

- Hip acts as a fulcrum between body weight and hip abductors, a dynamic equilibrium is developed with a goal of keeping the pelvis level and preventing Trendelenberg lurch
- Note – the lever arm from centre of motion (COM) of femoral head and the abductors is less than that between COM and body weight – thus placing the abductors at a mechanical disadvantage

6.11.5.1 Importance of Restoration of COM

Example: adult cases of developmental dysplasia of the hip (DDH) for THR

- High hip centre is less favoured in THR for DDH nowadays since ease of impingement and, hence, ease of dislocation, leg length discrepancy (LLD) produced and weak abductors
- Also needs special implants (e.g. cup usually small and high); and reasonable good bone stock

6.11.5.2 Importance of Restoration of Offset

- Abductors are at a mechanical disadvantage even in the normal hip; restoration of offset is even more important in the arthritic hip
- Less offset weakens abductors, more wear from increased joint reaction force, Trendelenberg lurch and need for walking aids
- Excess offset risks trochanteric bursitis and more stress to cement mantle (and the metal stem)

6.11.5.3 Efficacy to Restore Offset and Leg Length with Three Different Methods

- Increased neck length – does NOT provide an anatomical neck-shaft angle and, besides increase in offset, the leg length is increased
- Decreased neck-shaft angle – does NOT recreate the anatomical neck-shaft angle and it also affects both leg length and offset
- Medial shift of neck and increased neck length of the high-offset stem maintains the neck-shaft angle, does not affect leg length, and restores offset (the preferred method)

6.11.5.4 Drawback of Over-Correction of Offset

- Should be done carefully with recognition of the strength of the metal alloy used and fatigue limits of the stem design. The stresses within the femoral neck are increased with high offset stems, but without proper femoral component design and a risk of implant fracture present
- More stress on the cement mantle
- Trochanteric bursitis

6.11.5.5 Do We Still Osteotomise the GT?

- Trochanteric osteotomy is not routine in THR now in most centres, unlike in Charnley's days
- Charnley initially used this because – he initially wanted a neck-shaft angle of less than 135°; but this was not possible at his time as the less-than-adequate quality of metal used fractured with lower angles

6.11.5.6 Ways to Maximise the ROM

- Pre-operative ROM – most important factor (reason: in chronic stiff hips, extensor mechanics stiffen and periarticular fibrosis occur, e.g. if pre-operative <90°; most are less than 90° post-operatively; if pre-operative usually more than 140°, and can sometimes expect 120° or higher)
- Surgical technique
- Prosthesis design
- Proper patient rehabilitation

6.11.6   General Trends in THR

- Fewer and fewer cemented cups used nowadays in primaries
- In revisions, cementless fixation of both components become the standard for most surgeons
- Fixation of the femoral component is more controversial – contemporary cemented stems use a wide variety of design features and surfaces; on the femoral side, cementless fixation was shown to be effective in many settings
- Revision of femoral components mostly cementless, and most are extensive coated, although there is good evidence that rough-surface, tapered components can be effective in revision settings. Stem modularity also allows for greater intra-operative adaptability

6.11.7   Basic Principles in the 'Straight Forward' Primaries

- Charnley's principles: of low friction (low wear), will be discussed
- Know the four common wear mechanisms
- Know the pros and cons of the different types of articulating couples
- The cement 'weak link' and ways to improve on the cement mantle
- Know total joint tribology
- Other aspects: corrosion issues and the morse-tapers

6.11.7.1 General Things to Avoid

- Malposition of components
- High and lateralised acetabulum
- Unloaded structural grafts
- Expecting the graft to support more than half the cup (75% host bone contact preferred in cementless cups)
- Thin (<8 mm) polyethylene

6.11.7.2 General Things to be Encouraged

- Extensile approach: with wide exposures (no long-term result for the minimal incision technique which is in vogue nowadays)
- Optimisation of hip mechanics, e.g. COM, offset, etc. as previously discussed
- Optimise host–implant contact if cementless
- Cement the polyethylene if structural graft is going to occupy more than half the cup surface
- Use more durable polyethylene, e.g. high X-linked
- Pre-operative templating is a must
- Back-up plan especially in difficult primary
- Get necessary instrumentation
- Measure LLD pre- and intra-operatively, do not insist on equalisation in all cases (tell patient pre-operatively that we will not sacrifice issues such as soft-tissue tension in order to make leg length equal)
- Maximise component contact
- Envisage any expected difficulties in a pre-operative assessment meeting

6.12   Pre-Operative Assessment in THR

6.12.1 Introductory Statement

Before we discuss the details, the following points should first be stressed:

▨ Patient's expectations and temperaments

▨ Patient should be aware that there is no guarantee that any pre-operative LLD is always corrected post-operatively, although the surgeon will strive to equalise the leg length. Examples of the underlying reasons include: one should not sacrifice the balancing of soft-tissue tension in order to equalise leg length or when, intra-operative, one decides to go for a high hip centre

▨ The incidence of the different common complications should be told to the patient before signing the consent

6.12.2 History

▨ Hip status, degree of pain, whether ADL can be managed

▨ Nature of pain – e.g. vascular, spine

▨ Differentially diagnose referred pain

6.12.3 Past Health

▨ If RA – assess systemic control of the disease and the cervical-spine

▨ If history of radiotherapy (RT) for tumours – RT may impair bone ingrowth to cementless implants

▨ Heterotopic ossification (HO) risk and history of previous HO – arrange for prophylaxis

▨ Past health – childhood diseases and their treatment, old sepsis, any old injury with possible deformity

6.12.4 Physical Assessment

▨ Old incisions

▨ Overall lower limb alignment

▨ Gait

▨ Posture, e.g. pelvic obliquity; degree of lumbar lordosis can cause malposition of implants if significant deviation from normal

▨ Abductor powers – may need increased offset and/or rarely more constraints

▨ ROM and contractures – flexion and adduction contractures common

▦ LLD check very important – do not just rely on X-ray; differentially diagnose from apparent limb length discrepancy

▦ Clinical assessment of any excess anteversion or retroversion – if in doubt, sometimes use CT

▦ Other joints, which may in fact be the pain generator rather than the hip

6.12.5 Select Approach

▦ Usually of the surgeon's choice

▦ Trochanteric osteotomy is especially useful if wide exposure is needed in revision or if access to the region of high ilium is needed

▦ Anterolateral may be better in patients prone to post-operative dislocation, e.g. cerebral palsy (CP), or patients with flexion and adduction contractures

▦ Though some say if there is a previous posterior approach, another one should be avoided, not all experts agreed with this

6.12.6 Radiological Assessment

▦ Ensure X-ray taken in 15° IR – needed to most accurately predict stem size, neck length, offset and neck resection level

▦ Lowenstein lateral

6.12.7 Templating

6.12.7.1 Reasons to Template

▦ Help plan to restore normal hip biomechanics (very helpful if opposite hip normal)

  – Hip centre: most measure with respect to the teardrop, which is a constant bony landmark; some use the Muller ring to help

  – Offset: perpendicular distance from femur long axis to COM, – best to use normal hip to measure offset and assess level of neck cut

  – Leg length: from interischial line to LT (either upper or lower part of LT)

  – Others: (1) Neck shaft angle – significant variation among normal people. This not only affects offset, but if anatomical angle differs markedly from the proposed implant, can cause problems. (2) Special difficulties in some cases – e.g. degree of anterior bowing if any of the femur needs to be assessed if long-stem femoral compo-

nent planned, for example, to bypass stress-risers. (iii) In revision
THR, templating is even more important

▨ Help assess type of implant and any intra-operative precautions
needed

  – Calcar–canal ratio – type A is best for a cementless implant and
    type C best for cemented
  – Bone defects or losses, e.g. may need reinforcement ring

6.12.7.2 Difference Between Offset and Abductor Moment Arm

▨ The abductor moment arm is not the offset we referred to earlier; it is
measured by drawing a line between the anterior superior iliac spine
(ASIS) and posterior superior iliac spine (PSIS). A line is drawn from
a point one-third of the way from the PSIS to ASIS to the tip of GT.
This is said to approximate to the line of pull of the gluteus medius

6.12.7.3 Leg Length Assessment (Pre-Operative and Intra-Operative)

▨ Pre-operative measurement by both clinical (e.g. block test) and X-ray
(interischial line to LT)

▨ Intra-operative confirmation by a device placed between prominent
bone marks, e.g. ASIS (or iliac tubercle) to GT – measure before hip
dislocation and with trials in-situ, (if LLD >2 cm, consider SSEP and/
or wake-up test if large amount of lengthening may be needed)

6.12.7.4 Calcar–Canal Ratios

▨ Dossick described a method of classifying proximal femoral geometry
based on calcar–canal ratio; the diameter of the femur at the mid-portion of the LT divided by the diameter at a point 10 cm more distal.
Type A suits cementless <0.5, type C suits cemented >0.75 and type
B is in between

6.12.7.5 Templating the Acetabulum

6.12.7.6 Placing the Template

▨ Placed just lateral to the lateral edge of the teardrop, at 45° angle

▨ Ideal: cup completely covered by bone and spans distance between
teardrop and superolateral margin of the acetabulum

▨ The size that achieves the above with minimum removal of subchondral bone is selected (for cemented sockets, 2- to 3-mm space left for
cement)

▨ If the component medial edge is just lateral to teardrop, the horizontal and vertical distances from the teardrop should closely approximate those of the normal hip – Muller templates can help

6.12.7.7 Identifying COM
▨ The ideal position for the acetabular template and component is achieved by placing the inferomedial edge adjacent to the lateral margin of the teardrop. In most cases, this will restore the COM and can be checked using the Muller method

6.12.7.8 Tips for More Difficult Scenarios
▨ Protrusio – restore medial wall, achieve component lateralisation – added advantage is increase in offset and less impingement; try to get in a larger component with peripheral rim contact – get initial stability and/or antiprotrusio rings, especially if poor bone
▨ Lateralized acetabulum common [from large osteophyte especially in patients with diffuse idiopathic skeletal hyperostosis (DISH)]: proper removal using teardrop (transverse acetabular ligament marks the inferior border of the true acetabulum) as landmark, ensuring good coverage for cup. Incomplete removal result is not good, be it a cemented or cementless cup (inadequate host bone cover).
  Reaming technique – straight medial reaming to within a few millimetres of planned depth of reaming; this is to avoid superior placement of the component.
  How to tackle excess femoral anteversion – (1) use modular implants that can adjust version, (2) implants should be custom made; and (3) if use standard stem – can even need subtrochanteric osteotomy
▨ Superolateral defect and dysplastic hips: many hips migrate superolaterally – uncovers lateral margin of the acetabulum
  – Options – (1) High hip centre – small component 22-mm head; bone available may not be enough; danger of impingement on the anterior column and anterior inferior iliac spine with flexion and IR, also on the ischium in extension and ER, increased loading/wear. (2) BG favoured by Allan Gross. (3) Barrack sometimes put cup slightly more vertical and used an offset liner (not too commonly used method)

– Problems with hip dysplasia – (1) excess anteversion – use straight femoral stem and (2) posterior rotated GT – may need to osteotomise or even de-rotate GT

6.12.7.9 Femoral Component Templating [Always After Acetabulum Templating]

▦ Ensure X-ray taken in $15°$ IR – needed to most accurately predict stem size, neck length, offset and neck resection level
(If hip in fixed ER, determine COM of hip then transpose template to the opposite side hip for femoral templating)

6.12.7.10 Positioning the Template

▦ The femoral template is moved vertically until the centre of the femoral head template is at the same vertical height as the planned acetabulum COM. No matter what type of stem, the template should be kept centred along the neutral axis of the femur and not in varus or valgus

6.12.7.10.1 Various Implant Types

▦ Proximal-coated components – proximal fit and fill emphasised
▦ Extensive-coated cementless – fixation mainly distal, and a tight fit at isthmus is sought
▦ Cemented – need enough space (of 1–2 mm) for a proper cement mantle

6.12.7.10.2 Neck Cut

▦ Ideally, femoral bone stock should be maintained and neck cut usually planned to be between 1 cm and 2 cm above LT
▦ Pearl: anatomical stems in particular must have the neck cut made at a predetermined height to avoid anterior impingement of the tip of stem distally

What Happens with Improper Neck Cut

▦ The neck resection should be planned so as to utilise a neck length without a 'skirt' or thickened extension of the head, as this tends to impinge at extremes of motion; such impingement can cause decreased ROM and instability

6.12.7.10.3 Fine Tuning of the Offset

- Routine methods involve: manipulating neck-shaft angle and proximal geometry of implant used, medialising the take-off point of the neck of the stem, and increasing the use of implants with dual offset (or different offsets to choose from)
- More subtle methods:
  - Seat component lower
  - Use lower neck cut
  - Bigger head
  - Lateralised liner/build up the medial wall in protrusion

6.12.7.10.4 Other Aspects

- Difference between measured neck-shaft angle and the angle of our proposed implant – if it is more than a few degrees, an intra-operative adjustment be made or another implant can be used
  - Coxa Vara patients have higher offset: use of an implant with lower neck-shaft angle is suggested, or a lower neck cut could be made thus giving a longer neck (here, making the standard neck cut can lengthen the leg without necessarily restoring offset); use of high-offset components or implants with lower neck-shaft angle helps to preserve bone by minimising the need for low neck cut
  - Coxa Valga patients have low offset situation: if we want to use a component with a lower degree of valgus angle, a higher neck cut should be made and a shorter prosthetic neck used to maintain length and offset
  - Coxa Brevia, e.g. in old Perthes: here a standard cup that sometimes results in lengthening and helps restore normal length; however, some suggest a low neck cut and short neck to be used to avoid overlengthening

6.13   Cemented THR

6.13.1   Principles of Low Friction Arthroplasty

- Low frictional torque – use articulating couples with low coefficient of friction
- Small head – lessened volumetric wear; a smaller head creates a lower frictional torque than a bigger head (assume same biomaterial)

▨ Socket with maximal external diameter – distributes load over a wider area and decreases stress. Medialisation to diminish the joint force, but not excessive or protrusio will occur

6.13.2 The Coefficients of Friction of Different Articulating Surfaces
▨ Cartilage/cartilage 0.001
▨ Metal/cartilage 0.05
▨ Metal/bone 0.5
▨ Metal/metal 0.5
▨ Metal/tetrafluoroethylene polymer 0.02

6.13.3 About the Acetabular Component
▨ Simple hemispherical
▨ Must have a close fit to acetabulum to allow pressurisation of cement. (Notice the acetabulum in real life is not truly hemispherical and is in fact slightly elliptical)
▨ Pressure injection
▨ Allows pressurisation with transverse deepening of acetabulum

6.13.4 About the Femoral Component
▨ Proximal cement loading important
▨ Even now, it is difficult to be sure whether we need "controlled subsidence" such as Exeter stems
▨ Details of the different generations of cementation techniques have been discussed

6.13.5 More on the Femoral Prostheses
▨ Elastic moduli for all surgical metals are essentially about the same
▨ Can increase stiffness by increasing the cross-sectional area
▨ Increased stiffness is unphysiological, and creates stress shielding and bone/calcar resorption
▨ Large surface area of metal proximally
▨ Largest prosthesis that comfortably fits and yet produces a satisfactory cement mantle that is desirable
▨ Thick proximal cement mantle
▨ Short offset (40 mm)
▨ Valgus/neutral alignment (avoid varus)

▦ Lateral trochanteric displacement in an attempt to increase the abductor moment arm

6.13.6 Summary of Low Frictional (Low Wear) Arthroplasty Principle

▦ Socket:
  – Small head, thick plastic, transverse deepening, multiple holes, irrigation, flange on the acetabular component (help pressurisation)
▦ Stem:
  – Biggest stem that allows a good cement mantle, proximal pressurisation
  – (Neutral, 45 mm offset, and/or lateralise GT)

6.13.7 Disadvantage of Cemented Acetabular Cup

▦ Clinical result declines for acetabular side after the 10-year mark in long-term study
▦ Perhaps less indicated in avascular necrosis (AVN), RA, and DDH (Ranawart)
▦ Recent move/trend, especially within US to go with uncemented method, but in reality for elderly low-demand patients both cemented/cementless methods are equally satisfactory; usually decided by surgeon's preference and the local anatomy. There is more controversy with regard to the femoral side, since the results of cemented are better; for cementless, there are many designs and geometry, but a good one should prevent debris entering the effective joint space, as well as providing rotation stability. Some recent HA-coated stems produced less thigh pain; however, there are as yet no long-term results from this

6.13.8 Longevity of a Cemented Cup

The longevity of a cemented cup depends on:
▦ Quality of fixation, i.e. quality of cement penetration into the acetabulum (Ranawat)
▦ Many techniques to improve fixation: clean debris/blood with lavage, water balloon (Ling), holes with better digitation (Charnley), extension of lateral wall of polyethylene by use of flange allows better cement compression
▦ Proper orientation of cup (40° abduction, 15° anteversion, sometimes tailored to individuals)

- Design: metal-base designs are not good (Harris series: 20% need revision, 40% lucent lines at 11 years), the reason for which is unclear. Initially it was thought that they helped spread out the stress on subchondral bone; however, polyethylene with pegs/circumferential flange at the peripheral provide better fix
- Ranawat found poorer results with RA, ankylosing spondylitis (AS), dysplastic acetabulum and/or osteonecrosis (ON)
- Biomaterial: choice of bearings; polyethylene quality, and polyethylene thickness (thicker polyethylene decreases stress on polyethylene and on subchondral bone from finite element analysis)
- Host bone quality – poor and weak subchondral bone fares worse

6.13.9   Pre-Operative Patient Selection
- Think twice in RA/AS/dysplastics and/or ON
- Templating is important. Most companies provide templates for planning; should leave 2–4 mm space for cement

6.13.10 Choice of Material
- Polyethylene quality – choose polyethylene and a proper sterilisation technique that will reduce oxidative degradation. Also choose compression-moulded (0.05 mm/year) rather than machined polyethylene from extruded polyethylene bar stock (0.1 mm/year); future X-linked polyethylene results will be eagerly awaited

6.13.11 Intra-Operative Pearls
- Tricks to increase fixation – just discussed; both technique and implant design are important
- Goal: >80% covered cup, 15° anteverted, 40° abducted
- With regard to the prosthesis design – socket design needs to optimise fixation, and to increase surface area and torsional resistance – by peripheral pegs and grooves within the poly. The circumferential flange of polyethylene at the periphery of implant is used to increase pressurisation on the cement
- The cement mantle – concentric mantle of 3–4 mm within the prepared bed is our aim

6.13.12   Other Pearls

■ Good exposure, resect labrum, keep transverse acetabular ligament – help in cement pressurisation

■ Epidural and hypotensive anaesthesia – drier field obtained

■ Bed preparation – make the bone bed cancellous, but do not damage subchondral bone

■ Size of implant should be 2–4 mm smaller than last reamer used, but this depends on model used

■ Multiple fixation holes (some use combined large and smaller – large ones 10 mm depth and 6 mm wide)

■ Pulsatile irrigate and dry with sponge

■ Simplex cement is favoured by Ranawat, since it has superior intrusion properties, strength and better handling

■ Sustained external pressure during cementation

■ Trial implant to define the peripheral margins of the acetabular component, then mark the desired position prior to cement mixing

6.13.13   Measuring Linear and Volumetric Wear

■ Linear – mostly used since we use 2-D X-rays. Definition: the radiographic change in the socket thickness at maximum point of wear

■ Volumetric wear – notice the actual penetration of the head is in 3D. Definition: volumetric wear is calculated using simple trigometric formula based on the measured linear wear and square of the radius of the articulating femoral head – part of the reason Charnley used the 22 mm head

6.13.13.1   Monitor and Measurement of Wear

■ Charnley – reliability of the "wire marker" method to assess wear has been questioned by Amstutz

■ Compare recent and old post-operative X-ray (Livermore technique)

■ Compare change in head centre relative to centre of socket – using different computer software methods

6.13.13.2   Appendix

■ In practice, Ranawat found quite variable wear – depends on factors such as type of surface, head size, any metal backing, type of polyethylene used, etc.

■ 22-mm head wear rate: 0.07–0.15 mm/year reported

■ 28-mm head wear rate: 0.05–0.13 mm/year

6.14   Cementless THR

6.14.1   Key for Success in Cementless Fixation

6.14.1.1 Degree of Micro-Motion
- If there is more than 40 μm of micro-motion, the resulting interface is fibrous membrane
- If there is less than 40 μm of motion, membranous bone formation occurs without an intermediate fibrocartilage stage

6.14.1.2 Achieving Initial Primary Stability
- Press-fit components with supplemental screw fixation show better initial stability than pegs, screw and dual geometry components
- (A cadaver study of Ti mesh cups compared line-to-line fixation with screw versus 1-mm press fit; versus peg; versus 1-mm press fit with screw; versus 1.5-mm press fit – best stability was shown to be 1-mm press fit with two screws)

6.14.1.3 Intimate Contact: No Gaps and Press Fit
- Gaps as small as 0.5 mm result in less bone ingrowth and lower strength of fixation in animal models
- The optimal press-fit for initial stability is achieved by a 1- to 2-mm under-reaming, depending on design (e.g. in Ti-mesh designs)
- Drawback of more under-reaming – fracture acetabulum; and also inability to seat the component fully
- For cases in which press-fit cannot be achieved, two screws provide nearly the same degree of stability as achieved with press-fit cup – there is no advantage to using more than two screws

6.14.1.4 Pore Size
- A size of 100–400 μm is optimal for bone ingrowth
- In practice, ingrowth is reported to occur in 10–30% of available porous-coated areas with current designs. However, even this reported degree of ingrowth has resulted in excellent clinical results at 10 years

6.14.1.5 Implant Material
- The implant choice itself may affect bone growth
- Both Ti and CoCr can stimulate monocytes and osteoblasts to release inflammatory mediators in vitro. There is no difference in the amount

of ingrowth in terms of quality, but bone density is better quantitatively with Ti – as is the penetration
▦ A newer implant Tantalum is under investigation
▦ The Ti mesh has a modulus of elasticity that allows for flexibility of insertion using the press-fit technique. Caution is needed when this technique is extended to components of another design with a different modulus of elasticity

6.14.2 Causes of Failure of Cementless Cups
▦ Previous five factors not being paid attention to, most of which involve surgical technique and choice of implant
▦ Poor locking mechanism: examples – Mallory Head (hexlock increased the micro-motions), PCA (cracked liner rim), and HG 1 prosthesis (peripheral tines now replaced by rings)
▦ AML fails sometimes by catastrophic failure of the polyethylene
▦ Osteolysis, e.g. from backside (this wear mode may be lessened by better congruity between the acetabular liner and the shell) and use of screws and other factors contributory to osteolysis – large head, poor polyethylene, thin polyethylene, open cup with edge loading, etc.

6.14.3 Future
▦ Possible role of bisphosphonates
▦ Alternative bearings – e.g. high X-linked polyethylene (good wear resistance with hip simulator studies but no long-term clinical studies), compression-moulded polyethylene (beware of sensitivity, toxicity and oncogenesis); ceramic on ceramic articulations, but brittle. Role of HA – only good result if underlying implant surface is porous coat and not smooth since it gets dissolved with time
▦ Possible role of growth factors, e.g. transforming growth factor (TGF)-beta, bone morphogenetic protein (BMP) 7
▦ New materials under investigation, e.g. tantalum has better optimal pore size and increased porosity compared with mesh

6.14.4 Requirements for Proper Bony Ingrowth (Summary)
▦ Intimate contact – no gaps
▦ Good host bed – good vascular bone
▦ Little micro-motion – primary stability
▦ Surface area (of host bone contact) – 75%

- Proper component position – e.g. if cup is too open, edge loading occurs
- Good design – e.g. many demonstrate poor locking and fail early, e.g. PCA, Mallory head
- Good materials

6.15   THR Complications

6.15.1   Dislocation and Instability
- Component 'malposition'
- Soft-tissue tension problems
- Impingement
- Others:
  - Combinations of above
  - Excessive motion by patient
  - Late dislocaters; need to rule out sepsis

6.15.1.1 Component Malposition
A common error to avoid is having (1) too open an acetabular component (Fig. 6.6) that may predispose to dislocation (Fig. 6.7) or superolateral wear or (2) the combined anteversion of the acetabular and femoral component fall outside that of the normal range
- 'Safe zone' concept – acetabulum cup 15° (±10°) anteversion and avoid being too open less than 40–45°
- Expert's comment: need to individualise; what is suitable for one patient, may not for another
- Always check with trial components for stability before fixing the components

6.15.1.2 Soft Tissue Tension
- Charnley has the famous saying: – 'Soft-tissue tension is very important, sometimes even at the expense of trochanteric advancement, and despite lengthen the leg somewhat.'
- Check offset
- Proper hip position and hip centre
- Proper femoral neck length

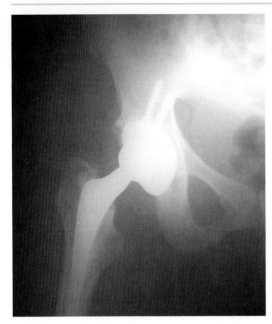

Fig. 6.6. Open orientation of the right acetabular cup, which may predispose to premature wear and dislocation

6.15.1.3 Impingement
- Two varieties: 'intra-articular' versus 'extra-articular'
- Examples of impingement: constrained liner, cups that are too horizontal, high hip centres, etc.

6.15.1.4 Combinations
- Be sure to correct all the causes intra-operatively
- Always remember there can be more than one cause for the hip dislocation

6.15.1.5 Other Causes
- Non-compliant patient
- Rule out sepsis as a cause of late dislocation

6.15.1.5.1 Treatment of Component Malposition
- Revise implant
- Sometimes constrained liner in selected cases

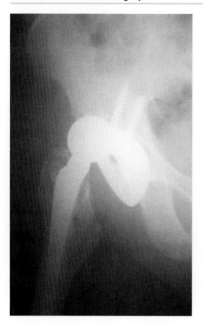

Fig. 6.7. Right hip dislocation in the patient in Fig. 6 post-operatively

6.15.1.5.2 Titrating Soft-Tissue Tension
- Restore hip centre
- Restore offset
- Restore abductor tension
- Sometimes even distal reattachment of the GT

6.15.1.5.3 Treatment of Impingement
- Find the cause (not always simple)

6.15.1.6 Recent Advances
- Use of bipolars
  - Advantage: sometimes considered in low-demand patients
  - Disadvantages: (1) larger diameter, biarticular (more volumetric wear); (2) acetabular erosion
- Use of large head
  - Advantages: (1) more stable; (2) ?less pain/migration

- Disadvantages: (1) wear issues; (2) patient's pelvis must be spacious enough to fit a large socket (since a minimum thickness of 8 mm of polyethylene must be obtained)
▪ Constrained locking socket (e.g. tripolar design from osteonics, and constrained liner from S-ROM)
  - Advantage: immediate stability
  - Disadvantages: (1) not all types with equal level of constraint; (2) if dislocate, will need open reduction

The current indication of constrained socket includes those patients whose cause of the dislocation remains unknown – patients with very weak abductors, CP patients, etc.

6.15.2 Other Complications Besides Dislocation
▪ Infection: discussed in Chap. 7
▪ Neurovascular complications: more common in difficult primaries. The reader is assumed to be familiar with the safe zones for screw placement in cementless THR
▪ Residual LLD: prevented by good pre-operative planning, using the appropriate implant, appropriate management of any bone defects, good soft-tissue tensioning and restoration of COM and offset
▪ Aseptic loosening and osteolysis: subject of osteolysis has been discussed

6.16   Difficult Primary THR

6.16.1   Section 1: Femoral Side

6.16.1.1 Developmental Dysplasia of the Hip (Fig. 6.8)
▪ Neck-shaft angle anomalies, e.g. vara/valga
▪ Offset problems, e.g. short femoral neck
▪ Hip centre, e.g. proximal position (Crowe 4)
▪ Version, e.g. commonly increased anteversion
▪ Soft tissues – femoral nerve may loop proximally, contracted hip muscles, and/or contractures
▪ LLD

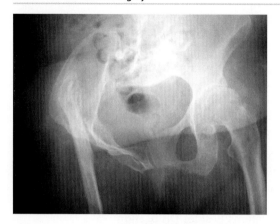

Fig. 6.8. Adult with old untreated developmental dysplasia of the right hip

6.16.1.1.1   Solution

- Hip centre: restore anatomical versus high-hip centre. Most prefer anatomical COM or near anatomical
- Exposure: especially if LLD – may need trochanteric slide especially if LLD is greater than 3 cm or for anterior transposition of a posterior located GT. The 2nd advantage is that it allows high iliac exposure of BG
- Subtrochanteric osteotomy: this allows distal and medial translation of socket position and compensates by shortening the femur at the diaphysis not metaphysis. The osteotomy level be made distal to the coating of a proximally coated implant (or within 2 inches of the lower end of the LT for extensive coated)

6.16.1.1.2   Indication of Subtrochanteric Osteotomy

- We use this approach for high riding hips when there is sufficient bone to perform a high hip centre that will require considerable femoral shortening. Also, if there is sufficient femoral neck bone to resect to compensate for an anatomical hip centre implant or when there is more than 45° anteversion, a subtrochanteric de-rotation can also be considered

6.16.1.1.3   Femoral Solutions

▨ Version way off the mark – can consider subtrochanteric de-rotation osteotomy (just discussed)

▨ Stems can be cemented (but must allow adequate offset and minimise impingement) or cementless (can be proximally, extensive-coated, modular, monolithic, or custom – avoid cementless if significant coxa valga because of possible calcar impingement)

6.16.1.2   RA and Juvenile RA

▨ Osteopenia – increased fracture risk

▨ Steroids – increased sepsis risk

▨ May increase bleeding if RA not burnt out since vascular

▨ Canal diameter – can be very narrow in juvenile RA, and wide in RA

▨ Anteversion – sometimes increased; use modularity

▨ Systemic complications – cervical-spine and organ systems

▨ Contracture release – often needed and capsulectomy often needed since very adherent

▨ Protrusio in RA is not uncommon

▨ In cases where there are too narrow/too wide canals, may consider avoiding cementless

6.16.1.3   Ankylosing Spondylitis

▨ More HO and stiffness (single dose of 700 rads within 24 h before operation may be given) – incidence reported varies a lot; 11% quoted in a recent paper

▨ Soft-tissue contracture – tenotomy and/or complete capsulectomy

▨ Pelvis:
  - Rigidly secure the pelvis with pegboard or similar supports to avoid intraoperative pelvic rotation
  - Beware of acetabular position especially if lumbar lordosis is lost – restore standing acetabular anteversion of 15–20°

▨ Lost lumbar lordosis – thus, non-ankylosed segments can act as fulcrum, neural complication can occur

▨ If head dislocation is difficult – may need in-situ neck cut – to avoid fracture

▨ Exposure – if difficult, may need trochanteric osteotomy/slide

▨ Implant – cemented or cementless possible (RT can affect bony ingrowth if uncemented implant – sometimes shield it)

- Hip hyper-extension is common and can lead to errors, predisposing to anterior dislocation
- Most surgeons feel that if spine and hip flexion deformity occur together, the hips should be tackled first
- New findings: in AS patients with severe kyphosis, doing THR first puts the prosthesis in an unstable position when the patient later resumes the usual posture. Thus, correcting spine first in severe combined (spine and hip) deformities may be considered

6.16.1.4 Osteogenesis Imperfecta

- OI – premature cartilage degeneration, protrusio, bowed femur, LLD, easy fracture, more malunion chance
- Femur reconstruction – may need incremental osteotomy to correct angular deformity and long stem
- Implants: e.g. cementless modular with adjustable neck lengths

6.16.1.5 Paget's Disease

- Bowed femur – may need osteotomy (and/or onlay allograft) to correct
- Brittle bone – fracture risk
- Optimise medical therapy – less hypervascular
- Risk of more blood losses – pre-operative donation, cell salvage, etc.; more blood loss if osteotomy is performed. (If diaphyseal osteotomy, stem should bypass the cut surface by 10 cm)
- Exposure – sometimes trochanteric slide

6.16.1.6 Pre-Existing Structural Deformities

- Distorted femoral canal (e.g. congenital, metabolic) – problems concerning length, version, angulation, canal width and patency)
- Previous hardware/canal stenosis – can act as stress risers
- Previous girdlestone – may have great metaphyseal bone loss and soft-tissue contractures
- Previous trochanteric fracture – if this occurs after medial displacement osteotomy, technical difficulties can be seen intra-operatively. Examples – screws may have been broken; stem insertion difficult, e.g. canal not patent; altered neck shaft and version; also higher loosening and infection rate. Excess scarring may need trochanteric osteotomy. The femoral stem should bypass the lowest screw hole by two canal diameters

▓ Tackling cement extravasation – for example, screw holes occluded by non-adherent conforming material, such as felt or dental dam, covered by mineral oil. Conversely, a modular fluted stem can bypass cortical defects, fill the distorted metaphyseal bone and restore proper version, with or without LLD. An extensive porous-coated stem can get fixation in the distally intact diaphyseal bone

6.16.1.7 Angular (Bowing)
▓ The decision whether to perform corrective femoral osteotomy – depends on pre-operative templating of extent of deformity

6.16.1.8 Take Down of Previous Fusion
Take down of previous fusion greatly affected by:
▓ The type of previous hardware used
▓ Quality and quantity of abductor muscles
▓ State of spine, especially ipsilateral knee and rest of lower limb,
▓ Previous operative report should be available
▓ Trochanteric osteotomy may be needed, and complete capsulectomy usually
▓ Neck osteotomy – careful preservation of posterior and superior acetabular bone stock (use AIIS, ischium and teardrop as guides)
▓ Depth of reaming established at the medial extent of the residual foveal soft tissue
▓ Femur – high speed drill to open canal, long IM rod, adequate offset, intra-operative X-ray, HO prevention
  – Complications of fusion take down are many: this includes sepsis, dislocation, HO, poor ROM, nerve palsies, etc.

6.16.2 Section 2: The Acetabular side

6.16.2.1 Shallow Acetabulum – Options
▓ High-hip centre (Harris)
▓ Anatomical centre with femoral head auto/allograft (Fig. 6.9) with and without flying buttress graft (gross)
▓ Medialisation – avoid overdone
▓ Cotyloplasty – done by the selected few trained for the procedure, danger of iatrogenic protrusio
▓ Oblong cup – more used in revisions however, and added options especially in revisions, e.g. impaction allografts, jumbo cups

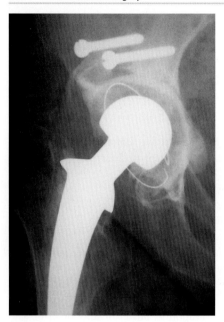

Fig. 6.9. Use of allograft in difficult primary total hip replacement

6.16.2.1.1   Armamentarium

▪ Femoral component – small, straight stem to accommodate the anteversion
▪ A modular femoral component that allows adjusting of the version is another option
▪ Cup should have an inner diameter of 22 mm or 26 mm and be able to be cemented or uncemented

6.16.2.1.2   Work-Up

▪ Pre-operative: LLD checks; location of neck cut decides on template (usually at level of LT because of problem of excess anteversion if neck is cut more proximal)
▪ Intra-operative: start with very small reamers – usually 36 mm – use a depth gauge and drill hole to decide how deep to ream. Stop reaming when 1 cm from inner cortex; then use trial cup; BG is needed if less than 70% of the host bone is covered by cup

- If BG used – needed at superior edge of the acetabulum or just inside it, and fixed with two screws; morsellised autograft may be added at the graft–host bone junction
- Before reduction, make sure tension is not excessive on the nerve; conduct wake-up test. Consider femoral shortening if it really is too tight

6.16.2.1.3   High Hip Centre

- Advantage: avoiding disadvantage of structural BG by inserting small uncemented cup into living host bone. Technique is easier
- Disadvantage: higher loosening chance, higher dislocation – from impingement against the ischium; thinner lining and smaller cup (leg length correction is still possible sometimes by long neck prosthesis or on the femoral side)
- Does not restore bone stock
- Current indication: "sometimes if there is adequate bone stock (especially if hip is stable and leg length correctable by a long neck implant) with a minimum to moderate LLD of 2–3 cm and an acceptable compromise to the anatomy"
- Note that the high hip centre principle uses a high and small socket, but not lateral.
  (Harris previously reported about problems with resorption, fragmentation and cup loosening)

6.16.2.1.4   The Option of Anatomical Centre
and Femoral Head Autografts (or Allografts)

- The shelf autograft if these is less than 70% coverage by host bone
- Principle sound since restores anatomical centre, bone stock, and leg length
- A cemented or uncemented cup can be used
- Good long-term results reported by Gross

6.16.2.1.5   Cotyloplasty

- Controlled fracture of the medial wall: this allows medial advancement of the socket – there are few people with experience of this technique and it should only be done by those trained to do it. Also risk of acetabular protrusio

- Centralisation – by reaming to the inner cortex and placing a small cup in a protruded position – reported in 1988, but later a high loosening rate was found

6.16.2.1.6   Oblong Cup
- Only advantage is that BG is not required
- This method will not replenish the bone stock

6.16.2.1.7   Subtrochanteric Osteotomy
- Especially in DDH cases
- Performed if hip is too tight for reduction of trial components and the nerve too tense, or if a wake-up test shows sciatic nerve weakness – then femoral shortening by a subtrochanteric osteotomy may be needed

6.16.2.2   Deep Acetabulum
- Acetabular Protrusio
  - DDx of causes of acetabular protrusio will be discussed. Do not forget that it can be iatrogenic after cotyloplasty – a non-popular option to tackle the shallow acetabulum: by the same token, too much medialisation can be risky, especially in patients at risk of developing protrusio, e.g. RA, porotics patients

6.16.2.2.1   Features of Acetabular Protrusio
- First described by Otto of Germany
- In the early days, it was most commonly caused by infection – e.g. TB/other microbes-gonococcus
- Now less sepsis, many secondary causes; primary cause is rare
- May be a 'normal' phenomenon between ages 4 years and 8 years (Br J Radiology)
- Treatment is age dependent
- Incidence unknown
- Natural history – most progress with decline in function and pain (predicted by Pauwel's theories of hip mechanics)

6.16.2.2.2   General Comments
- Key word: know the horizontal joint force of the hip
- Key concept: once the hip centre is too medial, progression is almost unavoidable (thanks to previous studies on finite element analysis)

(In inflammatory joint diseases such as RA, the mechanism equals destruction and weakening of bone; in other cases, it is mostly a qualitative defect of bone, e.g. metabolic bone disease such as osteomalacia)

6.16.2.2.3   Normal and Abnormal Hip Mechanics
- Three major factors contribute to hip joint force
    - Body weight
    - Distance of femoral head centre to midline
    - Neck-shaft angle
        Typical normal situation – usual hip joint force 69° from horizontal at stance phase of gait (Egan); others found that, in protrusio, it is usually 65° (McCollum)

6.16.2.2.4   DDx of Causes
- Secondary
    - Inflammatory– RA/AS
    - Non-inflammatory
        Metabolic (e.g. osteomalacia)
        Metastases
        Marfan's (i.e. CT disease, also Ehlers-Danlos)
        Old fracture/Paget's
        Infection (e.g. TB)
        Others, e.g. trisomy 18
- Primary – by exclusion, in fact rare (reported in some families; some say associated with chondrolysis)
    (Relative incidence: in 50% of osteomalacia patients, 15% of RA patients, one-third of patients with AS hips; and only 5% of patients with OA hip)

6.16.2.2.5   Radiological Assessment
- CE Angle more than 40°
- Medial wall medial to ilioischial line (3 mm in males, 6 mm in females, ± note any associated coxa vara)
- Grading system (Charnley):
    - Mild: 1–5 mm (with respect to ilioischial line)
    - Moderate: 6–15 mm
    - Severe: >15 mm

6.16.2.2.6   Blood Work
- ESR
- $CaPO_4$
- CBP
- ANF, RF
- Other investigations sometimes needed: synovial biopsy, especially if inflammatory in causation

6.16.2.2.7   Clinical Assessment
- History – family, syndrome
- Physical examination: neural – hip pain can first occur in as early as adolescence
- Decreased active and passive ROM of hip, especially abduction, sometimes Trendelenberg since abductors in lesser mechanical advantage with or without antalgic gait

6.16.2.2.8   Management Principles Depend on Age Group
- Young child
- Adolescent/young adult
- Middle age (younger than 40 years)
- Old age

6.16.2.2.9   Goal of Treatment
Restoration of bone stock and lateralisation of the hip centre

6.16.2.2.10 Role of Tri-Radiates Fusion in the Child
- In fact, an epiphysiodesis for the rare severe cases only
- Sometimes combined with valgus osteotomy in the older child

6.16.2.2.11 Valgus Osteotomy of Proximal Femur With and Without Soft-Tissue Releases for the Young Adult
- Previous: arthrodesis and resection have been described as treatment options
- Current ideas: valgus osteotomy can buy time in very selected cases, but there is less of a success rate if there is an increased age or if arthritis is setting in
- To tackle worries about LLD, some use a trapezoidal-shortening osteotomy. Worries of abductor high tension post-operatively are sometimes reduced by an open-wedge osteotomy of GT
- Assess need for soft-tissue release – e.g. iliopsoas, iliotibial band, etc.

6.16.2.2.12 Patient Selection

- Recent recommendation by Wenger: should not be performed in patients over 40 years of age, or in those who have significant OA changes
- Interesting in that pre-operative limited motion is not always a prelude to poor outcome
- Claims little difficulty to convert to THR

6.16.2.2.13 THR in the Aged Patient with Protrusio

- How to tackle the medial defect (guideline by Ranawart) – options:
  - Mild – 'no' BG may be needed
  - Moderate – cancellous BG, and some uses anti-protrusio cages to better distribute the stress
  - Severe – BG and cages
- Restoration of an anatomical (or more anatomical) hip centre
- How to remove the femoral head – corkscrew, in-situ neck cuts, break the vacuum, removal of osteophytes, sometimes extensile exposures

6.16.2.2.14 Appendix (on Medial Wall Reinforcement in THR)

- Medial cup placement caused high medial stresses, anatomical placement better
- In some studies, reinforce medial wall with cement and mesh not quite effective; metal-backed cages more effective – due to the superior stress distribution of the metal cup
- A metal-protrusio-ring device is more reliable; transfers stress from medial wall to the rim rather than flanged protrusio cup
- BG is optimum method for achieving lateralisation in protrusio – allograft of femoral head frequently used
- Approach most widely used is to fill with BG, then use porous-coated metal cup for acetabular reconstruction

6.16.2.3   Deformed Acetabulum

- Problems with conversion of a fused hip:
  - Exposure – trochanteric osteotomy helps identify the femoral neck and LT
  - Height and depth of socket – X-ray may be needed
  - Nerve injury – from change in tension
  - Leg length issues

- Heterotopic ossification – indocid; or give 700 rads
- Instability – e.g. post-operative because of abductor atrophy and prophylactic measures taken. Constraints?

6.17   Revision THR (Fig. 6.10)

6.17.1   Introduction: Consent
▨ When getting signed consent by the patient for primary THR, tell of the need for revision later, and inform that there may be a need to revise if there is progressive loss of bone stock from osteolysis (whether there are symptoms or not)

6.17.2   General Assessment: DDx of Septic and Aseptic Loosening

6.17.2.1 Investigations for Possible Septic Loosening
▨ Blood work
▨ Aspiration

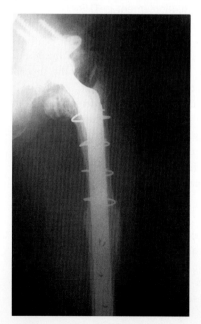

Fig. 6.10. A patient with revision total hip replacement done for aseptic loosening

▓ Bone scan and differential bone scan
▓ Clinical/radiological – periosteal reaction suggestive, for cavities – if due to mechanical causes tend to stabilise with time, and due to biological causes tend to excavate and can progress with time
▓ Intra-operative gram-stain
▓ Intra-operative frozen section and culture
  (Others, e.g. PCR)

6.17.2.2   Assessment of the Cementless Hip

▓ Signs of well-fixed stem – spot welds (common site between porous and non-porous coat junctions), no serial migration or subsidence
▓ Signs of micro-motion/loosen – serial migration/subsidence, pedestral at stem tip, shedding of beads, etc.

6.17.2.2.1   What Can One Figure Out if See (1) Broken Screw Versus (2) Backed out Screws?

▓ Broken screws imply the local bone stock is not bad
▓ Backed out screws imply either infected or osteolysis; hence, no bone for screw to hold upon (or very osteopenic to start with)

6.17.2.3   Assessment of the Cemented THR

▓ Acetabular cup: long-term result is not so good – most get loose at bone–cement interface
▓ Femoral side has better track record – definitely loose if see cement breakage, migration or complete bone–cement interface lines. Suggestive of loosening if progressive bone–cement interface lines detected
▓ The reader is assumed to know the Charnley's zones and Gruen zones in describing a loosened THR

6.17.2.4   Removal of Components: Cementless THR

▓ General comment – bony ongrowth (e.g. HA) easier to remove than good bony ingrowth
▓ Acetabular side – may use curved and thin osteotome; Zimmer has curved blade saws, etc.
▓ Femoral side – well-fixed cases may need extended trochanteric osteotomy
▓ Very difficult cases carbide saw the metal, removal of proximal part. Distal stem core it out like removal of broken screw

6.17.2.5   Removal of Component: Cemented THR

▨ Acetabular side – address the bone/cement interface

▨ Femoral side – look for debonding of metal–cement interface, otherwise attack bone–cement interface

▨ Sometimes use cement tap to help remove cement on femoral side; some instruments to help remove cement especially at cement plug areas at acetabular cup

6.17.2.6   Assess Bone Loss

▨ Judet view may help

▨ Some use CT to help assessment

6.17.2.6.1   Tackling Bone Loss on Acetabular Side

▨ Jumbo cup

▨ Oblong cup (when discrepancy between meridian and equator)

▨ Impaction bone grafting with help of wire mesh

▨ Medialise but not excessive

▨ ARR (acetabular reinforcement ring, e.g. Ganz)/Burch Schneider rings (Some use whole femoral allograft head in medial wall problem/protrusion)

6.17.2.6.2   Tackling Bone Loss on Femoral Side

▨ General comment – in cementless cases, those with no circumferential porous coat tend to get lysis at diaphysis; those that have get more lysis at GT or LT

▨ Options:
  – Implants with more distal fixation, e.g. PFMR (proximal femoral modular reconstruction)
  – Impaction bone grafting
  – Anatomical bow and long stem (e.g. S-ROM)
  – Severe bone losses: tumour prosthesis or custom-made prostheses or allograft–prosthetic composite

6.17.2.7   Soft-Tissue Re-Balancing

6.17.2.7.1   Role of Soft-Tissue Balance and Prevention of Dislocation

▨ Correct the tension and offset

▨ Correct the combined anteversion

▨ Beware of pelvic positioning

- Check impingement, e.g. neck short, osteophyte GT, femoral component too deep and/or undersized, on abduction the GT impinges

6.17.2.7.2   Implications of Early Versus Late Dislocation

- Early – most are early dislocation, e.g. soft-tissue imbalance or poor soft tissue, alignment and component malpositioned, impingement, etc.
- Late – think of (1) cup loose, (2) worn out liner, (3) sepsis

6.17.2.8   Special Risk if Acetabular Side Protrusio

- Can get adhered to the blood vessels of the pelvis (if really involved, double approach even including intra-abdominal approach to dig it out)
- May need a pre-operative angiogram
- This represents yet another lesson to intervene early for protrusio cases – since finite element analysis found that inexorable progression was inevitable due to the medial joint forces of the hip

6.18   Appendix

The following topics will be covered in the appendix:

- Primary and secondary OA hip
- Managing AVN hip
- Hip problems in the young adults

6.18.1   Hip OA

6.18.1.1   Dx of Primary OA Hip

- By exclusion

6.18.1.2   Epidmiology and Interesting Observation

- Studies concerning HK Chinese (study by Hoaglund of University of California) – extremely low primary OA hip (1%), and this low incidence stayed the same two decades later
- Occurs in Causasians 3–6 times as often as in Chinese, East Indians and Blacks

- Marked low rate for THR performed for primary OA hip: 1.3 per 100,000 versus 60 per 100,000 (Mayo Clinic data), versus Norway's 140 per 100,000
- It was observed in some studies that patients who had THR for primary OA hip seldom underwent TKR and vice versa
- Other predisposing factors – long leg OA; and some claims by many experts that 25–45% of cases are from hip dysplasia, while bearing in mind studies, for example, from Japan that low CE angle is common but primary OA uncommon for some uncertain reason

6.18.1.3 Pitfalls

- Hip dysplasia and patients with paediatric hip condition are common predisposing causes for hip arthritis (especially in countries where primary OA is uncommon). It is imperative to catch the window of opportunity to intervene by pelvic and/or femoral osteotomies depending on the underlying pathology if the patient is too young for THR, like in his or her twenties
- Two causes of acute deterioration of symptoms – (1) ruptured or torn labrum and (2) sometimes OA in some rarer case – can progress rapidly in terms of few months

6.18.1.4 Causes of Secondary OA

- AVN – sclerosis, lucency, flattening of head (will be discussed in detail in the next section)
- Paget's disease (Fig. 6.11) – bone enlarges, coarse trabeculation, cortex thickened
- Inflammatory arthritis – diffuse joint space narrowing, osteopenia, erosion
- Trauma remodelling – distorted contour with sclerosis and remodelling
- DDH – shallow acetabulum, increased acetabular index, sometimes hip subluxation or dislocation
- Slip – femoral retroversion, convexity of head–neck junction, short femoral head/short broad neck
- Perthes disease
  [Others: Charchot joint is less common in the hip, but sometimes affects the knee (Fig. 6.12) and elbow. Crystal arthropathy, like gout (Fig. 6.13), mostly spares the hip, but can cause OA in other peripheral joints]

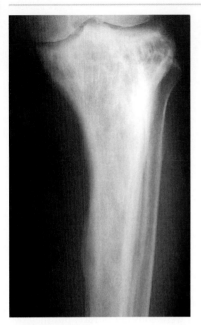

Fig. 6.11. Tibia X-ray of a patient with Paget's disease. Note the very coarse trabeculae and the expanded proximal tibia

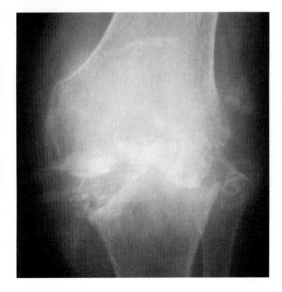

Fig. 6.12. Destroyed Charchot joint of the left knee

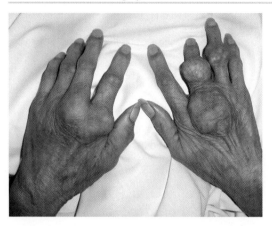

Fig. 6.13. This patient with tophaceous gout also has degenerative arthritis of both his feet

6.18.1.5 New Development (Role of Labral Lesions in Hip OA Pathogenesis with the Advent of Hip Arthroscopy)

- The hypothesis that labral pathology could conceivably contribute to the development of OA hip has yet to be confirmed
- Previously, acetabular labral lesions were considered rare; but they become more evident with increased use of hip arthroscopy and radial MRI
- The natural history of such lesions have not yet been defined, but may well be a possible predisposing cause of hip arthritis

6.18.2 Hip AVN

6.18.2.1 Introduction

- Occur in 3rd to 5th decades mostly, most spontaneous AVN occurring in the hip, although can occur in other areas such as the knee (Fig. 6.14)
- Most progress, and end up as OA hip. Of most series of total hip cases, 5–15% have an underlying cause of AVN

6.18.2.2 Natural History

- Most are progressive once symptoms appear and progress to debilitating disease
- Initially the disease is asymptomatic
- Only early intervention yields the best result

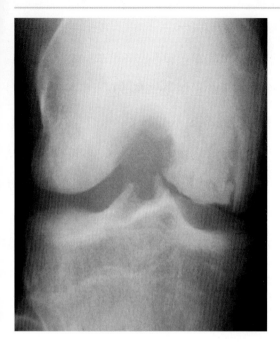

Fig. 6.14. This X-ray demonstrates osteonecrosis changes of the medial femoral condyle

▦ Hungerford found that most requires surgical intervention 2–4 years after Dx

6.18.2.3 Pathogenesis
▦ Bone at femoral head functions as a Starling resistor – the cortex is an inexpandable shell and blood vessels traversing it are thin-walled tubes
▦ As long as the driving pressure remains the same, flow is proportional to pressure within the shell. Any increase in pressure within the shell results in a proportional decrease in flow. There is no evidence of any compensatory mechanism to increase blood pressure in response to increased IM pressure. Anything that increased the marrow pressure – increased fat (steroids), nitrogen bubbles (Caisson disease), marrow diseases, fat emboli, intraosseous thrombosis – are all going to decrease the flow
▦ It has been reported that intraosseous bone marrow pressure – normal < 22 mmHg – can rise to very high in ON, e.g. up to 100 mmHg

6.18.2.4 Biomechanics and ON

▥ Principle 1: compression of the joint increases IM pressure on the convex side (the ball) of the joint but not the concave side reported in biomechanics journals
  - Explains why most cases occur at convex side – femoral head, humeral head, distal femur, talus
  - Hungerford says also contributory is that the 'anatomy of the joint dictates that the circulation on the convex side is more tenuous than on concave side'
▥ Principle 2: biomechanical forces on the ischaemic bone lead to collapse – (evidence): 'observation that, on the one hand, the area of ON corresponds exactly to the area of articular cartilage wear in OA; on the other hand, in impacted valgus fractured neck of femur cases, the area of collapse if ON ensues corresponds to the new WB area and not the anatomical zone that constituted the old WB area.'

6.18.2.5 Ficat Classification

▥ Normal X-ray appearance
▥ Sclerotic or cystic lesion, without subchondral fracture
▥ Cresent sign (subchondral collapse) and/or step off in contour of subchondral bone
▥ OA with decreased articular cartilage, osteophytes

6.18.2.6 Types of Classification

▥ Ficat – most used
▥ Steinberg – incorporates MRI (thought to be the most sensitive modality in Dx of AVN) – but the drawback of MRI is that it does not very accurately assess the status of the articular cartilage
▥ Marcus – correlates clinical, radiological and pathological information, including the state of articular cartilage
▥ Japanese investigational committee – stresses on the location
▥ Pennsylvania University – resembles classification by Marcus

6.18.2.7 Categories of Pathomechanics

▥ Direct cellular mechanism – e.g. RT, steroid, alcohol (steroids – lipid droplets in osteocytes enlarge and compress the cell, causing cell death)
▥ Extraosseous arterial mechanism: e.g. fractured neck of femur, (85% if displaced) and hip dislocation (damages the retinacular vessels).

Study of effect of arterial tamponade – animal study on hip blood flow (Launder J Bone Joint Surg 1981 [6]) (some claim, however, that the adult hip is more resistant to this effect)

- Extraosseous venous mechanism: it is not clear whether this is a cause or effect. Experiment from Johns Hopkin's Hospital: obstruction in vein flow causes only temporary decrease in blood flow, then rapid return to normal
- Intraosseous extravascular: e.g. hypertrophy of fat cells/steroid, Gaucher's; and possible role of intraosseous oedema haemorrhage
  Mechanism here is that an increase in compartment pressure tends to collapse the thin-walled vessels and causes decreased blood flow
- Intraosseous intravascular: e.g. sickle cell anaemia, dysbaric, intravascular coagulation (recently proposed – Schwartzman phenomenon – this involves the concept that an immune complex deposition may lead to arteriolar haemorrhage and ON), possibly fat emboli (hyperlipidaemia, steroids, alcohol). and possible role of increased platelet and hypofibrinolysis

6.18.2.8 Pathological Changes

- The softened necrotic cancellous bone is unable to withstand physiological forces and collapses, signalling usually the onset of symptoms
- A 'cleavage plane' occurs between the articular surface – which is nourished by the joint fluid – and the necrotic bone beneath it. (At this time, the avascular fragment will 'ballote' with compression, much like a tennis ball will compress and then resume its shape)
- Collapse of the articular cartilage is visible when the fragment no longer assumes its original shape, and the head flattens
- Near the end stage, the articular surface becomes dissociated from the cancellous bone and cleaves off as a large fragment. This is called 'delamination' representing late advanced stage and OA begins
- Once the articular surface collapses, salvage of congruent hip is almost impossible

6.18.2.9 Variables Influencing Our Management

- Stage – pre-collapse means stage 1 or 2 in most classification systems
- Size – first stressed by Steinberg; ON angle is useful concept – measure the angle subtended in (AP and frog lateral) <160° small, >250° large

- Age – one-quarter to one-third of the patients are very young (< 25 years); need to avoid THR and consider other options, e.g. vascularised BG, trapdoor procedure, surface replacements and/or osteotomy
- Severity of associated underlying disease (in two-thirds of cases)
  5th element added by Sugioka – site of the lesion (see later discussion)

6.18.2.10 Non-Operative Treatment
- Implantable bone stimulators (some studies have been shown to stimulate osteogenesis; reported in 1989) – this method has not been approved by the FDA
- Protected weight bear
- Long-term results not good

6.18.2.11 Aim of Operative Treatment
- Relieve pain
- Preserve head
- Prevent further joint deterioration
- Early intervention important

6.18.2.11.1 Method 1: Core Decompression and/or BG [Ficat's Stage 1, 2]
- Rationale based on an increase in intraosseous pressure in the femoral head resulting from venous congestion and other pathways (Hungerford)
- Immediate pain relief in most series
- Must be done before head collapse or stage 3
- Most agree that it does play an insignificant role in stage 3 (only 20% success rate)
- Complications in 1%; need protected WB for 6 weeks
- One study in 1996 included 1200 hips of which 741 had clinical success at 'all' stages – although much less effective in stage 3

6.18.2.11.2 Method 2: The Two Main Groups of Osteotomies (Rotational and Angular)
- Varus (F/E) osteotomy and valgus (usu extension) osteotomy
- Sugioka's transtrochanteric rotational osteotomy (in fact a combination of three osteotomies)

Rationale: the biomechanical effect of moving the necrotic fragment of the femoral head from the WB area to a less WB area (note the posterolateral area is most WB area) and also help decompress venous pressure

6.18.2.11.3 Ideal Candidate

▦ Best for small to medium lesions (<30% femoral head and combined necrotic angle less than 200°); mostly for stages 1, 2 and early stage 3

6.18.2.11.4 Indication of Sugioka's Osteotomy

▦ Be done early: stage-2 disease and the intact portion must be in such a position and of such size that, after rotation, the intact portion of the femoral head takes up at least 36% of the WB surface

▦ Not effective for those in medial third or NWB areas

6.18.2.11.5 Details on Sugioka Osteotomy (Fig. 6.15)

▦ In fact, a rotational flap of proximal femur, based on the vascular pedicle of the medial circumflex femoral vessels – the condition of the vascular pedicle dictates operative success or not – not the post-operative X-ray

▦ Involves three osteotomies:
  – GT
  – Inter-trochanteric passing from superolateral to inferomedial on AP
  – The 'secondary' osteotomy – that passes from the proximal flare of the LT inferolaterally to the inferomedial portion of the primary osteotomy
    (The purpose is to leave the LT with the femoral shaft as a medial buttress for the proximal fragment to rest on.)

▦ Also, the operation involves concomitant soft-tissue release, e.g. of short rotators, piriformis, iliopsoas, etc.; no attempt is made intra-operatively to expose or identify the vessels of the pedicle

6.18.2.11.6 Clinical Outcome

▦ 15-year-long follow-up of 295 hips by Sugioka; 80% did not need further operation

▦ The same good result, however, was not reproduced by papers from the States, e.g. Cabanela at Mayo Clinic; may be due to the complexity of operation, patient selection, etc.

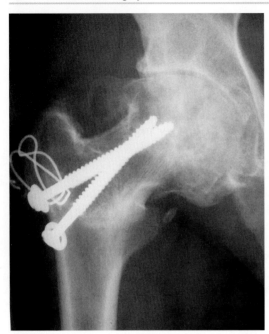

Fig. 6.15. Right hip postoperative X-ray after Sugioka type of osteotomy

6.18.2.11.7 Method 3: BG (Non-Vascularised and Vascularised)

▨ Many believe that articular cartilage integrity is an important factor in the successful treatment of AVN by vascularised/non-vascularised BG methods

▨ Aim at providing some kind of structural support to prevent collapse

▨ Hungerford stress a complication rate of 5% and donor site morbidity of 25% for vascularised BG

▨ Example of non-vascularised BG method:
  – Add cortical BG after core decompression
  – Cancellous through window in femoral neck; some Japanese studies used similar method by cortical bone instead – claims reasonably good outcome
  – Osteochondral graft – had hip dislocated posteriorly, removed necrotic bone and overlying cartilage, replaced by iliac crest graft and osteochondral graft. Meyers claimed good result (trapdoor method)

6.18.2.11.8   Method 4: Vascularised BG (Up to Stage 3, Never if OA+)

- Results of Urbaniak:
  - Patients with pre-collapse ~90% success with vascularised BG at 5-year mark
  - Patients with stage-3 disease – 77%
  - Stage 4 and 5 – 5-year rates were 57% and 68%

    (More recent studies suggested that, unlike stage-5 disease, some with stage 4 have cartilage like a 3, although some are as bad as 5 – with differing prognosis. Thus, it is with stage-4 disease that assessment of the state of the articular surface is especially important).

    Main indication – stage 3 since Urbaniak's results for stage 3 are significantly better than core decompression (though results for pre-collapse are better still, not without complication and the use of core can be considered if pre-collapse)

6.18.2.11.9   Method 5: Surface Replacement Type of Arthroplasty

- Cons: not many clinical studies, and no long-term results. The avascular process may go on after replacing surface
- Pros (Amstutz): less dislocation, less wear, less osteolysis, maintains bone stock, less LLD, and can be converted to THR
- Hungerford thinks that this procedure is not preservative but conservative – buy some time especially if patient is very young

6.18.2.11.10   Method 6: Formal Arthroplasties – Unipolar; Bipolar; THR

6.18.2.11.11   Problems of THR for Hip AVN

- Proposed reason: mineralisation defect secondary or independent of steroid-use
- Necrotic bone at calcar may affect bone remodelling around prosthesis

6.18.2.11.12   Outcome of THR done for AVN Hip

- Results in general are poorer than those done for OA as a primary
- Increased frequency of early revision – underlies need for hip salvage procedure before THR
- Higher failure rate even when young age and activity level are controlled for

▩ Example: L Dorr 45% failure reported in 1991
▩ Some report better results with modern cement technique or cement-less stems but short-term. A recent 10-year follow-up study revealed 17% revised in 1993

6.18.2.11.13   Conclusion
▩ Success rate after various procedures are variable – partly because of inability to very accurately determine the stage of the disease when intervention is initiated
▩ Patients with stage-4 disease has the widest variation in the appearance of the articular surface. MRI has been shown to be inadequate in assessing the articular cartilage – new studies aim at directly looking at articular cartilage by arthroscopy or direct visualisation (surgical joint dislocation) for more accurate evaluation and staging
▩ To draw any valid conclusion of efficacy of treatment; it is important to know the shape and quality of the femoral articular cartilage before initiating treatment
▩ Hungerford says that, in the last two decades, there has been much progress in salvage rather than on preservative procedures
▩ New BG substitutes and growth factors need further clinical trials and form part of his on-going researches

6.18.3   List of Young Adult Hip Problems
▩ Symptomatic patient with no radiological anomalies
▩ Asymptomatic hip with radiological anomalies
▩ Symptomatic and with the following X-ray anomalies:
  – X-ray pattern that will benefit from periacetabular osteotomy (PAO)
  – X-ray pattern that may benefit from femoral osteotomy
  – X-ray pattern that may benefit from valgus extension osteotomy (VEO)
  – Possible role of proximal femoral osteotomy in AVN hip

6.18.3.1   Painful Mobile Hips with Normal X-Ray
▩ Labral tear: can be sudden in onset, with or without a catching sensation; sometimes gives way and with or without mild effusion. Physical examination: may have positive acetabular stress test produced by hip flexion and IR. Definitive Dx may need radial MRI or hip arthroscopy

that may be both diagnostic and therapeutic. Cause of tear can be primary or secondary to predisposing causes like hip dysplasia
- Extra-articular causes (snapping hip): try to get the patient to reproduce the snap (e.g. source can be from psoas tendon or trochanteric bursitis, etc.)
- Referred pain: e.g. from spine, SIJ, knee

6.18.3.2 Asymptomatic Hip with Radiological Anomalies

6.18.3.2.1 Differential Diagnoses
- Early AVN of the femoral head
- Dysplastic hip
- Old neglected DDH (or residual changes despite treatment of childhood DDH)
- Old childhood hip disorders. There is some suggestion that persistent femoral retroversion after childhood SCFE may predispose to OA

6.18.3.2.2 Clinical Features of Hip Dysplasia (Fig. 6.16)
- Can be an incidental finding and completely asymptomatic, some of these cases can be observed
- PAO can be considered if the patient is starting to get disability from the hip condition. An adequate abduction range on physical examination is needed to allow the equivalent degree of acetabular reorientation
- The majority of patients with hip dysplasia has a slooping acetabulum on AP pelvis X-ray and signs of deficient acetabular coverage on the Faux Profile view
- PAO may be considered if the affected leg can be abducted and the hip reduces concentrically under anaesthetic on fluoroscopic screening
- Proximal femoral osteotomy has a lesser place in young adult hip dysplasia

6.18.3.3 Hips that May Benefit from PAO
- Acetabular dysplasia with decreased centre-edge angle, but the joint is not subluxated and still concentric
- Advantage of PAO: if done properly, not only postpone the need for THR, but abolish the need altogether. In other cases, good symptomatic relief in 80% cases for 10 years is expected

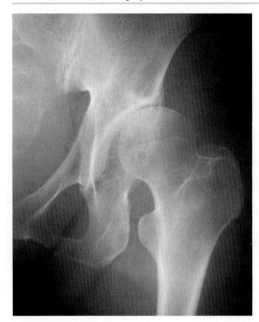

Fig. 6.16. Relatively young patient with left hip dysplasia

- Complications of PAO: fracture line extends beyond the peri-acetabular area, neurovascular injuries, deep learning curve. In future, some of the complications may be lessened by surgical navigation techniques. However, experts like Ganz seldom need the navigation techniques

6.18.3.4 Hips that May Benefit from Chiari
- The natural history of hip dysplasia is that once subluxation occurs, the likelihood of progression is much increased
- PAO is not indicated in hips that are no longer concentric, e.g. hip dysplasia patients with significant subluxation requires a Chiari, not PAO
- Salvage options include Chiari operation and the shelf procedure, especially if the patient is young. However, some experts feel that the graft used in the Shelf operation may resorb with time

6.18.3.5 Possible Role of Proximal Femoral Osteotomy

- AVN: discussed in the section on AVN hip
- Coxa Vara
- Hips that may benefit from VEO will be discussed

6.18.3.6 Hips that May Benefit from VEO

- Those hips with a flattened or mushroom shaped femoral head may be indicated for VEO (Fig. 6.17)
- This procedure if successful can be a good buy time procedure as 70% of patients may not need THR at the 10-year mark.

  Prerequisite: by adducting the femoral head, the WB zone needs to move from the antersuperolateral position to a fulcrum between the medial part of the head and the osteophytes deep in the acetabulum. A significant degree of flattening of the head is required. However,

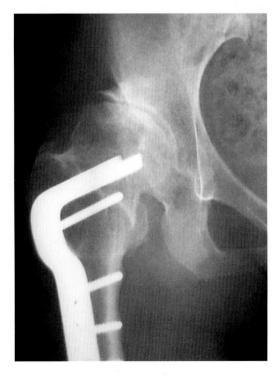

Fig. 6.17. Postoperative X-ray of the right hip after valgus extension osteotomy

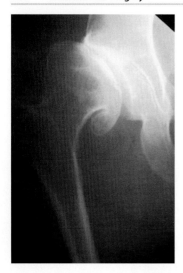

Fig. 6.18. X-ray of a degenerated hip with too huge capital drop osteophyte which may prevent successful performance of valgus extension osteotomy

those with an extra large capital drop osteophyte (Fig. 6.18) may hinder this change in fulcrum rather than a blessing. A frank gap should appear superolaterally with the hip in marked adduction and some flexion before VEO can be considered. Significant limitation of adduction is a contraindication

General Bibliography

Insall J, Scott N (eds) (2001) Surgery of the knee (vols 1, 2), 3rd edn. Churchill Livingstone, Edinburgh

Callaghan J, Rosenberg A, Rubash H (eds) (1998) The adult hip (vols 1, 2). Lippincott Williams and Wilkins, Philadelphia

Wright T, Goodman S (2001) Implant wear in total joint replacement, 1st edn. American Academy of Orthopaedic Surgeons, Rosemont, Illinois, USA

Macnicol MF (1996) Osteotomy of the hip. Mosby-Wolfe, Philadelphia

Selected Bibliography of Journal Articles

1. Ip D, Tsang WL et al. (2002) Comparison of two total knee prostheses on the incidence of Patella Clunk Syndrome. Int Orthop 26:48–51
2. Coventry MB (1985) Upper tibial osteotomy for osteoarthritis. J Bone Joint Surg Am 67:1136–1140
3. Maquet D (1985) The treatment of choice in osteoarthritis of the knee. CORR 192:108–112
4. Laskin RS, O'Flynn et al. (1997) The Insall Award. Total knee replacement with retention of the posterior cruciate ligament in rheumatoid arthritis. Problems and complications. CORR 345:24–28
5. Alexander C (1965) The aetiology of primary protrusio acetabuli. Br J Radiol 38:567–580
6. Launder WJ, Hungerford DS et al. (1981) Haemodynamics of the femoral head. J Bone Joint Surg Am 63:442–448
7. Naudie DD, Rorabeck CH et al. (2004) Sources of osteolysis around total knee arthroplasty: wear of the bearing surface. Instructional Course Lectures 53:251–259
8. Bozic KJ, Harris WH et al. (2004) The high hip centre. CORR 420:101–105
9. Harris WH (2003) Results of uncemented cups: a critical appraisal at 15 years. CORR 417:253–262

7 Orthopaedic Infections

7.1   Septic Arthritis

7.1.1   Part 1: Paediatric Age Group

7.1.1.1   Definition
- Septic arthritis is a bacterial infection in the synovium and joint space producing an intense inflammatory reaction with polymorphonuclear neutrophil (PMN) migration and release of destructive proteolytic enzymes (from the PMN and sometimes the bacteria)
- One in three patients have residual loss of function, avascular necrosis (AVN) and growth disturbances common in children
- Incidence is about the same as for osteomyelitis in children
- The hip joint is commonly affected in neonates and the knee more than hip in the older child

7.1.1.2   Age and Organism
- Neonate: staphylococcus, streptococcus and maternal organism; take obstetrics history (Hx) → can be associated with streptococci, gonorrhoea, syphilis, gram-negative bacilli, etc.
- Infants younger than 2 years: it was previously reported that haemophilus influenzae was a 'very' important cause – this is not so now in the UK since immunisation has become available. Currently, staphylococcus is a more likely cause than streptococcus
- Older child: staphylococcus is also a more likely cause than streptococcus

7.1.1.3   Hx and Physical Examination
- Neonate and/or infant: high index of suspicion since very commonly missed in these cases. Septic arthritis is thought of in any child with septicaemia, especially if there are suggestive signs: pseudoparalysis most important and abnormal joint posture, pain (less obvious) on motion/palpation, and/or asymmetrical buttock crease; bulge in the buttock perineum. Knee and elbow more easy to diagnose since superficial
- Older child: more often severe pain is observed, along with effusion and refusal to move the joint, fever and tachycardia

7.1.1.4 Investigations

■ Erythrocyte sedimentation rate (ESR) and C-reactive protein (CRP) are very useful but lack specificity, although sensitive. Seeing a trend is important. Levels of white blood cells (WBCs) are less so, though usually on the high end

■ Joint aspiration for Gram stain, culture, cell count and biochemistry is most important for diagnosis (Dx); do not jump to mention bone scans/magnetic resonance imaging (MRI)

■ Ultrasound (USS)-guided aspiration of deeper joints useful, especially the hip – USS positive immediately in general after infection, and many days before X-ray changes

■ X-ray: (acute) soft tissue swelling, joint distended/swell capsule (late changes): joint destruction, osteoporosis, metaphyseal involvement

7.1.1.5 Special Investigation

■ Bone scan: pressure inside joint sometimes causes hypo-uptake in femoral head, may be useful in suspected combined osteomyelitis and septic arthritis; sometimes if multiple joints are affected (10% of cases; but this is the figure for adults), and useful in those immuno-suppressed from whatever cause that may mask symptoms and signs

■ MRI: can see not only joint effusion, but see changes if associated osteomyelitis

■ CT: few indications [but useful in adults in exotic joints such as sternoclavicular joint (SCJ)/sacroiliac joint (SIJ) and/or pubic symphysis, especially in addicts]

7.1.1.6 Differential Diagnosis

■ Acute osteomyelitis: can be very similar, but careful examination finds that joint motion is allowed by the child; however, the two conditions can co-exist, especially in the hip and shoulder joints

■ Juvenile 'idiopathic' arthritis: initially can be monoarticular, but there is little pain and effusion is positive

■ Transient synovitis: clinical and aspiration

■ Perthes: USS sometimes useful in DDx

■ Post-traumatic effusion: Hx of trauma

■ Cellulitis and/or bursitis (children: prepatella bursitis more than olecranon)

■ Acute rheumatic fever

- Others: HSP (rare form of hepatorenal dysfunction in children associated with purpura), haemophilia, juvenile rheumatoid arthritis

7.1.1.7 Two Main Treatments to Be Given at the Same Time
- IV antibiotics: decrease systemic effect/toxaemia (30–50% blood culture positive)
- Open drainage and debridement: still the mainstay (in the older child with knee sepsis, can perform arthroscopic lavage. Hip sepsis often treated by open drainage)

7.1.1.8 Disadvantage of the Method of Repeated Aspiration
- Pus too thick for adequate aspiration
- Instillation of antibiotics irritant to cartilage
- Tension will recur
- Pain with each procedure
- Uncertain results

7.1.1.9 Open Hip Drainage
- Anterior Smith-Peterson approach used most
- Adequate debridement
- Drain in-situ
- If hip unstable, splint in a partially abducted and/or flexed posture with or without formal immobilisation if very unstable
- IV then oral antibiotics – for total of 6 weeks

7.1.1.10 Rare Organisms
- Streptococcus pneumoniae, E. coli, proteus, salmonella (sickle cell patients), serratia marcescens, clostridia welchii, neisseria, staphylococcus albus, aerobacter, bacteroides, paracolon bacillus.
  [Look out for unusual microbes in immunosuppressed patients or penetration of joint by foreign body (FB), or foreign body inside joint]

7.1.1.11 DDx Reasons for Negative Culture
- Partial antibiotics treatment (Rn)
- Poor culture technique
- Inadequate anaerobic cultures (some inject the aspirated fluid into blood culture bottles as well)

- Forgot blood culture, or forgot to aspirate
- Changing prevalence of organisms, and their culture characteristics
- Overall, 30% of cases result in negative culture

7.1.1.12 Best-Guess Antibiotics
- Neonate: cloxacillin and gentamicin
- 6 months to 2 years: cloxacillin or cephalosporin; cefuroxime
- Over 2 years: cloxacillin or cefuroxime
  Adjust, later according to sensitivity

7.1.1.13 Outcome
- Recover: (a) not deformed and (b) mild coxa magna
- Coxa brevia (with deformed head), coxa vara or coxa valga (physeal closure)
- Slip of epiphysis: coxa vara/valga
- Destroyed head: small remnant or dislocated

7.1.1.14 Late Reconstruction and Recurrence
- Late reconstruction of coxa vara by valgus osteotomy sometimes useful
- Overall recurrence 20%
- If it does not recur in 6 months, there is less than 10% chance of further infection relapse, and less than 5% if it does not recur by 1 year

7.1.2   Part 2: Adult Septic Arthritis

7.1.2.1   Predisposing Factors for Orthopaedic Infections
- Immunosuppressed/diabetes mellitis (DM)/chronic renal failure
- Rheumatoid arthritis (RA)
- Steroids
- Drug addicts
- Underlying abnormal joint
- Trauma
- Iatrogenic – increase in long revision operations for total knee replacement (TKR), total hip replacement (THR)
- Recent joint sepsis – can also spread to other joints, 10% multifocal

7.1.2.2 Clinical Features

▦ Usually typical, less tricky to diagnose than in neonates; may be more subtle in the partially treated

▦ Dx also by joint aspiration – besides sending aspirate for crystals

▦ Multifocal septic foci can occur in the chronically ill and immunosuppressed

7.1.2.3 Common DDx in Adults

▦ Osteoarthritis (OA)

▦ Crystal arthropathy

▦ RA

▦ Trauma

▦ Osteomyelitis/combined sepsis

▦ 'Septic Bursitis'

7.1.2.4 Anomalies of Aspirate in Affected Joints

▦ WBC: >50,000/cc

▦ 80% PMN

▦ Low sugar

▦ Gram-stain positive in two-thirds (two-thirds of which revealed Gram-positive organisms)

▦ Negative test for crystals

7.1.2.5 Appendix on Other Investigations

▦ ESR >20 in 95% cases

▦ Blood culture positive in 30–50%

▦ X-ray: may see joint swelling, later juxta-articular osteoporosis, later destruction and metaphyseal changes

▦ Tc bone scan good in detecting infection in peripheral joints, cannot differentially diagnose RA from sepsis

▦ CT: useful in IV addicts with sepsis in unusual regions → SCJ, SIJ and pubic symphysis

▦ MRI: selected cases only

7.1.2.6 Other Finer Points

▦ Start gentle mobilisation in approximately 1 week and pain is less; sepsis of hip less common in causing dislocation, although possible, e.g. infected Austin Moore hemi-arthroplasty, THR

▓ Prognosis worse in those left more than 1 week untreated, and presence of factors is predictive of poor prognosis: Gram-negative infection (in total joint, sometimes make re-implantation impossible); positive blood culture, more than one joint affected; serious co-morbidity, old age, prior osteoarthritis/abnormal joint

▓ Poor prognosis indicator after Rn started: effusion persistent, high WBC, positive synovial fluid culture

▓ Refer to the section on sepsis in total joints

▓ Refer to section on infected joints after open reduction and internal fixation (ORIF) for fracture, with implants in-situ

▓ Common culprit microbes in addicts: staphylococcus aureus, pseudomonas, serratia marcesens

▓ Salmonella in sickle cell anaemia, and pseudomonas in those whose sole stepped on a nail

▓ Septic bursitis – can have pain in full flexion due to tissue stretching, give drain and 2 weeks of antibiotics

7.2   Osteomyelitis

7.2.1   Chronic Osteomyelitis: Principles (Fig. 7.1)

▓ 'The bacteria is nothing, the environment is everything' – Louis Pasteur

▓ Important principles after Cierny: clean wound – live wound – stable wound – (Wound Revitalization)

7.2.2   Cierny/Mader Classification

▓ Anatomic aspects:
   – Types 1= medullary, 2=superficial, 3=localised, 4=diffuse

▓ Physiological aspects:
   – Host – normal healthy
   – Host – immune compromise
     Local factors → scar, arterial insufficiency, venous stasis, lymphoedema
     Systemic factors → DM, steroids, RA, age smoke, renal failure, liver failure, crystal arthropathy, acquired immunodeficiency (AIDS) patients

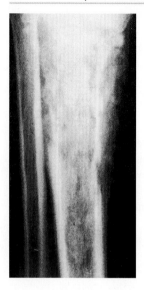

Fig. 7.1. A tibia with chronic osteomyelitis changes

7.2.3   General Portals of Entry
- Blood-borne: mostly in children and IV addicts
- Extension from surrounding infected area
- Direct inoculation: as in open fracture and after surgery

7.2.4   Explanation of the Cierny-Mader Classification
- Medullary: haematogenous osteomyelitis
- Superficial: e.g. ulcer with exposed bone
- Localised: e.g. cortex and medullary canal involvement
- Diffuse: e.g. cortical involved with extension to the medullary canal. 'All un-united fracture and total joint infections with osteomyelitis are included here'

7.2.5   Debridement Technique
- Atraumatic
- Skin incision and prior scar
- Expansile
- 'Pants-over-vest' incision
- Extra-periosteal dissection

- Reaming for intramedullary (IM) infection
- Oval cortical window and trough
- High-speed cutting tools
- Limit devitalisation
- Segmental resection
- Pulsatile lavage
- Antibiotics depot and dead space management
- Staged reconstruction protocol

7.2.6   Type-Specific Strategies

7.2.6.1 Type 1: Medullary

- Dx by use of X-ray and/or MRI, debride canal, hardware removal (but reaming during exchange nailing in the setting of infection in the presence of IM nail may also be useful)
  6 weeks of antibiotics post-operatively

7.2.6.2 Type 2: Superficial

- X-ray and/or MRI to check for any deeper canal involvement
- Debride surface with high-speed burr → until punctate, Harvesian bleeding from debrided surface ('paprika sign')
- Soft tissue cover needed (free flap/local)
- 2 weeks of antibiotics post-operatively at least
- If really superficial, usually one operation needed

7.2.6.3 Type 3: Localised

- X-ray and CT of help
- CT: assess remaining bone and potential portals to assess medullary canal
- Debride canal
- May need high-speed burr for troughs, sometimes polymethyl methacrylate (PMMA) beads
- Several weeks (at least 2) of antibiotics after operation
- Soft tissue cover
- After soft tissue cover, return for bead removal, and definitive osseous reconstruction (6 weeks post-operative antibiotics after the 2nd stage)

7.2.6.4   Type 4: Diffuse
■ These are infected non-unions or chronic septic joints
■ X-ray and CT/MRI all frequently used
■ Resection of the infected region frequently involved
■ Stabilisation needed [e.g. IM fixation/external fixation (EF)]
■ Soft tissue cover mostly required
■ 6 weeks of antibiotics post-operatively

7.3   Managing Septic Non-Union

7.3.1   General Principles
■ Adequate and thorough debridement to viable and healthy bone. Sometimes also need to be adequately debrided – remove non-viable muscles, debris
■ Repeated debridement frequently necessary
■ Soft tissue cover brought in early (preferably in less than 1 week if bed not contaminated, and flap needed). Notice that: (1) muscle flaps preferable as they help fight infection, are better cover for tibia and are good base for later split-thickness skin graft (SSG); (2) emergency soft tissue cover is sometimes needed, e.g. if joint is exposed, bare tendon, etc.
■ Eliminate dead space and IV antibiotics
■ Skeletal stabilisation always, EF is useful if large wound in nursing and raise flaps
■ Later Rn of bone defects – vascular BG considered if bone defect more than 6 cm and bed not contaminated. Alternative is the Ilizarov procedure

7.3.2   Pearls
■ Soft tissue healing very important or infection persists
■ Pasteur: the bug is nothing, the environment is everything
■ Especially in trauma open fracture wound, frequently polymicrobial

7.3.3   Classification of Tibia (and Fibula) Bone Defect [May]
■ Both T/F intact, less than 3 months rehabilitation expected
■ BG needed; 3–6 months rehabilitation expected
■ Tibial defect <6 cm, fibula OK; 6–12 months rehabilitation expected

- Tibial defect >6 cm, fibula OK; 12–18 months rehabilitation expected
- Tibial defect >6 cm, fibula not intact; more than 18 months rehabilitation needed

7.3.3.1 Cierny-Mader Classes
(Here Referring to Osteomyelitis of Tibia)

- Medullary, e.g. IM nail, removal of nail and reaming
- Superficial, e.g. in presence of plate and screws – contagious focus
- Local, e.g. local full thickness dead bone, can be removed but reassess stability
- Diffuse, e.g. needs inter-calary resection and unstable situation
- Host: A – normal, BL – local compromise, BS – systemic compromised, BSL – unfavourable both local and systemic factors → if operate, may make host worse

7.3.3.2 Systemic Factors

- DM, nutrition, RF, Hypoxia, Immune, crystal arthropathy, extremes of age

7.3.3.3 Local Factors

- Lymph drainage affected, venous stasis, vascular insufficiency, arteritis, effect of radiotherapy, fibrosis, smoking, neuropathy

7.3.4   Diagnosis

- Clinical features: pain, swelling, drainage
- Cultures: blood and bone. More often positive in acute cases
- X-ray: may see non-union, sometimes sclerosis, sometimes sequestrum, periosteal reaction
- Scan: e.g. Gallium binds to transferrin; Tc scan detects the increased blood flow
- CT: see sequestra, and areas of increased bone density
- MRI: assess the longitudinal extent of the lesion, and soft tissue status

7.3.5   Treatment

- Surgical (adequate debridement, dead space and soft tissue management, fracture stability restoration. Amputation as last resort)
- Antibiotics

- Nutrition
- Smoking should cease

7.3.6   Vascularised Bone Graft Results
- Only 70% unite if aetiology is infection
- Rises to 90% union for other aetiologies
- In recent years there has been more success with better wound Rn and local antibiotic beads; early flaps coverage
- Vascularised bone graft mostly for bone defects more than 6 cm, and satisfactory non-contaminated soft tissues
- Three usual steps – debridement, soft tissue management and obliterate dead space, and bone stability → EF, BG after healing of soft tissues
- Sometimes see vascularised bone graft hypertrophy, – bone scan hot, but sometimes complicated by fatigue fracture
- Muscle flaps – decrease dead space, bed for SSG, soft tissue cover, fight sepsis and increase chance of wound viability. Examples: local flaps like gastrocnemius flap; free flap like gracilis, latissimus dorsi, rectus flap, etc.

7.3.7   Summary of Key Concepts
- Multiple adequate debridement to healthy bone and assess whether limb is salvagable
- Maintain stability
- Find and eradicate the microbe – intravenous antibiotics and sometimes beads to fill dead space
- Soft tissue – get cover early, e.g. compound fracture tibia
- Late reconstruction, e.g. bone defect, etc.

7.4   Spinal Infections

7.4.1   Pyogenic Spinal Infections (Fig. 7.2)
- Pyogenic – acute (and/or subacute, chronic subtypes); mostly (50% in adults, 90% in children) from staphylococcus; sometimes delayed Dx. Location at paradiscal and disc (since lacks vascularity); in addicts, tends to occur more in younger individuals and in males. Rn is IV antibiotics after CT-guided biopsy and/or operation (if especially de-

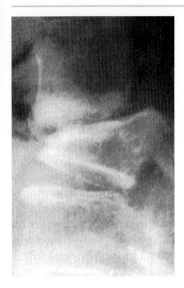

Fig. 7.2. An addict with a partially treated recent pyogenic spondylitis

layed with neural compression, too much destruction and instability, epidural abscess forming) and treat the cause (DM, steroids)
- Lumbar most common, cervical in IV mainliners injecting their upper limbs; adults nowadays more gram-negative sepsis – such as pseudomonas, E. coli, and/or anaerobes
- Previous claim of spread from Batson's plexus was doubted since very high pressure was needed for retrograde flow. Now, most believe it starts in paradiscal at endplate. As the cartilaginous end plates of child matures, blind-loops of vascular anastomosis remain – low-flow conduits provide a footing for septic emboli and bacterial seeding
- Minimum 4 weeks of IV antibiotics; for those treated conservatively, need brace, add chin extension in upper thoracic infection and cervical ones may need halo device. (Brace for 3 months). Overall 75% success rate with modern Rn

7.4.2 Non-Pyogenic Granulomatous Infections
- Tuberculosis [TB; 10% involves skeleton, and 5% the spine (Fig. 7.3); other peripheral joints are also affected (Fig. 7.4)]

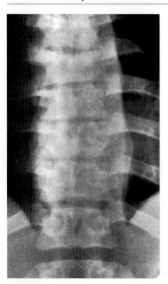

Fig. 7.3. Paravertebral shadow in a patient with tuberculosis of the spine

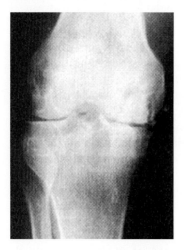

Fig. 7.4. Tuberculosis of the right knee joint

- More insidious course – abscess more common; only one-third with chest TB; one-third with positive histology taken intra-operatively and one-third culture positive
  - Useful adjuncts in Dx: CT-guided biopsy, polymerase chain reaction (PCR)- more and more used since culture not always positive
- Three subtypes: peridiscal, anterior, central
  - Peridiscal most common – even here, disc involved late (unlike pyogenic) and spreads to adjacent vertebrae via the anterior longitudinal ligament (ALL). Central types located in body cause collapse and deformity, DDx of neoplasm. Anterior type with scalloping of a few adjacent vertebrae (spreads in children rapidly, since it strips the periosteum)
- Unlike pyogenic, which is the most common in lumbar spine, TB is most common in thoracic spine, although lumbar is a close second (cervical is uncommon but spread is dangerous, and cervical pyogenic sepsis is not rare in mainliners that inject upper limb)
- Cause of neurology: chronic cases more from bony deformity/arachnoiditis; acute from pus, oedema, abnormal tissue, etc.
- Hong-Kong (HK) operation in addition to giving drugs is shown to prevent deformity and, hence, results in less of a chance of delayed Pott's paraparesis

7.4.2.1 Physical Signs of TB Spine
- Lumbar/fullness in femoral triangle
- Sacral TB/spreads sometimes to peri-rectal area
- Thoraco-lumbar cases may form psoas abscess
- Most common thoracic disease may see a paravertebral soft tissue shadow on X-ray (thoracic-level narrower spinal canal and prone to neurological deficit) and TB at T-spine level sometimes shows adhesions to the diaphragm
- Cervical is less common but can present as torticollis, spread to prevertebral area and to mediastinum to cause tracheal compression and is potentially dangerous
- Other signs: sinuses, scars of old lymph-node biopsy or thoracic surgery; see rib removal and BG on T-spine and/or lumbar X-ray; Pott's paraplegia
- Neural involvement varies a lot among series: 10–70%, being less in lumbar disease with obvious reason

- One-third of cases have associated extra-skeletal sites
- DDx of destructive lesion of sacrum present with palpable mass on *per rectal* examination: chordoma, chondrosarcoma
  (Posterior element involvement by TB rare; addicts occasionally have a more rapid clinical course)

7.4.2.2 Indications for Surgery
- Spinal instability
- Prevent deformity
- Progressive neurology
- Sometimes unable to get Dx using closed technique
- Failed medical Rn
  (Goal is to eradicate infection, relieve pain, prevent deformity and prevent recurrence and decompression)

7.4.2.3 Choice of Graft in Anterior Approach
- Rib graft if fusing not many levels, and in thoracic-spine
- Tricortical iliac crest graft
- Fibula – if need to span more segments – slower union since less cancellous, but stronger than above
- Allograft – not popular since risk of disease and infection
- Instrumentation: cages not usually recommended; occasionally add on posterior instrumentation to protect the anterior graft

7.4.3   Other Non-Pyogenic Granulomatous Infections
- Includes: other mycobacteria; fungi, aspergillus
- Many are immunocompromised and/or malnourished (assess by albumen/lymphocyte counts/transferrin, etc.)
- In every case of pyogenic/non-pyogenic infections, send some tissue for histology

7.4.3.1 Other Main Category: Epidural Abscess
Epidural abscess (Fig. 7.5) is dangerous since it can spread up and down, and is toxic to the patient. It is more common from pyogenic infections that were not properly treated or for which Rn was delayed. In general, it occurs in areas with more epidural fat: i.e. rare in cervical spine (except addicts)

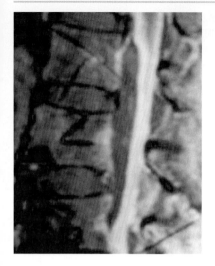

Fig. 7.5. Epidural abscess seen in this sagittal magnetic resonance image. Epidural abscess is toxic to the patient

- In cervical spine most occur anteriorly; while tend to locate posteriorly in the T-spine and L-spine
- Signs of myelopathy/radiculopathy should arouse suspicion in a patient with vertebral osteomyelitis. Danger: can communicate with retro-peritoneal space, mediastinum, and retro-peritoneum via the intervertebral foramen
- Natural course through five stages: LBP, raiculopathy, weakness, paralysis, toxaemia/death
- Meningitis is included in the differential Dx

7.4.3.2 Other Category: Subdural Abscess
- Very rare
- Only about 50 cases reported in the literature
- Less tender to percussion clinically
- Neurology due more to ischaemia and compression
- More in DM and pregnant individuals (liquefaction necrosis, less inflammation)

7.4.3.3 Other Category: IM Abscess
- Said to occur sometimes even in otherwise healthy subjects
- Rare

7.4.3.4 Other Category: Post-Operative Infections

- 1% after simple lumbar discetomy
- Increase to 4–5% chance in more complex fusion and surgery that involves instrumentation
- Contrast MRI sometimes helpful in assessment
- Many adopt quite an aggressive approach
- Superficial wounds may be left to granulate
- Deep sepsis:
  - When to remove implants will be discussed
  - How to deal with the BG
  - Local debridement (by layer) and haemostasis
  - Dead space eradication
  - Adequate duration of IV antibiotics if osteomyelitis
  - Use of flaps by plastic surgeons sometimes in bringing in vascularity, cover deep wounds and get rid of dead space

7.4.3.4.1 When to Remove Implants in Post-Operative Sepsis

- Failed instrumentation
- Fusion solid
- Refractory sepsis
- Left in place if early, especially if deemed essential for stability
  How about the grafts packed in?
- Many allow them to remain in place (especially if adherent)
- Other experts recommend removal of loose grafts and washing and replace

7.4.4   Appendix

7.4.4.1   Pitfalls in Dx

- Only one-quarter of pyogenic sepsis cases are blood culture positive
- First X-ray changes detected as late as 2–4 weeks, e.g. loss of disc height, blurred end plates sometimes soft tissue shadow
- In TB, look in X-ray for loss in psoas shadow – indicates retroperitoneal abscess, also look for retropharyngeal oedema, and widened mediastunum

7.4.4.2 Differential Diagnosis of TB from Pyogenic Spondylitis

- Patient nature, e.g. mainliner more pyogenic
- Pyogenic more often acute course, very painful even in the pain-tolerant mainliner
- More systemic upsets and ill, fever in pyogenic
- TB more insidious course, may be night sweats, ESR/WBC may be normal, TB chest associated in one-third of cases only

7.4.4.3 Radiological DDx

- Features favouring TB: body destruction, psoas abscess, usually some sclerotic areas due to chronicity
- Features favouring pyogenic: paradiscal, no sclerotic areas, paravertebra soft tissue possible, but no psoas abscess
- Not uncommonly, differential diagnosis impossible even with help of X-ray and/or MRI

7.4.4.4 Role of Nuclear Scan in Pyogenic

- Low sensitivity of indium scan for picking up Dx of pyogenic spine infections makes the use of gallium scan useful here – and it is in turn better than Tc, since previous changes occur earlier and resolution is reflected by follow-up scans earlier (gallium's specificity is 85% versus 75% with Tc scan)
- But why scan at all if we have MRI? – useful in cases where we suspect or want to rule out multifocal lesions (5% of cases)

7.4.4.5 Biopsy

- Some authorities go for CT-guided biopsy first, although some surgeons go in for operation and biopsy at the same time
- Advisable to hold our hands with antibiotics/anti-TB drugs before biopsy done (unless in dire circumstances)

7.4.4.6 Role of MRI

- In pyogenic: lower T1 due to replacement of the marrow fat
- High T2 image due to oedema
- Disc: spared until late in TB, involved mostly in pyogenics
- Abscess common in TB, soft tissue rather than abscess being the feature in earlier pyogenic infections– late cases can have epidural pus
- Gadolinium may help DDx infection from post-operative changes

7.4.4.7 Radiological DDx from Non-Infected Causes

▪ DDx from tumour: tumours rarely involve the disc, have different signals and less marked oedema in tissue planes

▪ DDx degeneration: here the disc has low signal, due to water loss

7.4.4.8 Summary of MRI Assessment

▪ Look for adjacent vertebrae being affected

▪ Disc space

▪ Impingement and involvement of the cord

▪ Paravertebral soft tissue and psoas abscess
(Level of fusion frequently has to be decided intra-operatively by appearance and experience, not from MRI findings alone)

7.4.4.9 General Pearls

▪ DDx more difficult in partially treated cases before referral

▪ Avoid the mention of the use of cages in examinations (although some experienced surgeons may resort to the use of cages in TB that required several levels excision and fusion, and BG found on table not to be stable enough; this is the exception rather than the rule. Cages should be avoided in pyogenic infections)

▪ MRC study commented: (a) all will fuse sooner or later, but those with Hong Kong operation show less deformity (and possibly are less likely of subsequent neurological deficit) and (b) one-third of cases have negative histology and one-third negative cultures

▪ In the ill patient, avoid anterior approach and try posterolateral drainage of pus (e.g. costo-transversectomy in the case of TB thoracic spine)

7.4.5   Highlight of Salient Points on TB Spine

7.4.5.1 Introduction

▪ The findings of the MRC trial are important

▪ Most commonly affected level – TL junction, especially L1

▪ 3% of TB cases have musculoskeletal involvement; half of these affect the spine

▪ All ages are affected (case report of congenital one from umbilical vein and foetal intake of amniotic fluid)

▪ Risk factors for TB in general – immunocompromised patient, e.g. AIDS, steroid, poor nutrition, drug addicts

7.4.5.2 Pathogenesis

- Delayed hypersensitivity (bone destruction by caseous necrosis)
- Selective involvement of the anterior vertebral column and collapse causes varying degrees of kyphosis
- Early or late paraparesis is another dreaded complication

7.4.5.3 Features in the Affected Child

- Stripping of ALL can cause rapid spread
- Abscesses tend to be larger and amount of bone destruction greater, but neural complications are comparatively lower than in adults
- Anterior growth apophysis can be destroyed causing affected anterior growth – since posterior elements are seldom affected in the usual case
- Retropharyngeal upper mediastinal paraspinal abscess can cause upper airway obstruction – classic inspiratory stridor (Millar asthma)

7.4.5.4 General Clinical Features

- Back pain
- Gibbus (or step)
- Abscess
- Paraparesis
- Constitutional upset
- Look for neurological deficit (in both early and late disease)

7.4.5.5 Causes of Death

- Systemic disease
- Cerviocomedullary disease from abscesses or instability can cause quadriplegia and even sudden death
- Stridor and respiratory obstruction in the child – from retropharyngeal and upper mediastinal paraspinal masses

7.4.5.6 Special Situations

- Cervical-dorsal region: asthma-like syndrome when the child lies down at night, from huge soft tissue mass around the bronchus
- Cervical spine: little role of conservative care since paraplegia is common [prefer anterior spinal fusion (ASF) and debridement]
- T-spine in child: 'aneurysmal syndrome' – abscess lifts up the loose periosteum; local effects may mimic an aortic aneurysm

7.4.5.7 Atypical Presentation

- Posterior elements (spine) – disease of the neural arch, picture is like spinal cord compression rather like cauda equina; not always easy to diagnose by means of simple X-ray
- Sacoiliac joint – pain from buttock to knee and/or abscess. Investigation: CT/MRI – determine site of abscess and plan accordingly
- Epidural abscess – pachymeningitis, arachnoiditis; can be lower limb spastic paresis or picture-like spinal cord tumour. Dx – MRI (if not available, cerebrospinal fluid myelogram: shows streaking of contrast)
- Lumbar spine: some authorities prefer conservative; but, if vertebral, destruction can cause early loss of lordosis or even reverse lordosis, with LBP in a 20-year long-term study
- Lumbosacral junction disease – tend to operate in these cases since kyphosis is likely
- Mutli-level disease is uncommon and has sometimes been mistaken for metastases in the past

7.4.5.8 Pathogenesis of Paraplegia

- Early onset – due to pus, disc, subluxation, sequestrum, pachymeningitis (presence of myelitis indicates poorer prognosis)
- Late onset – kyphus, bone bridge, proximal spinal stenosis
- Interestingly, the deterioration in neurology was more related to canal compromise than amount of kyphosis
  [Note that in many (60%) late cases of paraparesis, there is evidence of disease reactivation]

7.4.5.9 X-ray Appearances

- Frequently involves two adjacent vertebrae and their adjoining disc
- Anterior part of vertebra may be scalloped
- Fusiform paravertebral abscess shadow can be present, sometimes loss of psoas shadow

7.4.5.10 CT Scan

- Can see the details of bony destruction and soft tissue calcifications
- (Bone scan is less useful since, although it is sensitive, it is not specific)

7.4.5.11 Role of MRI
■ Helps in Dx of early disease
■ Helps to pick up multicentric lesions before plain X-ray changes get obvious
■ Can show TB arachnoiditis and extradural or intradural spread of the abscess if present
■ Mostly T1 hypodense, T2 hyperintense (gadolinium enhancing)
■ Rim enhancement with contrast is common since sequestrum in centre remains hypointense – but not specific for TB and can be mimicked by pyogenic infection and neoplasm

7.4.5.12 Role of Biopsy
■ Neither clinical nor radiological imaging criteria are absolutely pathognomonic – hence biopsy is usually needed to confirm the Dx

7.4.5.13 Pearls in Definitive Dx
■ CT-guided, fine-needle biopsy or video-assisted, thoracoscopic surgery – less invasive way to get a biopsy or drain an abscess. High cytology yield of 88% reported
■ Although the bacterial count is lower than lung lesions (and bacilli are not seen in 50% of histological lesions), the histological features of epitheloid granuloma, Langerhan's multinucleated giant cells and caseation are sufficient in Dx

7.4.5.14 Adjuncts in Dx
■ PCR [and enzyme-linked immunosorbent assay (ELISA)] – amplifies mycobacterial DNA. May be useful in difficult cases
■ MRI – ring enhancement with contrast, lost cortical margin (show the compression of neural structures well in, for example, late kyphus, etc.)

7.4.5.15 Main Goals of Rn
■ Eradicate infection
■ Preserve and restore neural integrity
■ Prevent and correct deformity

7.4.5.16 Anti-TB Drugs
- Some are bactericidal – kill active bacteria, e.g. rifampicin
- Some are sterilising – kill intermediate and slow bacteria, e.g. rifampicin and pyrazinamide
- Most anti-TB drugs are bacteriostatic
- Combination therapy helps to suppress the development of drug resistance

7.4.5.17 'Short Course Chemotherapy'
- Involves 2 months of rifampicin/INAH/pyrazinamide daily; then 4 months of rifampicin/INAH

7.4.5.18 Operative Indications
- For Dx
- For intractable pain
- For tackling neurological compression
- For preventing or correcting deformity
- For prevention or tackling penetration to other organs

7.4.5.19 Rationale of the HK Operation
- Dramatic prompt improvement in general condition
- Removes disease focus (sequestra, disc, caseous, and non-viable bone) and necrotic tissues
- Anterior strut graft for support and graft is in compression
- Less kyphosis
- Prevents paraparesis (and Rn-established paraparesis)
  Helps prevent the rapid spread of disease in children

7.4.5.20 MRC Trial (HK Operation Versus Debridement; Korea – CT and POP)
- Favourable status definition
  - Full physical activity
  - Clinical and radiological quiet
  - No sinus/abscess
  - No neurology (myelopathy)
  - No modification of allocated regimen

7.4.5.20.1 Radiological Fusion

- At 1 year, 70% Hong Kong operation versus 23% in debridement group (versus chemotherapy only 6%)
- At 10 years, less of a difference – 97% versus 90% (even chemotherapy-only group 73%, but this will imply that one-quarter of patients in this group were still not fused)

7.4.5.20.2 Angle of Kyphosis and Amount of Vertebral Loss

- HK operation results in less kyphosis (17-year prospective study in TB spine in child – only one kyphus, versus 60% in debridement cases)
- In MRC trial, mean increase in kyphosis 12°, many had 50° (5%)
- Less vertebral loss in those who had HK operation, versus some 30–40% with more than one vertebra loss in debridement and CT (chemotherapy) group

7.4.5.20.3 Effect of Duration of Paraplegia Before Decompression on Recovery

- Less than 9 months duration: complete recovery common
- More than 9 months duration: two-thirds with partial recovery (Hodgson 1960)

7.4.5.20.4 Effect of Growth After ASF in Child

- Study in Spine (1993) – patient of average age 7.6 years, no progression at 6 months
- Study in Spine (1997) – patient of average age 5 years, deformity can increase up to 10 years
- Conclusion – beware of using ASF in very young children, especially if multiple segments are involved; also in T-spine (some cases need A+P surgery; Spine 1997)

7.4.5.21 Difficult Scenarios

- Reactivation in old age with extensive destructive disease
- Lumbosacral disease
- Severe angular kyphosis in healed/latent disease – with associated cardio-pulmonary compromise

Principles – decompress, stabilise, and correct deformity. Approach depends on the region affected, e.g. anterior/costovertebrectomy/post-inter-body

7.4.5.22 Comments on Kyphosis Correction

▨ In multilevel disease, where three or more levels are involved: deformity can reach 100°; to achieve any significant correction of such severe and rigid deformity without neurological loss, the procedure has to be done gradually

7.4.5.23 Some Recent Trends

▨ With the advent of spinal instrumentation in the past decade, supplementing fusions with anterior or posterior instrumentation has been tried by some to improve and maintain deformity correction. [According to workers such as Oga, biofilm may be less likely to form with tuberculous infection even in the presence of an implanted device]

7.4.5.24 Some Important Bring-Home Messages

▨ TB spine can only be said to have definitely healed up when solid fusion has been obtained

▨ This important point was not stressed enough in the MRC report

▨ Another point not explored enough in MRC trial: with a very prolonged follow-up (much greater than 10 years) in 60 patients treated in Hong Kong University with conservative Rn, nearly half with late paraparesis and neural loss from progressive kyphus and cord compression, and atrophy and scarring responded poorly despite decompression and BG, and there was no good solution

▨ The conclusion of MRC that radical surgery "did not improve the chances of a favourable outcome apart from less late deformity" should be taken with a grain of salt. (Also, the lack of solid fusion can cause continued deterioration and neural loss)

▨ Chemotherapy is the most effective Rn, but radical operation causes earlier fusion, and less delayed deformity

▨ For multiple vertebral involvement cases, A+P surgery is advised, as well as ASF+posterior spinal fusion (PSF) since ASF alone in these cases work less well for the very young child (<7 years)

▨ After the work of Oga, some had advocated the use of pedicle posterior instrumentation in the earlier stages of thoracic/thoracic-lumbar disease

7.4.5.25 Conclusion

■ ASF is a demanding technique, but results in less back pain, less kyphosis, more rapid fusion, and possibly less likely to have late paraparesis in TB spine

■ Conservative: near ALL with an element of kyphosis is more likely to result in back pain; and fusion is slow even if it eventually occurs. Chemotherapy is the only Rn in countries with very limited resources

7.5   Infection in Presence of an Implanted Device: General Guidelines

(With infection after scoliosis surgery as an example)

7.5.1   Incidence

■ One study concerning infection after TSRH – 6%
■ Hong Kong study on infection after TSRH, 2% at 2 years
■ Incidence much lower for short-segment fusions – 0.2% (due to possibly shorter operation time)

7.5.2   Mechanism

■ Intraoperative seeding – many a times low virulence microbes
■ Blood spread
■ Fretting – micromotion among the components of the implant
  – Predisposing factors – DM, steroids, obesity, chronic sepsis Hx, smoker, prolonged hospitalisation, longer operation time, high blood loss
  (Definition of 'high' blood loss and 'long hours' >1 500 cc and >3 h)

7.5.3   Pathology

■ Glycocalyx: membrane surrounding the microbes
■ Some say these are mainly soft tissue and not bony infections
■ Contributory factor sometimes from dead space (though Harrington rod with fewer dead space)
■ Titanium with perhaps some inhibition on these low virulence organisms
■ Can be associated with implant loosening and spine not fused

7.5.4   Clinical Features

- Back pain
- Fluctuating mass
- Draining sinus

7.5.5   Managing Late Infection After Scoliosis Surgery

- Removal of implant (especially if fused)
- Debridement – include glycocalyx
- Primary wound close

7.5.6   Use of Prophylactic Antibiotics

- Most use 2–3 doses for prevention
- Johns Hopkin's experience – an extra dose if long operation (>4 h) or if more blood loss (>2000 cc)

7.5.7   Use of Antibiotics in Definitive Rn

- For 6 weeks, or until normal ESR
- Can sometimes change to oral after initial intravenous therapy

7.5.8   Common Clinical Scenarios

- Infected open fracture with metallic implant remaining in-situ
- Infected total joint implants (will be discussed). Refer to the works of Gristina
- Spine cases – infection after scoliosis surgery has just been discussed, but note the special case of TB (see papers by Oga)

7.5.9   Conclusions from Studies from Case Western (Animal Model)

- Established infected non-union is of course difficult; in this study, bacteria was injected into an animal (hamster) partial osteotomy model:
  - Highest infection rate in inadequately fixed fractures that are mal-aligned
  - Poor fixation is worse than no metal – FB affects host defence and fracture motion causes more tissue damage
  - Presence of metal did not necessarily increase the infection rate; rigid fixation (not loose implant and proper fixed fracture) can further reduce the infection rate

- Chance of infection depends also on the adherence and glycocalyx formation
- Cases of mixed growth: gram-positive bacteria can increase the infection rate with gram-negative organism; but presence of gram-negative organism seems to produce less effect

7.6   Infected Total Joint Replacements

(Key: prevention is better than cure)

7.6.1   Methods of Prevention

■ Methods:
- Vigorous Rn of early post-operative superficial and deep infections
- IV prophylactic antibiotics most important
- Others: include lamina air flow, closed body exhaust suits, careful tissue handling and perhaps antibiotic-cement for high risk patients. Minimise traffic in operating theatre

7.6.2   Formation of Bacterial Biofilm

■ Race to the surface – both the body's fibroblast and the bacteria try to get a foothold to the implanted device
■ Some bacteria are prone to produce glycocalyx which protects the frequently semi-dormant bacterial colonies from the body's defence cells and from antibiotics with formation of the bacterial biofilm. A typical example of bacteria-forming biofilms is staphylococcus epidermidis
■ The reader is highly recommended to read the works of Gristina

7.6.3   The Culprit Bacteria

■ Staphylococcus aureus (include MRSA)/epidermidis (65–70%)
■ Gram-negatives (e.g. biofilm-forming pseudomonas)
■ Anaerobes
■ Polymicrobial – especially in cases with Hx of wound discharges
■ Others (high chance of limb loss if gas gangrene, though uncommon)
(Note: it is not correct to say MRSA is 'more virulent' than ordinary staphylococcus aureus; it is more bacterial resistant)

7.6.4   Diagnosis

■ Dx is based on a combination of clinical, radiological and pathological studies in most cases

■ Dx is not straight forward in many cases since the biofilm shields the bacteria from identification of body's defence cells, including WBCs (hence even bone/white cell scans can be negative). Also, common to find the bacteria in a semi-dormant state with much reduced doubling times; thus gram-stain and culture of joint fluids are frequently negative

7.6.5   Clinical Pointers to Dx

■ Pain most common: DDx needed

■ Others: local warmth, swelling, loss of initial motion – but more in cases of acute sepsis

■ Signs: discharging sinus, wound erythema, effusion (sometimes present)

7.6.6   Investigations

■ X-ray: occasionally may find even periosteal reaction and subchondral bone resorption

■ Aspiration (sometimes need repeated aspiration), gram-stain of these aspirates pick up rate low, but can send for WBC count and biochemistry. More recently – PCR studies (very sensitive, sometimes even false positives)

■ Multiple passes in hip aspiration result in more chance of contaminants; may need fluoroscopy

■ Bone scan – Tc alone is not sensitive enough; indium white cell scan has higher sensitivity (increase from 35% to 85%), and newer ones include marrow scans, and even monoclonal antibody scans

■ Intraoperative frozen sections will be discussed shortly – helpful if find more than five polymorphs per high power field according to Mirra

■ Resort to synovial biopsy only if all prior investigations are inconclusive

7.6.7   Intra-Operative Dx

- Intra-operative frozen section: favoured by many current studies (5/HPF very suggestive but DDx is rheumatoid and osteolysis. If use 10/HPF as criteria, 95% accurate according to some studies)
- Intraoperative cultures – some experts advise that, if in doubt, wait for culture, debride and treat as for infected case with two-stage reconstruction
- Intraoperative cultures and frozen sections should be taken from all suspicious areas and not only from the membranes (e.g. of patella, tibial, femoral components in the case of TKR)

7.6.8   Classification – Gustilo et al

- Early post-operative infection – infected after less than 4 weeks; debride, retain components but exchange the polyethylene liner
- Late chronic infection – infected more than 4 weeks post-operatively, removal of implant, most use two-stage reconstruction
- Acute haematogenous infection – seeding of previously functioning prosthesis; either debridement and salvage (versus) removal
- Positive intra-operative culture: two or more positive intra-operative cultures, use appropriate antibiotics

7.6.9   Surgical Decision Making: Patient and Disease Factors

- Patient factors– high-risk groups and very high-risk groups
  - High risk: DM, psoriasis, steroids, immunocompromised
  - Very high risk: recent past soft-tissue infections, previous osteomyelitis highest risk

7.6.10   Disease Factor

- Bacteria that are virulent (e.g. staphylococcus, pseudomonas) difficult to eradicate
- Bacteria that form glycocalyx are more difficult to eradicate (they have won the race over the host cells 'for the surface'), e.g. staphylococcus epidermidis
- If infected by gram-negative bacteria, frequently lower success rate of re-implantation
- Sometimes atypical bacteria in the immunocompromised is not sensitive to prophylactic antibiotics, e.g. fungi
- Host bed important – less success if scarred

7.6.11 Literature on Retention of Prosthesis: Facts and Myths

▨ Debridement, retain prosthesis and liner exchange only in very strict selected cases since failure rate is reported to be 25–75%

▨ Criteria: recent studies found that the above may not work if there is intervention at more than 2 weeks post-operatively (although some researchers mention that retention may be tried if infection is diagnosed within 4–6 weeks post-operatively). Hence, early Dx and Rn is important. Less likely to succeed with virulent bacteria/gram-negative bacteria/polybacterial

▨ In the occasional elderly with many co-morbidities, a lesser procedure may just be done, with chronic antibiotic suppression – but this is usually not the "norm"

7.6.12 Importance of Adequacy of Debridement and Early Rn

▨ Early frequently means less than 2 weeks (although many say less than 4 weeks) – old definition of 3 months is obsolete

▨ Thorough synovectomy is very important

▨ There is currently an opinion that there is no role of arthroscopic debridement in Rn of an infected total joint (though some have tried this method)

7.6.13 Prosthesis Removal: 1 Stage Versus 2 Stages

▨ Less tendency nowadays to do one-stage re-implantation (but sometimes done in some centres in Europe) – and only in very, very selected cases with low virulence organism, good health of patient, no glycocalyx, etc.

7.6.14 What is the Gold Standard Nowadays?

▨ Most cases: removal of prosthesis, 6 weeks IV antibiotics (minimum) and two-stage re-implantation and usually interim cement spacer (antibiotic-loaded)/PROSTALAC (refer to publications by Clive Duncan's group)

▨ This classic two-stage reconstruction as initially suggested by Insall is highly recommended in most cases

7.6.15   Duration of IV Antibiotics and Minimum Inhibitory Concentration

- 6 weeks minimum (as also originally suggested by Insall)
- Some paper in the past, claimed that patient needs to prolong stay in hospital and maintain minimum inhibitory concentration at therapeutic level – not always done in every centre since high cost of prolonged hospital stay

7.6.16   Use of Antibiotic-Impregnated Cement

- Shown to have positive effect in success to eradicate infection
- Rate of elution differs with different antibiotics
- Do not use antibiotics that are readily inactivated by the exothermic reaction during cement setting
- Pelicose said to be better than simplex in re-implant since gets doughy earlier

7.6.17   Use of Cement Spacer and PROSTALAC

- Refer to Vancouver's experience and papers from Clive Duncan's group
- Spacers: the original concept comes from the instability after resection arthroplasty – functions include:
  - Provides local concentration of antibiotics
  - Maintains length and range of motion
  - Frequently also allows ambulation in these elderly subjects
    [PROSTALAC = the prosthesis of antibiotic-loaded acrylic cement]

7.6.18   Pearls During Re-Implantation Process: Cemented Versus Cementless

- Both cemented and cementless revisions have their proponents The 'best' choice lies in individual assessment of each particular case
- Antibiotic-loaded cement is usually used in revisions
- Type of antibiotics depends on sensitivity; if no organism identified, a few even use more than one antibiotic
- Be prepared to tackle bone defects
- Use of stemmed prosthesis sometimes needed in TKR. In THR, sometimes need long stem for the same token; possible use of allograft (essentially a piece of dead bone) with caution needed

7.6.19 Salvaging Failed Re-Implantation

■ Option 1: fusion – for those who have high chance of ambulation
  - Mostly successful in pain relief
  - But caution or even contraindication (C/I) if adjacent joints are stiff or if there is significant arthrosis
  - External fixator is cumbersome, although this may be a choice if surgeon wants one-go surgery with the debridement; IM device with highest union rate

7.6.20 A Word on Arthrodesis

■ Often mentioned, but not too often done in practice
■ Not easy to perform well in revision especially with bone loss. Notice it is important to regain leg length
■ Why is it important to regain leg length? If 2 cm short, it takes much more (3–4×) energy expenditure for the body to walk with the 'short limb gait'

7.6.21 Option 2: Resection Arthroplasty

■ Works by letting the body fill up the space with fibrous tissue – to retain a little stability
■ Indication as above – the non-ambulators, especially if the nearby joints are also problematic

7.6.22 Option 3: Amputation

■ Last resort
■ For:
  - Uncontrolled sepsis (e.g. gas gangrene)
  - Uncontrolled pain
■ Overall, needed in 3–5% of all infected joint replacements

7.6.23 Prognosis
(Even Given the Standard Two-Stage Reconstruction)

■ Poor if:
  - Delayed Dx
  - Immunocompromised host or with special risk factors
  - Host bed poor and scarred
  - Surgical debridement not prompt and inadequate
  - Virulent organism, gram-negatives, etc.

General Bibliography

Gristina A, Esterhai J, Poss R (eds) (1992) Musculoskeletal infection, 1992 edn. American Academy of Orthopaedic Surgeons, Rosemont, Ill., USA

Selected Bibliography of Journal Articles

1. Leong JC (1993) Tuberculosis of the spine. J Bone Joint Surg Br 75:173–175
2. Jung NY, Jee WH et al. (2004) Discrimination of tuberculous spondylitis from pyogenic spondylitis on MRI. Am J Roentgenol 182:1405–1410
3. Griffith JF, Kumta SM et al. (2002) Imaging of musculoskeletal tuberculosis: a new look at an old disease. CORR 398:32–39

Musculoskeletal Tumour Principles

Contents

8.1   Tumour Staging

8.1.1   Staging of Musculoskeletal Tumours (Enneking)

▨ Based on:
  – Histological grading
  – Site
  – Any metastases
    Prognosis depends on stage
    Staging helps plan treatment

8.1.2   Details of Enneking Staging

▨ Low grade (G1) intra-compartment (T1), no meastases (M0)
▨ Low grade (G1) extra-compartmental (T2), no metastases (M0)
▨ High grade (G2) intra-compartmental (T1), no metastases (M0)
▨ High grade (G2) extra-compartmental (T2), no metastases (M0)
▨ G1 or G2; T1 or T2; with metastases (M1)

8.1.3   More on Histological Grading

▨ G0 = benign histology (well differentiated and low cell to matrix ratio)
▨ G1 = low-grade malignant (few mitoses, local spread, moderate differentiation, low risk of metastases)
▨ G2 = high-grade malignant (mitoses frequent, poor differentiation, high risk of metastases)

8.1.4   More on the Anatomical Site of Tumour

▨ T0 = intracapsular
▨ T1 = intracompartmental (e.g. confined to the involved bone or involved joint capsule)
▨ T2 = extracompartmental (spread beyond the boundaries of the compartment from which the tumour arises)

8.2   Work-Up of a Patient with Suspected Musculoskeletal Tumour

■ History and physical:
- If suspicion of metastases to bone from a distant primary, check thyroid, breast, prostate, kidney and lung; do a rectal examination and check for signs of metastases elsewhere
- If suspicion of primary malignant growth from bone, note the age of the patient [some tumours occur in those of particular age groups, e.g. giant cell tumour (GCT) mostly occurs after closure of epiphysis] and the site of the tumour [e.g. different tumours have predilection for different sites, for instance: (i) in the case of long bones, Ewing's tumour often occurs in diaphysis, and osteosarcomas mostly at metaphysis; while (ii) in the case of the spine, osteoblastomas are commonly found in the posterior elements]

8.2.1   Blood-Work
■ Blood-work: blood picture (suspected haemic malignancy), erythrocyte sedimentation rate (ESR; usually elevated, very high in myeloma), liver function test (can be deranged if metastases), alkaline phosphatase (if bony origin, can be due to bony destruction/increased bone turnover), Ca/PO_4 (some tumours/metastases can have hypercalcaemia), tumour markers [e.g. prostate-specific antigen (PSA) if suspect metastases from prostate] and serum protein electrophoresis (monoclonal band in myeloma)

8.2.2   Other Investigations
■ Magnetic resonance imaging (MRI): can detect skip lesions, extent of bony malignancy, any involvement of other compartments and/or neurovascular structures; helps to plan biopsy tract and definitive resection
■ Computed tomography (CT): helps assess the extent of bony destruction by the tumour in areas such as the flat bones of the pelvis or acetabulum, and the spine, etc, to help plan reconstructive surgery (if still feasible), e.g. 3D CT reconstruction in planned total hip replacement for metastases involvement of the acetabulum, etc. CT also helps in the staging of some tumours, e.g. CT thorax

■ Others: X-ray and biopsy will be discussed separately; bone scan is useful to detect other lesions in the skeleton, and ultrasound is sometimes used in screening for metastases in solid organs such as the liver. Positron emission tomography (PET) scan is sometimes used to help search for an occult primary

8.2.3   Radiological Investigations

■ Way to describe the radiology of bone tumours:
  – Location (e.g. diaphyseal, meta-diaphyseal, metaphyseal, epi-meta-physeal, epiphyseal)
  – Zone of transition – fast-growing malignancies with ill-defined zone of transition
  – What the tumour does to the bony skeleton (e.g. bony destruction can be geographic, moth-eaten, permeative, etc) and sometimes there are characteristic radiological features of the matrix (e.g. ground glass appearance used to describe fibrous dysplasia, calcification common in chondroid lesions)
  – How the body's bony skeleton reacts to the tumour (e.g. intense sclerosis around an osteoid ostoma)
  – Other features of individual tumours (e.g. onion skin periosteal reaction in Ewing's sarcoma, etc.)

8.2.4   Interventional Radiology

■ Angiogram: use of angiography is useful before tumour resection of very vascular tumours (be it bony tumours or soft-tissue sarcomas), pre-operative embolisation sometimes very helpful to increase chance of resectability of the tumour

8.3   Principles of Tumour Biopsy

■ Need to know the probable stage and diagnosis before performing biopsy since many regard it as the last step in staging of the patient
■ Biopsy incision should be longitudinal – never transverse – and biopsy tract should be excised during definitive resection
■ Should preferably be done by the same surgeon who will later perform the tumour resection

▓ Do not cross compartments or dissect around neurovascular bundles to lessen seedling. If biopsy has to make bone window, oval shape is preferred to prevent stress riser and subsequent fracture
▓ Meticulous haemostasis
▓ Send samples for cultures
▓ Drains should go out through the wound

8.3.1   Common Types of Biopsy

▓ Frozen section – advantage in determining adequacy; check margins; send for culture in case of an infective cause and sometimes immediate diagnosis (always culture the tumour and biopsy the infection); sometimes immediate diagnosis is possible
▓ Closed aspiration and/or trucut – Advantages: cheap, no delay and few risks. Disadvantages: inadequate sample, improper placement, solid tumour difficult to aspirate, need experienced pathologist and aspiration does not allow for immunohistochemical analysis unlike trucut biopsy
▓ Open biopsy – Advantages: more material and absolute haemostasis. Disadvantages: risk of spread; delay in initiation of adjuvant therapy; sepsis; cost and/or longer operative time

8.3.2   Axiom Concerning Tumours in General

▓ Always culture the tumour and biopsy the infection
▓ Always take tissue for culturing bacteria, acid-fast bacilli, and fungus whenever an incisional biopsy is performed

8.4   Types of Surgical Margins

▓ Intra-lesional: through the tumour; hence, not therapeutic
▓ Marginal: high recurrence up to 50%; dissection is through the pseudo-capsule of tumour or the reactive zone
▓ Wide margins: lower recurrence around 10%; dissect further away leaving a cuff of normal tissue
▓ Radical margins: removal of the entire compartment
▓ Amputation: needs to be regarded as a form of reconstruction, used especially when limb salvage is not possible or deemed contraindicated

8.5   Indication of Limb Salvage

■ The saved limb must be functional, e.g. not insensate, etc.
■ Local control of the lesion must at least be equal to amputation, and satisfactory margin must be attainable with the type of tumour in question
■ Relative contraindications (decision has to be considered on individual basis): presence of pathological fracture, occasionally skeletal immaturity

8.5.1   Common Methods of Limb Salvage
■ Endoprosthesis
■ Allograft-prosthesis composite
■ Vascularised bone graft and/or allograft
■ Joint reconstruction and arthrodesis sometimes used if growths near major joints

8.6   Principle Behind 'Neoadjuvant' Chemotherapy

■ Advantages:
  – Early and immediate action of the agents on the tumour
  – Efficiency of tumour kill by the agent(s) can be assessed during resection and reduces tumour bulk and vascularity (90% kill rate to be labelled effective)
  – Effects can persist from 2 months to 2 years
  – Longer disease-free survival
■ Disadvantages:
  – In children, premature physis closure and stunted growth
  – Delays the timing of definitive surgery
  – Others: hair loss and other side effects of individual agents, etc. (P.S. usually adjuvant chemotherapy starts once the wound has healed)

8.7   Use of Radiotherapy

▪ Uses: (a) palliation for metastases and (b) pre-operative debulking of the tumour; Possibly results in less chance of seeding during operation
▪ Mechanism of action:
  – Formation of highly active intracellular free radicals that can stop cell division by causing damage to DNA
  – Energy absorbed by complex molecules causing disruption of chemical bonds
  – Diminish vascular supply to tumours by sometimes destroying tumour vessels
  – Normal tissues believed in general to have more reparative power than tumour cells
    (Note: not all tumours are radiosensitive; the fast growing and less differentiated ones are usually more responsive)

8.7.1   Adverse Reactions of Radiotherapy
▪ Creates new malignancy
▪ Inflammatory changes to irradiated bystander organs, e.g. cystitis, hepatitis
▪ Pigmentation, subcutaneous fibrosis, hair loss, muscle atrophy, lymphoedema

8.8   Benign and Malignant Soft-Tissue Tumours

8.8.1   General Hints for Possible 'Malignancy'
▪ Old age (>50 years)
▪ Deep seated (deep to the deep fascia)
▪ Large size (>5 cm)
▪ Behaviour – rapid growth, pain includes night pain, involvement of nearby structures, ulcer, lymph-node enlargement

8.8.2   An Idea of General Incidence
▪ Occurs in lung more than colon more than breast more than soft tissue more than bone (the above are incidences of new cases by site)

- Site of soft-tissue sarcomas: much more common in upper and lower extremities, than in areas like the chest wall, and rare in the retroperitoneum
- Although not very common, the incidence is higher in children, e.g. rhabdomyosarcoma

8.8.3   Possible Aetiology
- Radiotherapy (RT): sometimes implicated (but RT as a form of treatment of sarcoma is regarded as 'low' risk). Definition of RT-induced growth: (1) within the field of radiation; (2) with latency of more than 2 years and (3) sarcoma confirmed by histology
- Biological: viruses, e.g. Kaposi sarcoma
- Predisposing pre-existing lesion, e.g. chronic lymphoedema → lymphangiosarcoma
- Genetic factors, e.g. *NF 1* gene in neurofibromatosis (NF) – these patients have a ten times greater chance of developing malignant nerve-sheath tumours

8.8.4   General Comments
- Soft-tissue tumours usually come from primitive cells, e.g. smooth muscle differentiation can occur in an area normally devoid of smooth muscle
- Other examples: 'fibrous, fibrohistiocytic, adipose, smooth muscle, striated muscle, vascular, synovial, neural differentiation', etc.

8.8.5   Histological Analysis and Diagnosis
- Histology
- Points to remember about immune histochemistry: stain for actin/desmin if muscle origin is suspected; stain for S100 if nerve origin is suspected; stain for keratin/vimentin if epithelial origin is suspected
  - Sometimes use special marker, e.g. MIC-2/Ewing
- Electron microscope is less used; unless, for example, in search for Z-band in rhabdomyoblast and in some cases of round cell tumours
- Chromosome studies, e.g. 11–22 translocation occurs in 95% of cases of Ewing's (although many/all tumours with chromsomal aberrations, but consistent change in some growths helpful) – other example as in infantile fibrosarcoma/alveolar rhabdomyosarcoma

- Molecular genetics (and cytogenetics): make use not of chromosome, but the product they produce – abnormal protein formed by the gene; e.g. N-myc oncogene amplification in neuroblastoma (in cytogenetics, need fresh, non-necrotic tissue, minimal non-neoplastic elements, sterility and no bacteria)
- 'Flow cytometry and digital image analysis' are not of much use here

8.8.6   Formulating a Treatment Plan
- Know the:
  - Location(s) – sometimes skip lesions – deeper growths more likely to be aggressive
  - Size – larger usually more aggressive
  - Histological type – important for prognosis
  - Histological grade – important in prognosis
  - Depth
  - Status of the resection margin

8.8.7   Any Role of Excision Biopsy
- Never for extra-compartmental growths
- Excision biopsy not recommended in general unless pretty sure it is benign
- Some experts say that the main reason for this is that half of these deep-seated growths have viable satellites

8.8.8   Biopsy in Suspected Soft-Tissue Sarcomas
- Ultrasound-assisted biopsy of more superficial soft-tissue tumours is useful (can better select the right place to put the needle)
- For the more deeper seated growths with any chance of it being malignant, the current standard of care is to do incisional biopsy first; for example, one can plan better and sometimes needs adjuvant therapy before the definitive resection

8.8.9   Mayo Clinic's Histology Assessment
- The Mayo group uses 'cellularity, cellular atypia, and mitosis activity' mainly, and/or pleomorphism and necrosis (for this feature, get away from the surface, old scars and ulcers)
- Most people just say 'low' or 'high' grades

- Mayo four grades:
  - Grade 1: Low cellularity/atypia, no necrosis, <5–10 HPF
  - Grade 2: Moderate cellularity/some atypia, no necrosis, <5–10 HPF
  - Grade 3: More cells, mitosis <10 HPF
  - Grade 4: Mitosis >10 HPF, (or pressure necrosis)

8.8.10 Correlation of Histological Grading and Behaviour

- Group 1: correlation good; examples adult fibrosarcoma, leiomyosarcoma, malignant peripheral nerve sheath tumour (MPNST), certain (myxoid) malignant fibrous histiocytoma (MFH)
- Group 2: correlation poor – one typical example is that once we see Ewing – always 'grade 4' histology
  Other examples: infantile fibrosarcoma, Ewing, 'synovial sarcoma', some MFH (e.g. angiomatoid types), etc.

8.8.11 Points from the History and Examination

- History: pain (duration, nature), trauma heterotopic ossification (HO)
- Physical examination: size, depth, consistency, mobility, local neurovascular involvement, joint motion, lymph node, transillumination and/or other organs
- More likely malignant if >5 cm fixed and deep

8.8.12 Role of X-ray

- Soft-tissue shadow
- Bony erosion/pressure effects
- Calcification as in:
  - Haemangioma, synovial (osteo)chondromatosis, tumoral calcinosis, myositis ossificans, and HO

8.8.13 Role of CT

- Useful when there is: cortical destruction, identification of calcification or ossification
- Second main use in detecting pulmonary metastases: resolution down to a few millimetres

8.8.14 Important Role of MRI

- General advantages: multiplanar, more resolution and no radiation
- Can define the presence, site, extent; sometimes differentiate benign/malignant; help staging; and in some cases even characterise the nature of the growth
- Post-treatment evaluation

8.8.15 MRI Clue to Benignity

- Margin: more circumscribed in benign growths
- Signal pattern: more homogeneous if benign
- Size <5 cm
- Not cross compartment
- No adjacent structures affected (neurovascular structures/bone/joint)

8.8.16 Benign Cases Sometimes with Malignant Features on Histology

- Desmoid: heterogeneous and infiltrating
- Myositis ossificans – if in acute/subacute stage → irregular margin and reactive oedema
- Abscess, even organising haematoma
- Haemangioma
  Many of these cases need clinical correlation and consideration of the patient's age, site and history

8.8.17 Finer Points About MRI

- Signal: majority are low T1 high T2
  - Bright T1 in: fat (lipoma, some liposarcoma) or blood (some haemangioma, tumour with haemorrhage, haematoma)
  - Low T2: fibrous (scar, desmoid – but these may enhance with contrast), metal/foreign body, air, haemosiderin – shortening effect/pigmented villonodular synovitis (PVNS), haematoma, giant cell tumour of tendon sheath (GCTTS)
  - Low T1 + T2: e.g. PVNS/GCTTS

8.8.18 MRI Examples of Cases that Really Can Make a Definitive Dx on MRI Alone

- Group 1: haematoma/PVNS/GCTTS
- Group 2: haemangioma (presence of fat; shape if dilated/tortuous, heterogeneous and irregular, sometimes calcify – phlebolith)

- Group 3: desmoid (fibrous tissue, infiltrative, fascia plane, low T1 and T2; but enhance with gadolinium)
- Group 4: nerve tumour (only diagnose with certainty if the 'target' pattern is seen, i.e. low signal centre, high signal peripheral); the 'target'-like MRI pattern arises due to the fact that, in the centre part of the lesion, there is less collagen, but in the periphery of the lesion more myxoid elements. These tumours tend to be located along the course of the peripheral nerve, are well circumscribed and have a high signal on T2 of MRI
- Group 5: lipoma/liposarcoma (isointense with fat in all sequence; thin septation, liposarcoma can be heterogeneous as only some part may have fat signal) – liposarcoma is 'not' derived from fat; sometimes with thick septae/nodular areas. More confident in making MRI Dx of myxoid liposarcoma – it is more common, especially in popliteal fossa, the myxoid component resembling fluid
- Group 6: cyst (sharp margin, low T1, with gadolinium not enhancing except for the rim)

8.8.19 Features of Some Common Malignant Soft-Tissue Sarcoma

8.8.19.1 Malignant Fibrous Histiocytoma
- More in elderly, most in upper limb/lower limb
- DDx: carcinoma, lymphoma, possible melanoma
- Previously thought it might be derived from histiocytes – in fact fibroblastic differentiation
- Gross: lobulated, area of necrosis and haemorrhage
- Histology: high-grade pleomorphic, cartwheel pattern, much mitosis and/or giant cells
- Prognosis: size and depth (some myxoid variants as well)

8.8.19.2 Liposarcoma
- 50% of cases belong to 'myxoid' liposarcoma
- More in adult, deep seated, mostly upper and lower limb (especially thigh)
- Gross: lobulated, sometimes cystic component
- Histology: signet-ringed fat cells in vascular/myxoid stroma, and or round cells
- Other types refer to pathology texts

8.8.19.3 Malignant Nerve Sheath Tumour

- Two main types: sporadic and associated with NF
- P53 mutation in both types
- NF cases: 2–4% life time risk; latency of 10–20 years however
- Gross: haemorrhage and necrosis
- Histology: high grade
- Only 50% are S100 +; needs the use of ultra-structural analysis and history of tumour in a nerve distribution + NF patient to help Dx
- Histology: sometimes nuclear palisade, perivascular growth of cells, etc.
- Subgroup from those with NF; younger, more males
- DDx: synovial sarcoma, leiomyosarcoma, fibrosarcoma, etc.

8.8.19.4 'Synovial' Sarcoma

- 20- to 30-year age group, 10% of all soft-tissue sarcomas
- Most in upper and lower extremities (especially knee) – close proximity to joints/hence the misnomer
- Not inside joint
- Calcification frequent
- Gross: solid, lobulated; nearby nests common
- Needs wide excision

  Four types: anaplastic, monophasic fibrous, monophasic epithelial, biphasic, i.e. spindle cell and glands – sometimes in fact look like endometrium. Look for keratin staining; stroma can be hyaline or osteoid like
  DDx: fibrosar, MPNST, malignant haemangiopericytoma
  Survival: 5 year 30–60%; 10 year 10–20%
  Prognosis is worse with older age, large sized and anaplastic sarcomas and more mitosis

8.9   Discussion on Individual Bone Tumours

8.9.1   Bone-Producing Tumours

8.9.1.1   Osteoid Osteoma

- Painful lesions mostly in children and adolescents usually. Pain is worse at night (relief with aspirin) and/or painful scoliosis if at spine
- Can be found in any bone formed by endochondral ossification; more common in tibia and femur and/or spine

- Natural history is towards healing over years, but operation usually performed for pain
- X-ray: shows lytic nidus with nearby sclerosis, may need CT and/or tomogram to see nidus (diameter < 1 cm)
- Traditional treatment by excision of nidus and intact rim of reactive tissue. Newer innovation is by percutaneous radiofrequency probes reported recently with promising result

8.9.1.2 Osteoblastoma (Figs. 8.1, 8.2)

- Essentially a large-sized osteoid osteoma-like lesion – with also osteolytic area though surrounded by less intense sclerosis
- Pain is less than with osteoid osteoma and has less of a response to aspirin. More common in the posterior elements in the spine (50%). Overall, less common than osteoid osteoma. Patients are mostly less than 30 years old
- Treatment: en bloc resection if possible, since intralesional excision with chance of recurrence. Malignant change possible but rare

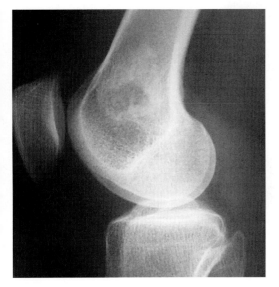

Fig. 8.1. Osteoblastoma located at the distal femoral condyle

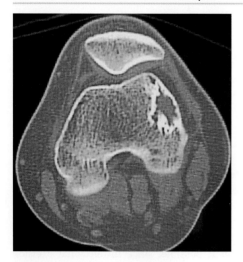

Fig. 8.2. Computed tomography scan of the distal femur of the patient in Fig. 8.1

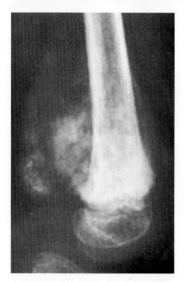

Fig. 8.3. Osteosarcoma of the distal femur with formation of osteoid tissue

8.9.1.3 Osteosarcoma (Fig. 8.3)

▪ Primary malignancy from bone with histological findings of osteoid seams formation in the stroma

▪ Rare: 1 in 200,000. Most patients are affected in the 1st and 2nd decades. Osteosarcoma is mostly located around the knee (metaphysis of distal femur and proximal tibia, i.e. fast growing area of the bone). Most in fact have micro-metastases at presentation, hence the principle of treatment is to combine surgery (limb salvage versus amputation) with chemotherapy. Limb salvage is only possible if nerves can be preserved, adequate muscle/soft tissue left intact, there are reasonably wide margins, and either preserve or reconstruct vessels

8.9.1.3.1 Types of Osteosarcoma

▪ Conventional osteosarcoma

▪ Some resemble osteoblast – osteoblastic osteosarcoma

▪ Some (2%) resemble fibrous dysplasia; very radiodense and little osteolysis (usually) – well-differentiated intraosseous osteosarcoma (regarded as the parosteal equivalent, though here it is inside the medulla)

▪ Some are purely lytic – telangiectatic osteosarcoma

▪ Parosteal – well differentiated on the surface, mostly at the posterior aspect of the distal femur

▪ Periosteal

▪ Those secondary to other pre-existing lesions, e.g. Paget's disease, etc.

8.9.1.3.2 Clinical Features

▪ Most present with pain and/or mass; pathological fracture is rather rare

▪ X-ray: one-third is lytic, one-third is osteoblastic, one-third is combined. Periosteal reaction with sunray spicules is quite common (Codman's triangle); look for bony cortical erosion with extension outside compartment. Screen for the common pulmonary metastases

▪ RT mainly for palliation and for disease at inaccessible sites

▪ Use of chemotherapy treatment is important since osteosarcoma is now regarded as a systemic disease

8.9.1.3.3 Prognosis

▪ The more proximal the worse the prognosis

▪ The larger the size of tumour the worse prognosis

- With old age the prognosis is worse
- Telangiectatic and secondary type have a worse prognosis; the classic type and parosteal variety fare better
- With a low percentage of tumour kill by neoadjuvant chemotherapy, prognosis is worse
- Prognosis is worse with multiple macroscopic metastases at presentation
- Recent papers found that pathological fracture may not adversely affect prognosis

8.9.1.3.4 Features of Telangiectactic Osteosarcoma

- Many view it as high-grade intramedullary osteosarcoma that had undergone total, or near total aneurismal bone cyst (ABC) change
- Represent 4% of all osteosarcomas, completely lytic on X-ray; and occur at any age, although mostly in their twenties. Many Paget's osteosarcoma changes are of this type
- Pain, rapid swelling, high destruction (mostly also in distal femur and proximal tibia)

8.9.1.3.5 About 'Low-Grade' Osteosarcoma

- Realisation that a subgroup of low-grade growths is important since these may respond poorly or not at all to chemotherapy! However, having said that, these 'low-grade' ones like the parosteal variant, and the so-called fibrous-dysplasia like the osteosarcoma variant; we must assess and grade their stroma carefully, since if stroma is high grade, even the less malignant parosteal ones can de-differentiate

8.9.2   Cartilage-Producing Bone Tumours

8.9.2.1   Osteochondroma (Exostosis)

- Can affect any bone formed from endochondral ossification
- Constitutes half of all benign bone tumours, direction is away from the growth plate, moving towards diaphysis with growth
- Can be single or multiple (multiple exostoses or diaphyseal aclasis), most present before 2nd decade
- Can be sessile/pedunculated; excise if symptomatic or interfere with joint function. Excision preferably after skeletal maturity since less recurrence
- X-ray: medullary cavity of stalk continuous with the parent bone

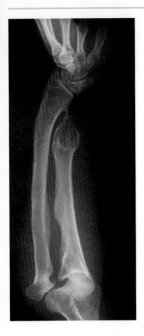

Fig. 8.4. Multiple exostoses affecting the forearm causing bowing

8.9.2.2 Multiple Exostoses (Figs. 8.4, 8.5)
▪ Autosomal dominant
▪ Most present with bowing of forearm or lower limb, due to differential growth between radius/ulna and tibia/fibula
▪ May cause leg length discrepancy, and deformities may need osteotomy, exostosis excision and Ilizarov correction
▪ 20% overall malignancy risk
  (DDx of Trevor's disease from simple exostosis)
▪ Trevor's disease differs from the usual exostoses – osteochondroma on Epiphyseal side of the growth plate

8.9.2.3 Enchondroma (Fig. 8.6)
▪ Most are located in the medullary cavity, although a periosteal subtype arises at the periosteum
▪ Most common site is at the small bones of the hands and feet; long bones are occasionally affected; persons affected are in their 1st to 5th decades

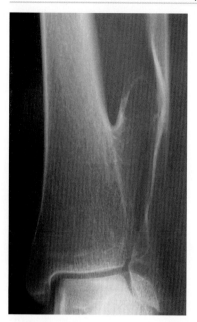

Fig. 8.5. Multiple exostoses affecting the ankle causing bony deformity

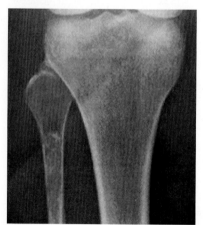

Fig. 8.6. Enchondroma of the proximal fibula

▨ Sometimes multiple associated with haemangiomata (Mafucci disease) or asymmetrical involvement of many long bones of the body with possible deformity and leg length discrepancy (Ollier's disease)

▨ 75% Cases solitary, can be incidental finding or present as pathological fractures

▨ X-ray: endosteal scalloping commonly seen, affected bone may be expanded, and there may be areas of calcification

▨ Treatment:
  – For less active cases, may try curettage and grafting, but there is 50% recurrence, which has to be weighed against the morbidity of wide excision
  – Periosteal form needs excision with an adequate margin

▨ Prognosis:
  – Mafucci is associated with nearly 100% malignant change
  – Ollier's disease associated with 50% chance of malignant change. Osteotomy and/or lengthening by Ilizarov may be required for deformity and/or leg length discrepancy

8.9.2.4 Chondroblastoma

▨ Most common in the skeletally immature, arising from chondroblast. Most important feature is its epiphyseal location, although occasionally may expand into the metaphysis

▨ Location in the body commonly at proximal part of the femur, humerus or the tibia

▨ X-ray: eccentric lucent area at the epiphysis in an immature skeleton is the hallmark. Little reactive changes of the nearby bone, small areas of calcification may occur

▨ Treatment:
  – Mostly treated by curettage and grafting with 20% recurrence and/or cryotherapy
  – Beware not to break into the joint during curettage lest spillage of chondroblasts into the joint

8.9.2.5 Chondromyxoid Fibroma (Fig. 8.7)

▨ Typically eccentric metaphyseal lesions of the long bones especially lower limb. Contains variable amounts of myxoid, chondroid and fibroid elements

▨ Most present as chronic pain or incidental finding

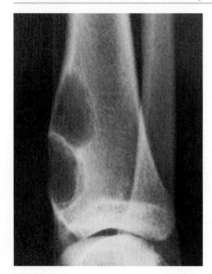

Fig. 8.7. Patient with chondromyxoid fibroma of the distal tibia

- X-ray: the eccentric lesion usually thins the overlying cortex; margins are well defined and may have a sclerotic rim
- Mostly occurs in youths 10–20 years old at the metaphysis of long bones, but rarely in flat bones of older subjects
- Natural history: locally invasive, not metastatic
- Histology: plump/stellate cells, dense nuclei, long cytoplasmic process, and/or areas that look like chondroblastoma, aneurysmal bone cysts
  - Small and no cortex destruction – may try curettage and BG (care not to spill some into the soft tissues or nodules form)
  - Others – en-bloc excision
- Most surgeons will wait until skeletal maturity before operation
- Prognosis:
  - Good prognosis if excised, to guide against malignant change

8.9.2.5.1 Chondrosarcoma (Fig. 8.8)
- Can be de-novo or secondary to pre-existing benign cartilaginous tumour
- Majority middle to old age, most commonly at pelvis, femur, ribs
- Present usually as a mass or pain. Search for any lung metastases

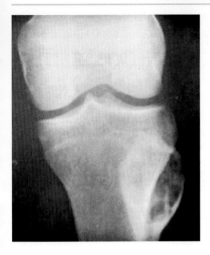

Fig. 8.8. Chondrosarcoma around the knee in this elderly woman

▪ X-ray: typically lucent lesion with central calcification and cortical destruction and expansion. Can be intramedullary as in malignant change after Ollier's; or surface as in malignant change from a previous exostosis

▪ Treatment:
  – Essentially a surgical disease requiring wide marginal excision since RT and chemotherapy are usually resistant. RT may be useful in tumours at inaccessible sites

▪ Prognosis:
  – Only 20% of high-grade tumours survive 5 years
  – 70–80% of low-grade tumours survive 5 years

▪ Variants:
  – Mesenchymal: rare, age usually younger, cells more poorly differentiated, metastases to lung
  – Clear cell: affects ends of long bones and histology may look like renal clear cell tumour. Some thought this entity might be an aggressive variant of chondroblastoma

8.9.2.5.2 What Constitutes a 'De-Differentiated' Chondrosarcoma

▪ This entity refers to a high-grade sarcoma complicating a pre-existing enchondroma or low-grade chondrosarcoma

- The exact cell lines that these derive from is unclear. Some authorities, instead of labelling it as de-differentiation, even say it is a misnomer since, for example, enchondroma cells do not replicate and the sarcoma probably arises from a reparative process (resembles the case of bone-infarct-related sarcomas)
- X-ray: both lytic and radiodense areas are usually present (though it can be wholly lytic if late); a previous X-ray for comparison is useful
- Histology: sarcoma (various types) and nearby usually either enchondroma or low-grade chondrosarcoma
- Treatment: one may find it difficult to understand why this entity responds to CT and/or RT while other chondrosarcomas do not
- From the afore-said discussion, it is obvious – the sarcoma component in these de-differentiated chondrosarcomas have many possibilities; some are MFH like, etc.
- Hence, usually quoted treatment includes either amputation versus limb salvage or combined chemotherapy and surgery

8.9.3   Fibrous-Forming Bone Tumours

8.9.3.1   Fibrous Cortical Defect

- Common before skeletal maturity; more in males than in females
- Most are incidental findings
- X-ray: with lucency at the metaphyseal cortex, eccentric in location, and well-defined margin or zone of transition. With growth, appear to move towards diaphysis
- Natural history is towards spontaneously healing, which is sometimes triggered by pathological fracture
- Treatment: intracapsular curettage and bone grafting usually suffice

8.9.3.2   Fibrous Dysplasia (Figs. 8.9, 8.10)

- Usually regarded as harmatomatous fibrous and osseous tissue replacing the medullary area of long bones. The bony element is woven bone
- Lower limb more affected and bending/deformity of weight-bearing bones like the femur is not uncommon (Shepherd's crook deformity)
- Most are monostotic, and most occur/present before skeletal maturity; more in males than in females. X-ray: lucent lesion with ground glass matrix admixed with areas of sclerosis; cortex may be expanded

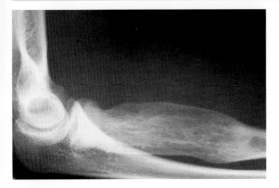

Fig. 8.9. Fibrous dysplasia affecting the proximal radius

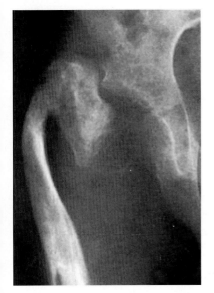

Fig. 8.10. Fibrous dysplasia with shepherd's crook deformity

- The polyostotic form (McCune-Albright Syndrome with Café-au-lait pigmentation with margins like the Coast of Maine can present with precocious puberty and chance of malignant transformation of 4%; more in females than in males) can present with pathological fracture
- Treatment: monostotic and symptomatic sites of polyostotic may need curettage and grafting. Deformities if significant may require osteotomy and/or lengthening/shortening procedures

8.9.3.3 Malignant Fibrous Histiocytoma

▮ Most occur in middle age males

▮ Present with pain, swelling or pathological fractures

▮ Most are primary, but may be secondary to fibrous dysplasia, Paget's, post-RT, etc.

▮ Common site is around the knee, with X-ray changes of moth-eaten lytic lesion at the metaphysis sometimes with soft-tissue extension

▮ Treatment: most need amputation or radical margin excision; neoadjuvant therapy is sometimes used

8.9.3.4 Fibrosarcoma

▮ Most are very malignant with early spread

▮ X-ray: most are lytic with poorly defined margins, sometimes soft-tissue extension and/or periosteal reaction

▮ Most require radical excision and adjuvant chemotherapy, since mostly radio-resistant

8.9.4   Reticulo-Endothelial Bone Tumours

8.9.4.1 Eosinophilic Granuloma (Fig. 8.11)

▮ One type of a group of disorders of histiocytes, previously known as histiocytosis X, now better termed Langerhan's cell histiocytosis. Aetiology of this group of disorders is unknown; likely to be a reactive proliferation of usually well-differentiated histiocytes to an unknown stimulus (the Letterer-Siwe variant is different since with poorly differentiated cells). The typical "Langerhan giant cells" on histology have grooved nuclei and much pale stained cytoplasm

▮ Mostly seen in children, but the typical triad of exopthalmos, skull lesions and diabetes insipidus is not always present

▮ Variant with visceral involvement is mostly seen in those younger than 3 years of age with poor prognosis

▮ Affects any bone, but most common in the skull and lower limb long bones, such as the femur, and spine

▮ X-ray: can be lucent or heterogeneous (loculated like) radiodensity with no/minimal sclerotic rim. In the spine, can cause marked collapse (vertebra plana); lesion in the skull described as punch out. Less commonly, presents as general osteoporosis with no definite bone lesion

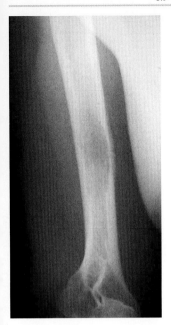

Fig. 8.11. Histiocytosis X affecting the humerus in this young boy

■ Most need curettage and grafting if only to ascertain Dx, although may heal spontaneously. Better prognosis if there is no extra-osseous involvement. Those with systemic organ involvement and Letterer-Siwe have poor prognosis. Systemic involvement may result in need for chemotherapy. RT is sometimes used for aggressive lesions and inaccessible disease

8.9.5 Ewing's Sarcoma (Fig. 8.12)
■ Cell origin is unknown
■ Pain and/or fever in young (5–30 years of age)
■ White blood cell count and ESR are usually elevated
■ Found more in lower limb than in pelvis/sacrum than in upper limb; sometimes even rib and scapula
■ Can also be extra-skeletal
■ X-ray: permeative (spread via Harvesian canals) with periosteal (onion skin) reaction, sometimes the soft-tissue component predominates

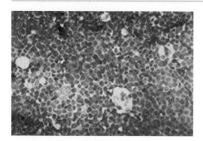

Fig. 8.12. Histology of Ewing's. Note the abundance of small round cells

- Chromosome 11/22 translocation (molecular studies)
- DDx: osteomyelitis and others – lymphoma, histiocytosis X, osteosarcoma, MFH, etc.
- Histological DDx: from PNET cells – by immunostain/neurosecretion granules
- Very young: add metastatic neuroblastoma in DDx
- Treatment: CT is traditional mainstay of treatment, but many add surgery, especially if can adequately excise the tumour if in expandable bones, careful with RT as adjuncts in children – growth changes, $2°$ malignancies, and 30% recurs
- Treatment trend: towards preoperative chemotherapy, followed by wide/radical surgical margin excision and limb salvage if possible. If radiosensitive, RT may be used as an adjunct in extensive disease
- Prognosis: worse if cells are not or are poorly sensitive to preoperative chemotherapy, pelvic lesions or metastatic disease already at presentation

8.9.6   Lymphoma of Bone
- Most occur in middle to old age and represent non-Hodgkin's lymphoma
- Occur mostly around the knee, presenting with a mass or pain
- X-ray: poorly defined lucent areas, although an occasional sclerotic area may occur; the true extent of the lesion may only be obvious on MRI. One cause of a wholly radiodense 'ivory' vertebra
- Treatment: wide local excision is recommended, but chemotherapy is needed if there is systemic involvement

8.9.7   Miscellaneous Bone Tumours

8.9.7.1   Haemangioma of Bone

- Most are found in the vertebra, although most are not symptomatic, and pain and pathological fractures are possible but not common. Other sites include the long bones, which may increase in length if very vascular
- Most lesions are made up of capillaries or carvernous spaces on histology
- X-ray of affected vertebra featured by coarse and vertical trabeculae due to destruction of the horizontal trabeculae. Skull lesions are lytic but resemble wheel spokes on CT
- Treatment: most vertebral lesions can be observed. Vertical striated vertebral lesions have to be differentiated from Paget's disease. Expanding vertebral lesions can consider embolisation followed by excision with or without RT. Lesions at long bones are best treated by excision and grafting

8.9.7.1.1 Vascular Tumour Classes

- Benign: haemangioma and variants (common in one of five autopsy findings of spine; do not all need treatment)
- Intermediate behaviour: haemangioendothelioma (can be multifocal, in axial or appendicular skeleton)
- Malignant: angiosarcoma of bone is very rare (<0.1% in large series); that of soft tissue is more common. There is only a 20% 5-year survival, despite adequate treatment

8.9.7.1.2 Angiosarcoma of Bone

- Very malignant, fortunately rare, bone lesions
- Two main clinical patterns:
  - Those with many lesions in one bone or two or more lesions in adjacent bones (angiosarcomata of bone is a rare scenario in which a malignant tumour of bone can affect bones on both sides of the joint. This is an exception rather than the rule). Better prognosis
  - Usually multiple or large single, very rapidly progressive and destructive lesions that spread also to the lungs and other bony areas. Poor prognosis
- Treatment: careful assessment of the true extent of the disease is important. Cases discovered early enough may be treated by radical ex-

cision or amputation. However, many cases are already widespread locally with metastases as many run a rapid clinical course

8.9.7.1.3 Aneurysmal Bone Cyst

▨ Mostly seen in the skeletally immature before 20 years of age

▨ Expansile lucent and cystic lesions can occur in long bones or especially in the posterior elements of the spine and flat bones such as the pelvis

▨ Can be primary, but in every case it is necessary to search for secondary causes, i.e. secondary to an underlying disorder that produces ABC changes, e.g. osteoblastoma, and the prognosis will obviously be different

▨ Investigations also include CT, in which typically fluid levels can be seen

8.9.7.1.4 General Features of ABC (Fig. 8.13)

▨ Introduction: ABC is the 'great masquerade' of bone lesions since it can in fact be associated with: GCT, giant cell reparative process, fibrous dysplasia, chondroblastoma, osteosarcoma, etc. The key is in the histology; search everywhere for a possible hidden primary lesion. To complicate issues, it has also been reported that traumatic subperiosteal haemorrhage and surgery itself can potentially produce aneurismal bone cyst

▨ ABC involves a destructive process that transforms a pre-existing bone lesion into an expanded collection of blood-filled spaces

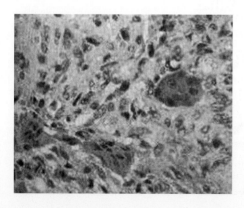

Fig. 8.13. Histology of aneurysmal bone cyst

■ 50% of ABCs have an associated underlying cause; treat the cause. Some had tried curettage and 50% recurred, then curettage was repeated

8.9.7.2 GCT of Bone (Fig. 8.14)

■ Most are seen in the skeletally mature skeleton, in which the expansile eccentric tumours are usually found near the epiphyseal region of the ends of long bones. Can also occur in flat bones such as the pelvis and the spine. The behaviour of these tumours can vary from benignity to aggressive behaviour with metastases to the lungs. Treatment needs to be individualised

■ Many conditions can give rise to giant-cell like pictures on histology and the gross specimen needs to be cut in many different areas if there is uncertainty (e.g. giant cell rich osteosarcoma, chondroblastoma and, in the hand, giant-cell reparative granuloma, etc.)

8.9.7.3 Multiple Myeloma

■ Featured by causing lytic-type destructive bone damage with little nearby sclerosis reaction, caused by malignant proliferation of plasma cells

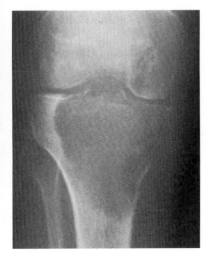

Fig. 8.14. Giant cell tumour shown here at the knee. Note its eccentricity

▨ Most common among primary bone tumours; usually occurs in middle to old age
▨ Affects both long and flat bones with red marrow
▨ Most present with diffuse bone pain, pathological fracture or symptoms of anaemia
▨ X-ray: irregular punch out lesions are common, especially in the skull; skeletal survey is recommended for assessment of the multiple lesions rather than bone scan as the latter can be either hot or cold
▨ Blood work: featured by markedly raised ESR; further investigations include Ig immunoelectrophoresis and urine for Bence Jonce proteins. Screen for hypercalcaemia. Bone marrow biopsy is useful in seeing the characteristic abnormal plasma cell proliferation
▨ Treatment:
  – Role of surgery: used in excision of solitary plasmacytoma, prophylactic nailing of long-bone lesions and selected cases with cord compression
  – Role of chemotherapy: may bring about remission or is used for palliation. Bisphosphonates can be used if hypercalcaemic
  – Role of RT: most is radiosensitive, can cause re-ossification of lytic defects; or can be for palliation
▨ Prognosis:
  Survival is usually lengthened by the use of chemotherapy to a median of around 2 years, with the cause of death usually from either haemorrhage or infection, since these patients are infection prone from the relative lack of immunoglobulins

8.9.7.4 Adamantinoma

▨ Rare bone tumour suspected to be epithelial in origin causing local destruction commonly at the tibial shaft in 90% cases
▨ Growth is rather slow as low-grade malignant; affects patients mostly in the 1st to 4th decades
▨ Most patients present with pain or swelling of subacute or chronic onset
▨ X-ray: lucent, eccentric, relatively well-defined lesion with thinned cortex; may appear lobulated at times. Soft-tissue extension possible in which case the true extent of the lesion can best be revealed by means of MRI

- Some authorities believe that the entity 'osteofibrous dysplasia' (which also occurs mostly in the tibia and in close association with adamantinoma) in fact can be the precursor lesion
- Treatment: wide margin excision is the rule as it is not commonly sensitive to RT or chemotherapy
- Most survive around 10+ years, depending on whether metastases have occurred (lymphatic or haematogenous)

8.9.7.5 Chordoma

- Rare tumour believed to have arisen from notochord remnants that failed to degenerate; hence most common either in the sacro-coccygeal area or at the cranio-cervical area of the axial skeleton
- The common scenario is either sacral pain or mass sometimes easier to feel on rectal examination, even sphincter disturbance. Those with less common skull-base tumours may have headache or local neurological deficits
- X-ray: featured by mid-line mass lesion typically at sacrum with destruction and soft-tissue shadow. The local bony anatomy after tumour destruction can be seen on CT, while MRI can be useful to assess the soft-tissue component and extent of neural structure involvement. Bone scan is less useful as it is often a cold scan
- Treatment: though wide local excision is desirable, it is seldom feasible in practice, and RT can be used as adjunct. Even in adequately resected cases, patients are often left with sexual and sphincter dysfunction. Prognosis is even poorer if there are already metastases to liver, lungs and other bony locations

8.9.8   Difficulties in Histological DDx of Bone Tumours

8.9.8.1 Conventional Osteosarcoma Versus Osteoblastoma

- Background: features of osteoblastoma
  - Many occur in spine – especially posterior element (in vertebral body alone? – not yet reported to our knowledge)
  - Rare (size varies)
  - An aggressive subtype with possible invasion of nearby bones reported
  - Isolated case reports with general toxicity or osteomalacic syndrome found in the literature

- DDx by site, behaviour and histology
  X-ray: less reliable unless it shows typical changes of conventional osteosarcoma (60%) and especially in long bones; but cannot rely on cortical integrity for DDx
- Histology: some osteoblastomas can produce lace-like osteoid patches; need DDx from osteosarcoma (especially if found in peripheral portion), since osteosarcoma can be permeative and maturing towards the periphery. Also (1) only in osteoblastoma can we see tumour cells line-up surrounding the osteoid seams; (2) there is more discrete demarcation between osteoblastoma tissue and nearby normal bone and (3) there is frequent mitosis and frank sarcomatous stroma in osteosarcoma

▨ DDx is important since even the aggressive osteoblastoma subtype is quite benign

▨ Treat conventional osteosarcoma along conventional lines (mostly neoadjuvant CT and limb salvage surgery if possible)

▨ Getting a good margin in spine is not easy for osteoblastoma; some have tried curettage, but 20% recurs (perhaps less with repeated attempts); otherwise radical excision is required, if technically feasible
  (Note: osteoblastoma turned into osteosarcoma has been reported but is very rare; aggressive osteoblastoma is sometimes associated with ABC and abundant 'epithelioid' osteoblasts)

8.9.8.2 DDx of Well-Differentiated Osteosarcoma and Fibrous dysplasia

▨ Sometimes this subtype can be radiodense with little lysis, and even the edges are more well defined than conventional osteosarcoma

▨ Fibrous dysplasia – can be mixed lytic/dense (depends on amount of dysplastic bone) with ground-glass appearance; sometimes even expanded cortex (cystic changes); sometimes one cortex is much expanded (protuberance)

▨ Histological DDx does not depend on infiltration behaviour, but on (1) fibrous dysplasia never having cell atypia and (2) no orderly osteoid seams – in fact it is said to be like 'Chinese characters'. NB. Beware, as both can have areas of cartilage

8.9.8.3 DDx of ABC Versus Telangiectactic Osteosarcoma

- X-ray: it is not possible to make a Dx of telangiectactic osteosarcoma on X-ray, but three in four have a periosteal reaction; while ABC continues to be a big masquerade in X-ray pattern from well defined to more permeative, most do not have a sclerotic rim
- Histology: in telangiectatic osteosarcoma, the specimen may sometimes lack osteoid but, if present, are lace-like (not seams of reactive bone as in ABC); abundant osteoclast-like giant cells are a feature (though quite common in ABC), cellular atypia and obviously malignant stroma

8.9.8.3.1 Enchondroma Versus Ollier Versus Low-grade Chondrosarcoma

- Enchondromas – always centrally located and stop growing after skeletal maturity (since many believe they are cartilage rests), with the exception of Ollier's which can continue to grow
- Since histological DDx of enchondroma and low-grade chondrosarcoma is typically difficult, it is important to show evidence in the latter that they continue to grow (especially if patient is skeletally mature) or permeate in between Harversian canals

8.9.8.3.2 Clinical/Radiological/Histological Evidence Needed to Diagnose "Low-Grade Chondrosarcoma"

- Clinical – there is still growth, especially if there is a soft-tissue mass (with enchondroma there is never a soft-tissue mass)
- X-ray – normal enchondroma (sites: more in hands/feet than in proximal humerus, proximal femur and tibia); as patient ages the central lucent patch starts to calcify to become radiodense rings and stipples. Becomes more dense when mature
- The mineralisation in chondrosarcoma is not a discrete continuous line. Also, enchondromas, though sometimes with mild endosteal erosion, never show cortical destruction or scalloping. In chondrosarcoma, cortical thickening can occur due to infiltration by tumour cells, involving the Harversian system
- Histological pointers of sarcoma: pleomorphism, high cellularity, separated not by bone by fibrous bands, and especially insinuating into the Harversian spaces

8.9.8.3.3 Osteochondroma Versus Peripheral Chondrosarcoma

- Standard teaching: if serial X-ray shows cartilage cap thickness of more than 2 cm, this suggests a malignant change. Normal cap thickness is 0.5–1.5 cm and, with old age, there is no perichondrium or cap
- Chance of malignant change is only 1% for peripheral exostosis, but 10% in multiple exostosis – need close follow-up
- Since pelvic exostosis results in a high chance of malignant change, some like to excise all prophylactically (sometimes also excise scapula ones) – the above policy not agreed by all, some surgeons like serial follow-up, and sometimes we are forced to adopt serial follow-ups if operation is refused by patient

8.9.8.3.4 Suggestion of Malignant Change in Exostosis

- Assess cartilage cap thickness by means of MRI: normal < 1 cm
- Some may have mottled calcification (not well defined) at the cap
- Developed soft-tissue mass – usual exostosis never develop soft-tissue mass
- Pain sometimes can occur even in usual exostosis with fracture of stalk, nerve impingement and inflammation from bursa

8.9.8.3.5 Features of Surface Chondrosarcoma

- Surface chondrosarcoma arises either from pre-existing exostosis or de-novo
- Most are low-grade lobulated growth and can invade nearby soft tissue
- Treatment is excision with adequate margin, since RT/CT is not usually effective (an occasional de-differentiated chondrosarcoma arising near a pre-existing chondroid lesion may respond to CT and/or RT)

8.9.8.3.6 Periosteal Chondroma

- No stalk
- From beneath periosteum
- As local thickening

8.9.8.4 DDx of Clear Cell Chondrosarcoma Versus Chondroblastoma

▦ Nature: chondroblastoma is a rare benign tumour of foetal type cartilage differentiation. Site: long bones – centre of lesion at epiphysis; or even in pelvis and calcaneus – but not the flat bones

▦ Clinical features: joint symptoms are not uncommon since location is usually at the epiphysis – stiffness and effusion

▦ Clinical: clear cell chondrosarcoma in older age patients (30–50 years) versus chondroblastoma in younger patients (mostly 15–25 years). Location is similar, but 60% of clear cell chondrosarcoma occurs at the head of the femur, and pain can occur in addition to the joint symptoms

▦ X-ray: very similar → lytic lesion at epiphysis in half of the cases extends to metaphysis; can have stippled calcification and sometimes grows to large size (4–14+ cm). No scelerotic rim, occasionally expands/destroys cortex. (In contrast, extension to metaphysis is very common in clear cell chondrosarcoma; one-third with calcification.) Histology:

▦ Chondroblastoma – chondroid matrix; lies stromal and has multinucleated giant cells. Stromal cell has round clear cytoplasm – like a fried egg – calcification of matrix around cells called chicken-wire (can have areas like chondromyxoid fibroma)

▦ Clear cell chondrosarcoma – cells slightly larger than in chondroblastoma, with clear cytoplasm, with foci of grade-1 chondrosarcoma. Many believe this entity was derived from the former

8.9.8.5 Comparison Between Spinal Chondrosarcoma and Chordomas

▦ Background: (1) spine usually involved with low-grade chondrosarcoma – 7% of total; can be a soft-tissue mass attached to vertebral body or cause neurology; (2) chodoma formed from notocord rests – hence, usually either at (a) skull base or (b) sacrum (other area of vertebral column reported)

▦ Similarities: (1) both can have lobulated appearance with 'chondroid'-like matrix; (2) both can affect the spine; and (3) there are two forms of histological chordoma variants: (a) those with chondroid-like matrix and (b) those 'de-differentiated' types that have much poorer prognosis

  – Tumour cell appearance – chondrosarcoma cells sit inside lacunae, while chordoma cells are in sheets (with bubbly cytoplasm)

- Matrix: (1) those chordoma with de-differentiated type have no chondroid matrix – easy to differentially diagnose (most of these can occur in sacrum), (2) those chordomas with chondroid matrix → DDx by immunostain since both the tumour cell and matrix stain for keratin (indicating epithelial origin) – the chondroid of chondrosarcoma does not

▪ Spine chondrosarcoma grows quite slowly, but excision is not easy; most die later of recurrences; an occasional case may try RT (most of these are low grade, and metastases are not common)

▪ Chordoma can spread to lung (in about 30%) and needs more aggressive treatment – planning depends on level of spine and nearby structures

8.10   Bone Metastases

▪ Common tumours (usually carcinomas) most likely to metastasise to bone are from: breast, thyroid, kidney, lung, prostate

▪ Bone is the 3rd most common site for metastases in general

▪ Common seeding in axial skeleton (Fig. 8.15) rather than appendicular skeleton is likely due to the persistence of the red marrow. In the axial skeleton, mostly the vertebral body is commonly involved. The

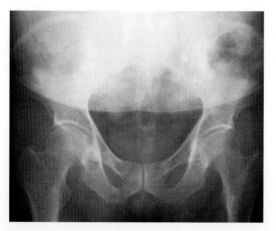

Fig. 8.15. Metastases from prostate carcinoma in an elderly man

pelvis and ribs are also commonly affected in axial skeletal involvement

■ Spread to the axial skeleton from the prostate for instance has been surmised to be facilitated to be via Batson's venous plexus that bypasses the lung in this system of valveless veins. However, some recent articles have cast doubt as to whether this is a major route judging from calculation of the pressure differences

8.10.1 Common Presentation

■ Pain
■ Pathological fracture or impending fractures
■ Spinal cord compression
■ Hypercalcaemia

8.10.2 Pain

■ Probably the most common symptom
■ Caused by stretched periosteum, nerve stimulation in the endosteum, and soft-tissue extension may involve neurovascular bundles

8.10.3 Work-Up

■ Known primary: if clinical pictures are obvious and bone scan, etc are typical, there is no absolute need for biopsy. (Bone scan is able to pick up lesion before X-ray does preceding it by a few months or sometimes up to 1 year. This is because lucent metastases must destroy 30–50% of the bone density in order to be detectable by X-ray)
■ Unknown primary:
  – Biopsy needed, but send also for bacterial and acid-fast bacilli culture besides sending specimen for histology
  – Other adjunct investigations include bone scan, tumour markers, chest X-ray, CT of the chest and abdomen, etc.

8.10.4 Treatment

■ Role of RT in palliation pain:
  – Can reduce pain and may reduce tumour growth
  – Common dose 20–40 Gray; half the cases expect complete pain relief
  – Complications include AVN, delayed wound healing, pigmentation and malignancy

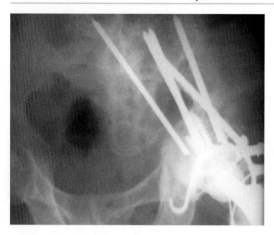

Fig. 8.16. Postoperative X-ray after left hip reconstruction of a destroyed left acetabulum

- Role of bisphosphonates in hypercalcaemia:
  - May be used to treat hypercalcaemia and may also decrease bone pain. Some studies claim that they may reduce the incidence of pathological fracture. If there is extensive destruction already, long-term administration may be required

    (P.S. Surgical intervention has a role not only in prophylactic nailing of long-bone metastatic lesions but in treatment of pathological fractures. Maintenance of a better quality of life is sometimes indicated even in patients with significant bony destruction provided they are fit for surgery. Figure 8.16 is an example of hip reconstruction in a patient with very extensive acetabular bone resorption)

General Bibliography

Levesque J, Maxx R, Bell R, Wunder J, Kandel R, White L (eds) (1998) A critical guide to primary bone tumours, 1998 edn. Williams and Wilkins, Philadelphia

Selected Bibliography of Journal Articles

1. Bacci G, Ferrari S et al. (2002) Osteosarcoma of the limb. Amputation or limb salvage in patients treated by neoadjuvant chemotherapy. J Bone Joint Surg Br 84:88–92
2. Kumta SM, Cheng JC et al. (2002) Scope and limitations of limb sparing surgery in childhood sarcomas. JPO 22:244–248
3. Wolfe RE, Enneking WF (1996) The staging and surgery of musculoskeletal neoplasms. OCNA 27:473–481
4. Rydholm A (1997) Surgical margins for soft tissue sarcomas. Acta Orthop Scand Suppl 273:81–85

Subject Index

Printing and Binding: Stürtz GmbH, Würzburg